THERAPEUTIC MODALITIES
IN SPORTS MEDICINE

WILLIAM E. PRENTICE, Ph.D., A.T., C., P.T.
Associate Professor of Physical Education,
Coordinator of Sports Medicine Specialization,
Department of Physical Education, and
Assistant Clinical Professor, Division of Physical Therapy,
Department of Medical Allied Health Professions,
The University of North Carolina,
Chapel Hill, North Carolina
Director, Sports Medicine Education and Fellowship Program
HEALTHSOUTH Rehabilitation Corporation and
American Sports Medicine Institute
Birmingham, Alabama

TIMES MIRROR/MOSBY
COLLEGE PUBLISHING

ST. LOUIS • TORONTO • BOSTON • LOS ALTOS   1990

Editor: Pat Coryell
Assistant editor: Loren Stevenson
Project manager: Mark Spann
Cover designer: Susan E. Lane
Production: Editing, Design & Production, Inc.

Cover photograph: © David Madison Photography

Library of Congress Cataloging-in-Publication Data

Therapeutic modalities in sports medicine / [edited by] William E.
  Prentice.—2nd ed.
      p.   cm.
   Includes bibliographies and index.
   ISBN 0-8016-3358-3
   1. Sports—Accidents and injuries—Treatment.   2. Physical
therapy.   I. Prentice, William E.
   [DNLM: 1. Athletic Injuries—rehabilitation.   2. Athletic
Injuries—therapy.   3. Physical therapy—methods.   QT 260 T398]
   RD97.T484   1990
   617.1′027—dc20
DNLM/DLC
   for Library of Congress   89-12230
                                                                  CIP

C/D/D   9 8 7 6 5 4 3 2   01/D/018

Contributors

Gerald W. Bell, Ed.D., A.T., C., P.T.
Associate Professor,
Department of Physical Education,
University of Illinois,
Urbana, Illinois

J. Marc Davis, A.T., C., P.T.
Athletic Trainer/Physical Therapist,
Division of Sports Medicine,
Student Health Service,
The University of North Carolina,
Chapel Hill, North Carolina

Craig Denegar, Ph.D., A.T., C.
Associate Professor of Physical Therapy,
Slippery Rock University,
Slippery Rock, Pennsylvania

Phillip B. Donley, M.S., A.T., C., P.T.
Professor,
Department of Health and Physical Education,
West Chester State College,
West Chester, Pennsylvania

Susan H. Foreman, M.Ed., A.T., C.
Assistant Athletic Trainer,
University of Virginia,
Charlottesville, Virginia

Daniel N. Hooker, Ph.D., A.T., C., P.T.
Coordinator of Athletic Training,
Division of Sports Medicine,
Student Health Service,
The University of North Carolina,
Chapel Hill, North Carolina

Clairbeth Lehn, A.T., C., P.T.
Athletic Trainer/Physical Therapist,
Division of Sports Medicine,
Student Health Service,
The University of North Carolina,
Chapel Hill, North Carolina

William E. Prentice, Ph.D., A.T., C., P.T.
Associate Professor of Physical Education,
Coordinator of Sports Medicine Specialization,
Department of Physical Education, and
Assistant Clinical Professor, Division of
Physical Therapy,
Department of Medical Allied Health
Professions,
The University of North Carolina,
Chapel Hill, North Carolina

Ethan N. Saliba, M.Ed., A.T.C., P.T.
Instructor, Currey School of Education,
Assistant Athletic Trainer,
University of Virginia,
Charlottesville, Virginia

John C. Spiker, M.Ed., A.T., C., P.T.
Athletic Trainer/Physical Therapist,
West Virginia University,
President, Morgantown Physical Therapy
Associates,
Morgantown, West Virginia

Preface

There is little argument that professional athletic trainers and physical therapists use a wide variety of therapeutic techniques in the treatment and rehabilitation of sports-related injuries. One of the more important aspects of a thorough treatment regimen often involves the use of therapeutic modalities. At one time or another, virtually all sports therapists make use of some type of modality. This may involve a relatively simple technique such as using an ice pack as a first aid treatment for an acute injury or more complex techniques such as the stimulation of nerve and muscle tissue by electrical currents. There is no question that therapeutic modalities are useful tools in injury rehabilitation. When used appropriately, these modalities can greatly enhance the athlete's chances for a safe and rapid return to athletic competition. Unfortunately, the sports therapists' rationale for using a particular modality is too often based on habit rather than on analysis of effectiveness. For the sports therapist, it is essential to possess knowledge regarding the scientific basis and the physiologic effects of the various modalities on a specific injury. When this theoretical basis is applied to practical experience, it has the potential to become an extremely effective clinical method.

What role should a modality play in injury rehabilitation? An effective treatment program includes three primary objectives: (1) management or reduction of pain associated with an injury, (2) return of full nonrestricted range of movement to an injured part, and (3) maintenance or perhaps improvement of strength through the full range. Modalities, though important, are by no means the single most critical factor in accomplishing these objectives. Therapeutic exercise that forces the injured anatomic structure to perform its normal function is the key to successful rehabilitation. However, therapeutic modalities certainly play an important role in reducing pain and are extremely useful as an adjunct to therapeutic exercise.

It must be emphasized that the use of therapeutic modalities in any treatment program is an inexact science. If you were to ask ten different sports therapists what combination of modalities and therapeutic exercise they use in a given treatment program, you would probably get ten different responses. There is no way to "cookbook" a treatment plan that involves the use of modalities. Thus what this book will attempt to do is to present the basis for use of each different type of modality and allow the sports therapists to make their own decisions as to which will be most effective in a given situation. Some recommended protocols developed through the experiences of the contributing authors will be presented.

The sports therapist continues to gain acceptance in the medical community as a highly qualified and well-educated paramedical professional concerned with the treatment and rehabilitation of injuries to athletes. It is essential for the programs educating student trainers and therapists to provide classroom instruction in a wide range of specialty areas including injury prevention, care and management, injury evaluation, and therapeutic treatment and rehabilitation techniques. Detailed instructions in the use of therapeutic modalities should be of primary concern to those who intend to pursue a career in sports medicine.

The use of therapeutic modalities in the treatment of athletic injuries by individuals with various combinations of educational background, certification, and licensure is currently a controversial issue. Formal classroom instruction in the use of therapeutic modalities is included in all physical therapy programs and is also provided in the majority of athletic training education programs. Physical therapists who are licensed to practice have been given permission to legally use modalities in their patient treatment programs. Likewise, some states have also granted licensure to athletic trainers, thus allowing them full use of therapeutic modalities. Specific laws governing the use of therapeutic modalities vary from state to state. How should modalities be used by athletic trainers who are not licensed by the state in which they are working?

The use of therapeutic modalities has traditionally been in the hands of physical therapists and athletic trainers. The laws of the various states place limitations on this use. The reader of this book should be careful that any use he or she makes of a modality is within the limits allowed by the law of his or her particular state. I do not intend for the reader to interpret anything in this book as encouraging him or her to act outside the scope of the law of his or her state.

The editor hopes that this text will be a useful tool in the continuing growth and professional development of all individuals concerned with and interested in the field of sports injury rehabilitation. The following are a number of reasons why this text should be adopted for use.

COMPREHENSIVE COVERAGE OF THERAPEUTIC MODALITIES IN A SPORTS MEDICINE SETTING. The purpose of this text is to provide a theoretically based but practically oriented guide to the use of therapeutic modalities for the individual who routinely treats sports-related injury. It is intended for use in advanced courses in sports medicine where various clinically oriented techniques and methods are presented.

The second edition of this text has been expanded to make the coverage of various modalities more comprehensive. In particular, the chapters on pain, basic principles of electricity, electrical stimulating currents, and massage have been expanded and updated using the latest information available. A new chapter has been added on the latest modality available to the sports therapist, the low-power laser. Also, an appendix has been added that will assist the sports therapist in the clinical decision-making process with regard to the use of the various therapeutic modalities.

This text begins with a discussion of pain, in terms of neurophysiologic mechanisms of pain and the role of therapeutic modalities in pain management. The modalities are then classified in a logical order in relation to the electromagnetic and acoustic spectra. Detailed discussions of various therapeutic modalities, including the infrared modalities, shortwave and microwave diathermies, ultraviolet therapy, ultrasound electrical stimulating currents, low-power laser, massage, and other specialized modalities are presented with emphasis on (1) the physiologic basis for use, (2) clinical applications, and (3) specific techniques of application. Although it is certainly true that therapeutic modalities are important and necessary tools that should be used in dealing with physical problems of all varieties, this text will deal specifically with why and how these modalities are best used in the treatment and rehabilitation of injuries related to sports. This text is the only one available that is oriented specifically toward the use of modalities in the treatment of sports-related injury.

BASED ON SCIENTIFIC THEORY. This text discusses various concepts, principles, and theories that are supported by scientific research, factual evidence, and previous experience of the authors in dealing with injuries related to sport. The material presented in this text has been carefully researched by the contributing authors to provide up-to-date information on the theoretical basis for employing a particular modality in a specific injury situation. Additionally, the manuscript for this text has been carefully reviewed by sports therapists, both athletic trainers and physical therapists, who are considered experts in their field to ensure that the material reflects factual and current concepts for modality use.

TIMELY AND PRACTICAL. Certainly, therapeutic modalities used in a clinical setting are important tools for the sports therapist. The availability of this text fills a void that has existed for quite some time in the educational program of the student sports therapist. Instructors have been forced to use a variety of randomly selected handouts and photocopied materials in those courses that attempt to provide the student with instruction in the theoretical basis and practical application of the various modalities.

During the preparation of this second edition, the editor received much encouragement from sports medicine educators regarding the usability of this text in the classroom setting. It should serve as a needed guide for the sports therapist who is interested in knowing not only how to use a modality but also why that particular modality is most effective in a given situation.

The authors who have contributed to this text have a great deal of clinical experience dealing with sports-related injury. Each of these individuals has also at one time or another been involved with the formal classroom education of the student trainer or therapist. Thus this text has been directed at the student of sports-injury rehabilitation who will be asked to apply the theoretical basis of modality use to the clinical setting.

PERTINENT TO THE SPORTS THERAPIST. This text deals specifically with the use of therapeutic modalities in the sports medicine setting. Several other texts are available that discuss the use of the physical modalities with patient populations other than athletes. The sports medicine emphasis makes this text unique.

PEDAGOGICAL AIDS. The aids this text uses to facilitate its use by students and instructors include:

Objectives   These goals are listed at the beginning of each chapter to introduce students to the points that will be emphasized.

Figures and Tables   Essential points on each chapter are illustrated with clear visual materials.

Summary   Each chapter has a summary that outlines the major points covered.

Glossary of Key Terms   Each chapter contains a glossary of terms for quick reference.

References   A list of up-to-date references is provided at the end of each chapter for the student who wishes to read further on the subject being discussed.

Appendix A   A complete list of manufacturers of therapeutic modality equipment is provided.

Acknowledgments

If you have never been involved in the production of a textbook, it is difficult to understand the magnitude of such an undertaking. Dozens of individuals have been involved with this project from its inception, and all have contributed in their own way, but a few deserve special thanks.

Loren Stevenson, my developmental editor at Times Mirror/Mosby, has been responsible for coordinating the efforts between the publisher and me. She has offered much encouragement, constructive suggestions, and extreme patience in the completion of this text.

When assembling a group of contributors for a project such as this it is essential to select individuals who are both knowledgeable and well respected in their fields. It also helps if you can count them as friends, and I want to let them know that I hold each of them in the highest regard, both personally and professionally.

The following individuals have invested a great amount of time and effort in reviewing this manuscript. Their contributions are present throughout the text. I would like to thank each one of them for all their valuable insight.

William S. Quillen, Ph.D., A.T., C., R.P.T.
United States Naval Academy
Bobby Patton, Ed.D., A.T., C.
Southwest Texas State University
Jay A. Bradley, M.Ed., A.T., C.
Indiana University—Purdue University at
 Indianapolis
Frank E. Walters, Ph.D., A.T., C.
Texas A&M University
Charles J. Redmond, M.Ed., A.T., C., R.P.T.
Springfield College

And finally, I would like to thank my wife Tena and my sons Brian and Zachary for being understanding and patient while I pursue a career and a life that I truly enjoy.

William E. Prentice

Contents

Pain and Mechanisms of Pain Relief

1

Phillip B. Donley and Craig Denegar

OBJECTIVES

Following completion of this chapter, the student will be able to:

- Define pain, its types, and its positive and negative effects.

- Describe the characteristics of sensory receptors.

- Describe an appropriate neurophysiologic mechanism for pain control for the therapeutic modalities used by the sports therapist.

- Describe how pain perception can be modified by cognitive factors.

The International Association for the Study of Pain defines **pain** as "an unpleasant sensory and emotional experience associated with actual or potential tissue damage, or described in terms of such damage."[14] Pain is a subjective sensation with more than one dimension and an abundance of descriptors of its qualities and characteristics. In spite of its universality, pain is composed of a variety of human discomforts, rather than being a single entity.[13] The perception of pain can be subjectively modified by past experiences and expectations. Much of what we do to treat athletes' pain is to change their perceptions of pain.[4]

Pain does have a purpose. It warns us that there is something wrong and can provoke a withdrawal response to avoid further injury. It also results in muscle spasm and guarding or protection of the injured part. Pain, however, can persist after it is no longer useful. It can become a means of enhancing disability and inhibiting efforts to rehabilitate the injury. Prolonged spasm, which leads to circulatory deficiency, muscle atrophy, disuse habits, and conscious or unconscious guarding, may lead to a severe loss of athletic ability.[10] Chronic pain may become a disease state in itself. Often lacking an identifiable cause, chronic pain can totally disable a patient.

Research in recent years has led to a better understanding of pain and pain relief. This research also has raised new questions, while leaving many unanswered. We now have better explanations for the analgesic properties of the physical agents we use, as well as a better understanding of the psychology of pain. However, new physical agents, such as the laser and microamperage electrical stimulators, and new approaches to older agents such as transcutaneous electrical nerve stimulators, challenge our understanding of injury and pain. Not even the mechanisms for the analgesic response to heat and cold have been fully described.

The control of pain is an essential aspect of caring for the injured athlete. The sports therapist has several therapeutic agents with analgesic properties from which to choose. The selection of a therapeutic agent should be based on a sound understanding of its physical properties and physiologic effects. This chapter will not provide a complete explanation of neurophysiology, pain and pain relief. Instead, it presents an overview of some theories of pain control, intended to provide a stimulus for the sports therapist to develop his or her own rationale for using modalities in the treatment of injured athletes. Ideally, it also will interest some in research to establish the physiologic and psychologic soundness of the use of agents for pain relief and to expand our understanding of pain. Several physiology textbooks provide extensive discussions of human neurophysiology and neurobiology to supplement this chapter.

Many of the modalities discussed in later chapters have analgesic properties. Often, they are employed to reduce pain and permit the athlete to perform therapeutic exercises. Some understanding of what pain is, how it affects us, and how it is perceived is essential for the sports therapist who uses these modalities.

TYPES OF PAIN

Pain has been categorized as either **acute** or **chronic.** Pain lasting for more than 6 weeks is generally classified as chronic. There is more research devoted to chronic pain and its treatment, but acute pain, or pain of sudden onset lasting less than 6 weeks, is a more likely problem for the sports therapist.

Referred pain, which also may be either acute or chronic, is pain that is perceived to be in an area that seems to have little relation to the existing pathology. For example, injury to the spleen often results in pain in the left shoulder. This pattern, known as **Kehr's sign,** is useful for identifying this serious injury and arranging prompt emergency care. Referred pain can outlast the causative events because of altered reflex patterns, continuing mechanical stress on muscles, learned habits of guarding, or the development of hypersensitive areas, called **trigger points.**

Irritation of nerves and nerve roots can cause **radiating pain.** Pressure on the lumbar nerve roots associated with a herniated disc or a contusion of the sciatic nerve can result in pain radiating down the lower extremity to the foot.

Deep somatic pain is a type that seems to be **sclerotomic** (associated with a **sclerotome,** a segment of bone innervated by a spinal segment). There is often a discrepancy between the site of the disorder and the site of the pain.

TISSUE SENSITIVITY

The structures most sensitive to damaging (noxious) stimuli are, first, the periosteum and joint capsule; second, subchondral bone, tendons, and ligaments; third, muscle and cortical bone; and finally, the synovium and articular cartilage. A variety of "silent" fractures produce little or no pain. Different anatomic tissues exhibit varying degrees of sensitivity to pain. Avulsion fractures tend to be quite painful, because they tear away the periosteum. Musculoskeletal pain is usually spread over a large area unless it is close to the surface. For example, a hamstring strain usually results in pain over the posterior thigh, whereas an acromioclavicular sprain usually localizes over the joint.

GOALS IN DEALING WITH PAIN

Regardless of the cause of pain, its reduction is an essential part of treatment. Pain signals the athlete to seek assistance and often is useful in establishing a diagnosis. Once the injury or illness is diagnosed, pain serves little purpose. Medical or surgical treatment or immobilization is necessary to treat some conditions, but physical therapy and an early return to activity are appropriate following many athletic injuries. The sports therapist's objectives are to encourage the body to heal through exercise designed to progressively increase the capacity for athletic work and to return the athlete to competition as swiftly and safely as possible. Pain will inhibit therapeutic exercise. The challenge for the sports therapist is to control acute pain and protect the athlete from further injury, while encouraging progressive exercise in a supervised environment.

PERCEPTION AND TRANSMISSION OF PAIN
Sensory Receptors

There are several types of sensory receptors in the body, and the sports therapist should be aware of their existence and the types of stimuli that activate them. Activation of some of these sense organs with therapeutic agents will decrease the athlete's perception of pain.

Six different types of receptor nerve endings are encapsulated in connective tissue and are found in the skin:

1. Meissner's corpuscles are activated by light touch.
2. Pacinian corpuscles respond to deep pressure.
3. Merkel's corpuscles respond to deep pressure, but more slowly than pacinian corpuscles, and also are activated by hair follicle deflection.
4. Ruffini corpuscles in the skin are sensitive to touch, tension, and possibly heat, and those in the joint capsules and ligaments are sensitive to change in position.
5. Krause's end bulbs are thermoreceptors that react to a decrease in temperature and touch.[18]
6. Pain receptors, called **nociceptors** or **free nerve endings,** are sensitive to extreme mechanical, thermal, or chemical energy.[3] They respond to noxious stimuli, in other words, to impending or actual tissue damage (for example, cuts, burns, sprains, and so on). The term *nociceptive* is from the Latin *nocere,* to damage, and is used to imply pain information.

These organs respond to superficial forms of heat and cold, analgesic balms, and massage.

Proprioceptors found in muscles, joint capsules, ligaments, and tendons provide information regarding muscle tone. The muscle spindles react to changes in length and tension when the muscle is stretched or contracted. The Golgi tendon organs also react to changes in length and tension within the muscle. See Table 1-1 for a more complete listing.

Some sensory receptors respond to phasic activity and produce an impulse when the stimulus is increasing or decreasing, but not during a sustained stimulus. They adapt to a constant stimulus. Meissner's corpuscles and pacinian corpuscles are examples of such receptors.

Tonic receptors produce impulses as long as the stimulus is present. Examples of tonic receptors are muscle spindles, free nerve endings, and Krause's end bulbs. The initial impulse is at a higher frequency than later impulses that occur during sustained stimulation.

Adaptation is the decline in generator potential and the reduction of frequency that occurs with a prolonged stimulus or with frequently repeated stimuli. If some physical agents are used too often or for too long, the receptors may adapt to or accommodate the stimulus and reduce their impulses. The accommodation phenomenon can be observed with the use of superficial hot and cold agents, such as ice packs and hydrocollator packs.

As a stimulus becomes stronger, the number of receptors excited increases, and the frequency of the impulses increases. This provides more electrical activity at the spinal cord level, which may facilitate the effects of some physcal agents.

TABLE 1-1   **Some Characteristics of Selected Sensory Receptors**

| Type of Sensory Receptors | Stimulus | | Receptor | |
	General Term	Specific Nature	Term	Location
Mechanoreceptors	Pressure	Movement of hair in a hair follicle	Afferent nerve fiber	Base of hair follicles
		Light pressure	Meissner's corpuscle	Skin
		Deep pressure	Pacinian corpuscle	Skin
		Touch	Merkel's touch corpuscle	Skin
Nociceptors	Pain	Distension (stretch)	Free nerve endings	Wall of gastrointestinal tract, pharynx, skin
Proprioceptors	Tension	Distension	Corpuscles of Ruffini	Skin and capsules in joints and ligaments
		Length changes	Muscle spindles	Skeletal muscle
		Tension changes	Golgi tendon organs	Between muscles and tendons
Thermoreceptors	Temperature change	Cold	Krause's end bulbs	Skin
		Heat	Corpuscles of Ruffini	Skin and capsules in joints and ligaments

Modified from Previte, J.J.: Human physiology, New York, 1983, McGraw-Hill, Inc.

A nociceptive neuron is one that transmits pain signals. Its cell body is in the dorsal root ganglion near the spinal cord. Afferent neurons or nerve fibers conduct impulses from the periphery toward the brain, while efferent fibers, such as motor neurons, conduct impulses from the brain toward the periphery. Approximately 25% of the myelinated Aδ and 50% of the unmyelinated C fibers contact nociceptors and are considered nociceptive, afferent neurons (Table 1-2).

     Once a nociceptor is stimulated, it releases a neuropeptide **(substance P)** that initiates the electrical impulses along the afferent fiber toward the spinal cord. Substance P also serves as a transmitter substance between the first-order afferent fiber and a second-order afferent fiber (Fig. 1-1) at the dorsal horn of the spinal column. Many nervous system transmitters conduct the excitation across the synapse and initiate an electrical impulse in the second-order nerve fiber. Such electrical impulses carry sensory messages (pain, warmth, touch) to sensory centers in the brain where they are integrated, interpreted, and acted upon.

Neural Transmission

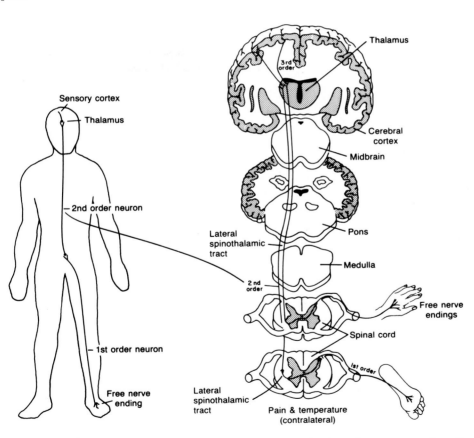

Figure 1-1. The lateral spinothalamic tract carries impulses of pain and temperature from the sensory receptors to the cortex.

TABLE 1-2   **Classification of Afferent Neurons**

Size	Type	Group	Subgroup	Diameter (Micrometers)	Conduction Velocity	Receptor	Stimulus
Large	A α	I	1a	12-20 (22)	70-120	Proprioceptive mechanoreceptor	Muscle velocity and length change, muscle shortening of rapid speed
	A α	I	1b				
	A β	II	Muscle	6-12	36-72	Proprioceptive mechanoreceptor	Muscle length information from touch and pacinian corpuscles
	A β	II	Skin			Cutaneous receptors	Touch, vibration, hair receptors
	A δ	III	Muscle	1-5 (6)	6(12)-36(80)	75% mechanoreceptors and thermoreceptors	Temperature change
Small	A δ	III	Skin			25% nociceptors, mechanoreceptors and thermoreceptors (hot and cold)	Noxious mechanical and temperature ($>45°$ C, $<10°$ C)
	C	IV	Muscle	0.3-1.0	0.4-1.0	50% mechanoreceptors and thermoreceptors	Touch and temperature
	C	IV	Skin			50% nociceptors, 20% mechanoreceptors, and 30% thermoreceptors (hot and cold)	Noxious mechanical and temperature ($>45°$ C, $<10°$ C)

The sensations of pain and temperature are transmitted along the Aδ and C fiber afferents. These fibers have different diameters (A δ are larger) and different conduction velocities (A δ are faster). The C fibers also are connected to more of the nonadapting nociceptors. These differences result in two qualitatively different types of pain, termed *fast* and *slow*.[3] Fast pain is brief, well-localized, and well-matched to the stimulus—for example, the initial pain of an unexpected pinprick. Slow pain is an aching, throbbing, or burning sensation that is poorly localized and less specifically related to the stimulus. There is a delay in the perception of slow pain following injury, but the pain will continue long after the noxious stimulus is removed. Fast pain is transmitted over the larger, faster-conducting A δ afferent neurons and originates from receptors located in the skin. Slow pain is transmitted by the C afferent neurons and originates from both superficial tissue (skin) and deeper tissue (ligaments and muscle).[3]

The various types of afferent fibers follow different courses as they ascend toward the brain. Most C afferent neurons enter the spinal cord through the dorsolateral tract of Lissauer and synapse in an area called the **substantia gelatinosa** with a second-order neuron. The second-order neuron crosses contralaterally to the lateral spinothalamic tract, where it travels up the spinal cord to the thalamus. Here it synapses with a third-order afferent neuron that sends its axon to the postcentral gyrus or the sensory cortex. Most analgesic physical agents used in sports medicine are believed to slow or block the impulses ascending along the C afferent neuron pathways.

Synapse
Transmission

For information to pass between neurons, a transmitter substance must be released from one neuron terminal (presynaptic membrane), enter the synaptic cleft, and attach to a receptor site on the next neuron (postsynaptic membrane). In the past, all the activity within the synapse was attributed to **neurotransmitters,** such as acetylcholine. It is now apparent that several compounds that are not true neurotransmitters can facilitate or inhibit synaptic activity. These compounds are classified as biogenic amine transmitters or neuroactive peptides. Serotonin and norepinephrine are examples of biogenic amine transmitters. About two dozen neuroactive peptides have been identified, including substance P, enkephalins, and β-endorphin.[3]

Serotonin and enkephalins may be active in descending (efferent) pathways thought to block the pain message.[5] Enkephalin is an endogenous (made by the body) opiate that inhibits the release of substance P. It is released from **interneurons,** enkephalin neurons with short axons. The enkephalins are stored in nerve-ending vesicles found in the substantia gelatinosa and several areas of the brain. When released, enkephalin may bind to presynaptic or postsynaptic membranes.[3]

Norepinephrine is a biogenic amine transmitter that is released by the depolarization of some neurons and that binds to the postsynaptic membranes. Analgesia increases with the inhibition of norepinephrine and decreases with its stimulation. An increased level of norepinephrine in the central nervous system usually is associated with decreased analgesia.[1]

Other endogenous opiates may be active analgesic agents. These neuroactive peptides are released into the central nervous system and have an action similar to that of morphine, an opiate analgesic. There are specific receptors located at strategic sites, called *binding sites,* to receive these compounds. **β-Endorphin** is a 31−amino acid peptide with potent analgesic effects. It is released by the anterior pituitary gland and elsewhere within the central nervous system.

NEURO-
PHYSIOLOGIC
EXPLANATIONS
OF PAIN
CONTROL

The neurophysiologic mechanisms of pain control through stimulation of cutaneous receptors have not been fully explained. Much of what is known and current theory are the result of work involving transcutaneous electrical nerve stimulation. However, this information often provides an explanation for the analgesic response to other modalities, such as massage, analgesic balms, and moist heat.

The models of the analgesic response to cutaneous receptor stimulation presented here were first proposed by Melzack and Wall[12] and Castel.[5] These models essentially present three analgesic mechanisms:

1. Stimulation from ascending A β afferents results in the blocking of impulses (pain messages) carried along A δ and C afferent fibers.
2. Stimulation along descending pathways in the dorsal horn of the spinal cord

results in a blocking of the impulses carried along the A δ and C afferent fibers.

3. The stimulation of A δ and C afferent fiber causes the release of endogenous opioids (β-endorphin) into the central nervous system, resulting in a narcotic-like suppression of the central nervous system and a generalized analgesic response.

These theories or models are not necessarily mutually exclusive. Recent evidence suggests that pain relief may result from combinations of dorsal horn and central nervous system activity.[2,7]

Blocking the Pain Impulses with Ascending A β Input

Pain modulation due to sensory stimulation and the resultant increase in the impulses in the large diameter (A β) *afferent* fibers was proposed by the **gate control theory of pain** (Fig. 1-2).[12] Impulses ascending on these fibers stimulate

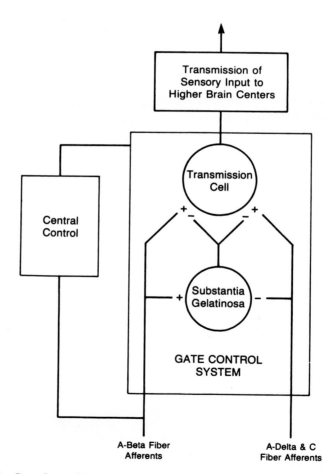

Figure 1-2. The Gate Control System. Increases A-beta input and stimulates the Substantia Gelatinosa which inhibits the flow of afferent input to sensory centers.

the **substantia gelatinosa** as they enter the dorsal horn of the spinal cord. Stimulation of the substantia gelatinosa inhibits synaptic transmission in the large and small (A δ and C) fiber afferent pathways. The "pain message" carried along the smaller-diameter fibers is not transmitted to the second-order neurons and never reaches sensory centers. The balance between the input from the small- and large-diameter afferents determines how much of the pain message is blocked or gated.

The concept of sensory stimulation for pain relief, as proposed by the gate control theory, has empirical support. Rubbing a contusion, applying moist heat, or massaging sore muscles decreases the perception of pain. The analgesic response to these treatments is attributed to the increased stimulation of large-diameter afferent fibers.

The gate control theory also proposes that A δ and C fiber impulses inhibit the substantia gelatinosa, facilitating the perception of pain. The sensation of pain does not diminish rapidly, because free nerve endings do not accommodate and the afferent impulses from them "open the gate" to further pain message transmission.

The discovery and isolation of endogenous opioids in the 1970s led to new theories of pain relief. Castel[5] introduced an endogenous opioid analogue to the gate control theory (Fig. 1-3). This theory proposes that A β impulses trigger a release of enkephalin from enkephalin interneurons found in the dorsal horn. These neuroactive amines inhibit synaptic transmission in the A δ and C fiber afferent pathways. The end result, as in the gate control theory, is that the pain message is blocked before it reaches sensory levels.

The gate control theory proposed a second analgesic mechanism, that involves descending efferent fibers. The central control, originating in higher centers of the central nervous system, could affect the dorsal horn gating process. Im-

Descending Pain Control Mechanisms

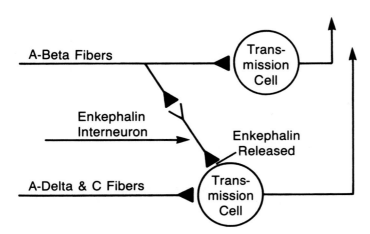

Figure 1-3. Presynaptic inhibition of dorsal horn synapse transmission due to A-beta fiber stimulation at enkephalin interneurons.

pulses from the thalamus and brain stem (central biasing) are carried into the dorsal horn on efferent fibers in the dorsal or dorsal lateral paths (or tracts). Impulses from the higher centers act to close the gate and block transmission of the pain message at the dorsal horn synapse. Through this system, it was theorized, previous experiences, emotional influences, sensory perception, and other factors could influence the transmission of the pain message and the perception of pain.

Castel offers an **endogenous opioid** model of descending influence over dorsal horn synapse activity (Fig. 1-4). Stimulation of the periaqueductal gray region of the midbrain and the **raphe nucleus** in the pons and medulla by ascending neural input, especially from A δ and C fiber afferents, and possibly central biasing, activates the descending mechanism. The periaqueductal gray region sends impulses along the efferent fibers in the dorsal lateral tract, which synapse with enkephalin interneurons. The interneurons release enkephalin into the dorsal horn, inhibiting the synaptic transmission of impulses to the second-order afferent neurons.

This model provides a physiologic explanation for the analgesic response

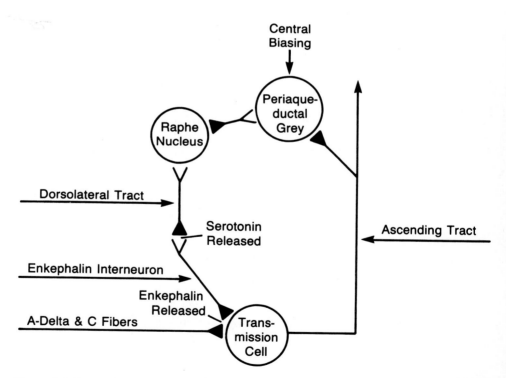

Figure 1-4. Descending inhibition. Activation of the periaqueductal grey and Raphe Nucleus results in impulse transmission along efferent fibers and the stimulation of enkephalin interneurons.

to brief, intense stimulation. The analgesia following acupressure and the use of some transcutaneous electrical nerve stimulators (TENS), such as point stimulators, is attributed to this descending pain control mechanism.

β-Endorphin

There is evidence that stimulation of the small-diameter C fiber afferents can stimulate the release of other endogenous opioids.[6,8,11,15-17,19-22] **β-Endorphin** (BEP) is a neuroactive peptide with potent analgesic affects. The term endorphin refers to an opiate-like substance produced by the body. One of the sources of BEP is the anterior pituitary gland. Here it shares the prohormone propiomelanocortin (POMC) with adrenocorticotropin (ACTH).

Prolonged (20 to 40 minutes) C fiber afferent stimulation has been thought to trigger the release of BEP from the anterior pituitary gland (Fig. 1-5).[5] Electro-acupuncture and TENS with long pulse widths (>200 μ) and low pulse rates (1 to 5 pulses/second) will cause the C fiber depolarization necessary for BEP release. Recent findings do not support the anterior pituitary gland as a source of BEP in low pulse rate, long pulse width TENS—induced analgesia.[9] These results and the recognition that BEP does not readily cross the blood—brain barrier[3] suggest that if BEP or other endogenous opioids are active analgesic agents, they are released from areas within the brain.

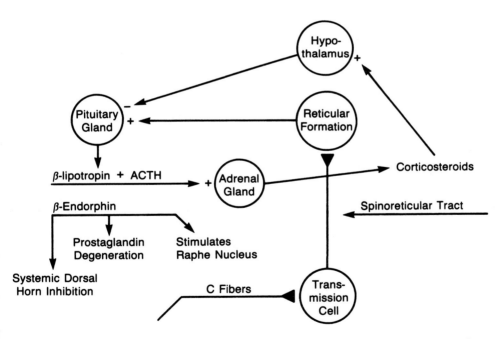

Figure 1-5. β-Endorphin Modulation. This mechanism proposes that C fiber afferent impulses, mediated by the reticular formation of the thalamus, stimulates the release of ACTH and β-endorphin by the pituitary. It is more likely that the analgesia following prolonged C fiber afferent stimulation results from endogenous opiads released in the brain.

Summary of Pain Control Mechanisms

The body's pain control mechanisms are probably not mutually exclusive. Rather, analgesia is the result of overlapping processes. It is also important to realize that the theories presented are only models. They are useful in conceptualizing the perception of pain and pain relief. These models will help the sports therapist understand the effects of therapeutic modalities and form a sound rationale for modality application. As more research is conducted and as the mysteries of pain and neurophysiology are solved, new models will emerge. The sports therapist should adapt these models to fit new developments.

COGNITIVE INFLUENCES

Pain perception and the response to a painful experience may be influenced by a variety of cognitive processes, including anxiety, attention, depression, past pain experiences, and cultural influences. These individual aspects of pain expression are mediated by higher centers in the cortex in ways that are not clearly understood. They may influence both the sensory discriminative and motivational affective dimensions of pain.

Many mental processes modulate the perception of pain through descending systems. Behavior modification, the excitement of the moment, happiness, positive feelings, focusing (directed attention toward specific stimuli), hypnosis, and suggestion may modulate pain perception. Past experiences, cultural background, personality, motivation to play, aggression, anger, and fear are all factors that could facilitate or inhibit pain perception. Strong central inhibition may mask severe injury for a period of time. At such times, evaluation of the injury is quite difficult.

Athletes with chronic pain may become very depressed and experience a severe loss of fitness. They tend to be less active and may have altered appetites and sleep habits. They have a decreased will to perform and often develop a reduced sex drive. They may turn to self-abusive patterns of behavior. Tricyclic drugs are often used to inhibit serotonin depletion for the athlete with chronic pain.

Just as pain may be inhibited by central modulation, it may also arise from central origins. Phobias, fear, depression, anger, grief, and hostility are all capable of producing pain in the absence of local pathologic processes. In addition, pain memory, which is associated with old injuries, may result in pain perception and pain response that are out of proportion to a new, often minor, injury. Substance abuse can also alter and confound the perception of pain. Substance abuse may cause the chronic pain patient to become more depressed or may lead to depression and psychosomatic pain.

PAIN MANAGEMENT

How should the sports therapist approach pain? First, the source of the pain must be identified. Unidentified pain may hide a serious disorder, and treatment of such pain may delay the appropriate treatment of the disorder. Once a diagnosis has been made, many physical agents can provide pain relief. The therapist should match the therapeutic agent to each athlete's situation. Casts and braces may prevent the application of ice or moist heat. However, TENS electrodes often can be positioned under a cast or brace for pain relief. Following acute injuries, ice may be the therapeutic agent of choice because of the effect of cold on the inflammatory process. There is not one "best" therapeutic agent for pain control. The sports therapist must select the therapeutic agent that is most appropriate for each athlete, based on the knowledge of the modalities and professional judgment. In no situation should the therapist apply a therapeutic agent without first developing a clear rationale for the treatment.

In general, physical agents can be used to:

1. Stimulate large-diameter afferent fibers. This can be done with TENS, superficial heat, massage, and analgesic balms.
2. Decrease pain fiber transmission velocity with cold or ultrasound.
3. Stimulate small-diameter afferent fibers and descending pain control mechanisms with acupressure, deep massage, or TENS over acupuncture points or trigger points.
4. Stimulate a release of BEP or other endogenous opioids through prolonged C fiber stimulation with TENS.

Other useful pain control strategies include the following:

1. Encourage central biasing through cognitive processes, such as motivation, tension diversion, focusing, relaxation techniques, positive thinking, thought stopping, and self-control.
2. Minimize the tissue damage through the application of proper first aid and immobilization.
3. Maintain a line of communication with the athlete. Let the athlete know what to expect following an injury. Pain, swelling, dysfunction, and atrophy will occur following injury. The athlete's anxiety over these events will increase his or her perception of pain. Often, an athlete who has been told what to expect by someone he or she trusts will be less anxious and suffer less pain.
4. Recognize that all pain, even psychosomatic pain, is very real to the athlete.
5. Encourage supervised exercise to encourage blood flow, promote nutrition, increase metabolic activity, and reduce stiffness and guarding, if the activity will not cause further harm to the athlete.

The physician may choose to prescribe oral or injectable medications in the treatment of the injured athlete. The most commonly used medications are classified as analgesics, antiinflammatory agents, or both. The sports therapist should become familiar with these drugs and note if the athlete is taking any medications. It is also important to work with the team physician to assure that the athlete takes the medications appropriately.

The sports therapist's approach to the athlete has a great impact on the success of the treatment. The athlete will not be convinced of the efficacy and importance of the treatment unless the therapist appears confident about it. The sports therapist must make the athlete a participant rather than a passive spectator in the treatment and rehabilitation process.

The goal of most treatment programs is to encourage early pain-free exercise. The physical agents used to control pain do little to promote tissue healing. They should be used to relieve acute pain following injury or surgery or to control pain and other symptoms, such as swelling, to promote progressive exercise. The sports therapist should not lose sight of the effects of the physical agents or the importance of progressive exercise in restoring the athlete's athletic ability.

Reducing the perception of pain is as much an art as a science. Selection of the proper physical agent, proper application, and marketing are all important and will continue to be so even as we increase our understanding of the neurophysiology of pain. There is still the need for a good empirical rationale for the use of a physical agent. The sports therapist is encouraged to keep abreast of the neurophysiology of pain and the physiology of tissue healing to maintain a current scientific basis for selecting modalities and managing the injured athlete.

SUMMARY

1. Pain is a response to a noxious stimulus that is subjectively modified by past experiences and expectations.
2. Pain is classified as either acute or chronic and can exhibit many differing patterns.
3. Early reduction of pain in a treatment program will facilitate therapeutic exercise.
4. Stimulation of sensory receptors via the therapeutic modalities can modify the athlete's perception of pain.
5. Three mechanisms of pain control may explain the analgesic effects of physical agents:
   a. Dorsal horn modulation due to the input from large-diameter afferents through a gate control system, the release of enkephalins, or both.
   b. Descending efferent fiber activation due to the effects of small fiber afferent input on higher centers including the thalamus, raphe nucleus, and periaqueductal gray region.
   c. The central release of endogenous opioids including β-endorphin through prolonged C fiber afferent stimulation.
6. Pain perception may be influenced by a variety of cognitive processes mediated by the higher brain centers.
7. The selection of a therapeutic modality for controlling pain should be based on current knowledge of neurophysiology and the psychology of pain.
8. The application of physical agents for the control of pain should not occur until the diagnosis of the injury has been established.
9. The selection of a therapeutic modality for managing pain should be based on establishing the primary cause of pain.

GLOSSARY

accommodation Adaptation by the sensory receptors to various stimuli over an extended period of time.

ACTH Adrenocorticotropic hormone. This hormone has antiinflammatory actions.

afferent Conduction of a nerve impulse toward an organ.

avulsion fracture A fracture in which a small piece of bone is torn away by an attached tendon or ligament.

β-endorphin A neurohormone derived from β-lipotropin and containing enkephalin. It is similar in structure and properties to morphine. β-endorphin has a half-life of 4 hours.[18]

β-lipotropin A pituitary hormone containing β-endorphin and enkaphalin and having opiate activity.[18]

bradykinin A chemical formed in injured tissue as part of the inflammatory process that vasodilates small arterioles.

central biasing A theory of pain modulation mediated in the raphe nucleus.

efferent Conduction of a nerve impulse away from an organ.

endogenous opiates Naturally occurring opiates.

endorphins Endogenous opiates whose actions have analgesic properties. They are neurohormones and not neurotransmitters (i.e., β-endorphins).[18]

enkephalin Neurotransmitter proteins that are pain-relieving molecules. They block the passage of noxious stimuli by servicing descending neurons to counter ascending signals. They inhibit the release of substance P and are produced by enkephalinergic neurons.[18]

enkephalinergic neurons Neurons with short axons that release enkephalin. They act as interneurons (internuncial neurons) and are found in the substantia gelatinosa, nucleus raphae magnus, and periaqueductal gray matter.[18]

focusing Narrowing attention to the appropriate stimuli in the environment.

interneurons Neurons contained entirely in the central nervous system. They have no projections outside the spinal cord. Their function is to serve as relay stations within the central nervous system.

joint capsule Ligamentous structure that surrounds and encapsulates a joint.

neurotransmitter Substance that passes information between neurons. It is released from one neuron terminal (presynaptic membrane), enters the synaptic cleft, and attaches (binds) to a receptor on the next neuron (postsynaptic membrane). Substance P, enkephalins, serotonin, methionine, and leucine enkephalin are neurotransmitters.[2]

nociceptive Pain information or signals or pain stimuli.

norepinephrine A neurotransmitter that may enhance pain. When it is inhibited, analgesia is increased. Increased levels in the central nervous system decrease analgesia.[2]

opiate receptors Neurons that have receptors that bind to opiate substances.[2]

periosteum A highly vascularized and innervated membrane lining the surface of bone.

polymodal nociceptors Small unmyelinated afferent fibers that have high threshold axons and respond only to cutaneous stimulation (i.e., pain, deep pressure, and temperature).[4] C fibers are examples of these.

prostaglandins Irritants that are synthesized locally during injury in tissues from a fatty acid precursor (arachidonic acid). They act with bradykinin to amplify pain by sensitizing afferent neurons to chemical and mechanical stimulation. Aspirin is thought to be capable of interrupting the process. Prostaglandins are powerful vasodilators. They induce erythema, increase leakage of plasma from vessels, and attract leukocytes to an injured area.[2]

raphe nucleus Part of the brain that is known to inhibit pain impulses being transmitted through the ascending system.

referred pain (referred myofascial pain) When nociceptive impulses reach the dorsal gray matter, they converge and their summation can depolarize internuncial neurons over several spinal segments, causing the individual to feel pain in distal areas innervated by these segments.

sclerotome A segment of bone innervated by a spinal segment.

sensitization Prolonged depolarization of nociceptive neurons that results in continuous stimulation. Most sensory receptors are rendered less sensitive after prolonged stimulation. This is not the case with nociceptive neurons.[4]

serotonin A neurotransmitter that may block noxious stimuli through descending neurons that block ascending neurons. It is found in the vesicles in nerve endings that bind when released to postsynaptic membranes. Its action is terminated by reuptake into presynaptic membranes. It is probably involved in both endogenous pain control and opiate analgesia. Increased levels of serotonin in the central nervous system are generally associated with increased analgesia.[2]

stimulus-produced analgesia (SPA) Pain relief created by stimulation of portions of the central nervous system, either directly or indirectly. Common methods are electrical stimulation, needle, pressure, or extreme cold applied to acupuncture points, trigger points, or motor points.[24]

substance P A peptide believed to be the neurotransmitter of small-diameter primary afferents. It is released from both ends of the neuron.[4]

substantia gelatinosa Located in the dorsal horn of

the gray matter; thought to be responsible for closing the gate to painful stimuli.

T cell Transmission cell or neuron in the dorsal horn of the cord that is an interneuron or internuncial neuron. Principal location may be lamina V.[23]

trigger point Localized deep tenderness in a palpable firm band of muscle. If the muscle is stretched, a palpating finger can snap the band like a taut string, which produces local pain, a local twitch of that portion of the muscle, and a jump by the patient. Sustained pressure on a trigger point reproduces the pattern of referred pain for that site.

REFERENCES

1 Adler, M.W.: Endorphins, enkephalins and neurotransmitters, Med. Times **110**:32-35, 1982.

2 Anderson, S., Ericson, T., Holmgren, E., et al.: Electroacupuncture affects pain threshold measured with electrical stimulation of teeth, Brain **63**:393-396, 1973.

3 Berne, R.M., and Levy, M.N.: Physiology, St. Louis, 1988, The C.V. Mosby Co.

4 Bishop, B.: Pain: its physiology and rationale for management, Phys. Ther. **60**:13-37, 1980.

5 Castel, J.C.: Pain management: acupuncture and transcutaneous electrical nerve stimulation techniques, Lake Bluff, Ill., 1979, Pain Control Services.

6 Chapman, C.R., and Benedetti, C.: Analgesia following electrical stimulation: partial reversal by a narcotic antagonist, Life Sci. **26**:44-48, 1979.

7 Cheng, R., and Pomeranz, B.: Electroacupuncture analgesia could be mediated by at least two pain relieving mechanisms; endorphin and non-endorphin systems, Life Sci. **25**:1957-1962, 1979.

8 Clement-Jones, V., McLaughlin, L., Tomlin, S., et al.: Increased beta-endorphin but not met-enkephalin levels in human cerebrospinal fluid after electroacupuncture for recurrent pain, Lancet **2**:946-948, 1980.

9 Denegar, C.R., Perrin, D.H., Rogol, A.D., et al.: Influence of transcutaneous electrical nerve stimulation on serum cortisol concentration, pain and range of motion (abstract), SEACSM Annual Meeting, Jan. 20, 1988. Reprint Int. J. Sports Med. (in press).

10 Kuland, D.N.: "The injured athletes" pain, Curr. Concepts Pain **1**:3-10, 1983.

11 Mayer, D.J., Price, D.D., and Rafii, A.: Antagonism of acupuncture analgesia in man by the narcotic antagonist naloxone, Brain Res. **121**:368-372, 1977.

12 Melzack, R., and Wall, P.: Pain mechanisms: a new theory, Science **150**:971-979, 1965.

13 Melzack, R.: Concepts of pain measurement. In Melzack, R., editor: Pain measurement and assessment, New York, 1983, Raven Press.

14 Merskey, H., Albe-Fessard, D.G., Bonica, J.J., et al.: Pain terms: a list with definitions and notes on usage, Pain **6**:249-252, 1979.

15 Pomeranz, B.: Brain opiates at work in acupuncture, New Scientist **73**:12-13, 1975.

16 Pomeranz, B., and Chiu, D.: Naloxone blockade of acupuncture analgesia: enkephalin implicated, Life Sci. **19**:1757-1762, 1976.

17 Pomeranz, B., and Paley, D.: Electro-acupuncture hypoalgesia is mediated by afferent impulses: an electrophysiological study in mice, Exp. Neurol. **66**:398-402, 1979.

18 Previte, J.J.: Human physiology, New York, 1983, McGraw-Hill, Inc.

19 Salar, G., Job, I., Mingringo, S., et al.: Effects of transcutaneous electrotherapy on CSF beta-endorphin content in patients without pain problems, Pain **10**:169-172, 1981.

20 Sjolund, B., and Eriksson, M.: Electroacupuncture and endogenous morphines, Lancet **2**:1085, 1976.

21 Sjolund, B., Terenius, L., and Eriksson, M.: Increased cerebrospinal fluid levels of endorphins after electro-acupuncture, Acta Physiol. Scand. **100**:382-384, 1977.

22 Wen HL, Ho WK, Ling N, et al.: The influence of electroacupuncture on naloxone: induces morphine withdrawal: elevation of immunoassayable beta-endorphin activity in the brain but not in the blood, Am. J. Clin. Med. **7**:237-240, 1979.

23 Willis, W.D., and Grossman, R.C.: Medical neurobiology, ed. 3, St. Louis, 1981, The C.V. Mosby Co.

24 Wolf, S.L.: Neurophysiologic mechanisms in pain modulation: relevance to tens. In Manheimer, J.S., and Lampe, G.N., editors: Clinical applications of tens, Philadelphia, 1984, F.A. Davis Co.

SUGGESTED READINGS

Bonica, J.J.: Pain research and therapy: past and current status and future needs. In Ng, K.Y., and Bonica, J.J., editors: Pain, discomfort and humanitarian care, New York, 1979, Elsevier.

Brena, S.F., and Chapman, S.L.: Chronic pain: an algorithm for management, Postgrad. Med. **72**(1):111-117, 1982.

Buchthal, F., and Rosenfalck, A.: Evoked action potentials and conduction velocity in human sensory nerves, Brain Res. **3**:1, 1966.

Burgess, P.R., and Perl, E.R.: Myelinated afferent fibers responding specifically to noxious stimulation of the skin, J. Physiol. (Lond.) **190**:541, 1967.

Byrne, M., Troy, A., et al.: Cross validation of the factor structure of MPQ, Pain **13**:193, 1982.

Casey, K.L., and Jones, E.G.: Suprasegmental mechanisms: an overview of ascending pathways: brain-stem and thalamus, Neurosci. Res. Program Bull. **16**:103, 1978.

Cattell, M., and Hoagland, H.: Response of tactile receptors to intermittent stimulation, J. Physiol. **72**:392, 1931.

Cosentino, A.B., Cross, D.L., et al.: Ultrasound effects on electroneuromyographic measures in sensory fibers of the median nerve, Phys. Ther. **63:**1789, 1983.

Digregorio, J.G., and Barbieri, E.J.: Pharmacologic management of pain, Am. Fam. Physician **27:**185-188, 1983.

Dubner, R., and Bennett, G.J.: Spinal and trigeminal mechanisms of nociception, Annu. Rev. Neurosci. **6:**381, 1983.

Fordyce, W.E.: Behavioral methods for chronic pain and illness, St Louis, 1976, The C.V. Mosby Co.

Fordyce, W.E.: A behavioral perspective on chronic pain. In Ng, L.K.Y., and Bonica, J.J., editors: Pain, discomfort, and humanitarian care, New York, 1980, Elsevier/North-Holland.

Fordyce, W.E.: Behavioral concepts in acute pain management, Mediguide Pain **3**(2):1-3, 1982.

Frankel, F.H., Wineburg, E., and Isele, F.W.: Hypnosis focusing consciousness to relieve pain, Aches Pains **4:**6-12, 1983.

Gammon, G.D., and Starr, I.: Studies on the relief of pain by counter-irritation, J. Clin. Invest. **20:**13, 1941.

Georgopoulos, A.P.: Functional properties of primary afferent units probably related to pain mechanisms in primate glabrous skin, J. Neurophysiol. **39:**79, 1976.

Gracely, R.H.: Psychophysical assessment of human pain. In Bonica, J.J., editor: Advances in pain research and therapy, vol. 3, New York, 1979, Raven Press.

Gracely, R.H.: Pain measurement in man. In Ng, L.K.Y., and Bonica, J.J., editors: Pain, discomfort and humanitarian care, New York, 1980, Elsevier/North-Holland.

Guyton, A.C.: Textbook of medical physiology, ed. 7, Philadelphia, 1986, W.B. Saunders Co., pp. 545-605.

Hancock, M.B., Foreman, R.D., et al.: Convergence of visceral and cutaneous input onto spinothalamic tract cells in the thoracic spinal cord of the cat, Exp. Neurol. **47:**240, 1975.

Hensel, H.: Thermoreception and temperature regulation, New York, 1981, Academic Press.

Hökfelt, T., Terenius, L., et al.: Evidence for enkephalin immunoreactive neurons in the medulla oblongata projecting to the spinal cord, Neurosci. Lett. **14:**55, 1979.

Hughes, J.: Search for the endogenous legend of the opiate receptor, Neurosci. Res. Program Bull. **13:**55, 1975.

Hughes, J.: Intrinsic factors and the opiate receptor system, Neurosci. Res. Program Bull. **16:**141, 1978.

Ishijima, B., Yoshimasu, N., Fukushima, T., et al.: Nociceptive neurons in the human thalamus, Confin. Neurol. **37:**99, 1975.

Izzo, K.L., and Aravabhumi, S.: Physical medicine and rehabilitation in treating chronic pain, Med. Times **110:**43-48, 1982.

Kanner, R.: Psychotropic drugs in the management of pain, Curr. Concepts Pain **1**(2):51-74, 1983.

Kerr, F.W.L.: Neuroanatomical substrates of nociception in the spinal cord, Pain **1:**325, 1975.

Kerr, F.W.L.: An overview of neural mechanisms of pain, Neurosci. Res. Program Bull. **16:**30, 1978.

Kerr, F.W.L., and Wilson, P.R.: Pain, Annu. Rev. Neurosci. **1:**83, 1978.

Kessler, R.M., and Hertling, D.: Management of common musculoskeletal disorders, Philadelphia, 1983, Harper & Row Publishers, Inc., pp. 51-74.

Klepac, R.K., Dowling, J., et al.: Sensitivity of the McGill Pain Questionnaire to intensity and quality of laboratory pain, Pain **10:**199, 1981.

Kuhar, M.J., Pert, C.B., and Snyder, S.H.: Regional distribution of opiate receptor binding in monkey and human brain, Nature **245:**447, 1973.

LaMotte, R.H., and Campbell, J.N.: Comparison of responses of warm and nociceptive C-fiber afferents in monkey with human judgments of thermal pain, J. Neurophysiol. **41:**509, 1978.

LaMotte, R.H., Ghalhammer, J.G., et al.: Peripheral neural mechanisms of cutaneous hyperalgesia following mild injury by heat, J. Neurosci. **2:**765, 1982.

Long, D.M.: External electrical stimulation as a treatment of chronic pain, Minn. Med. **57:**195, 1974.

Luce, J.M., Thompson, T.L., Getto, C.J., and Byney, R.L.: New concepts of chronic pain and their implications, Hosp. Pract. **14:**113-123, 1979.

Macaiewicz, R.: Central pain pathways, Mediguide Pain **3**(4):1-4, 1982.

Mayer, D.J., and Price, D.D.: A physiological and psychological analysis of pain: a potential model of motivation. In Pfaff, D.: Physiological mechanisms of motivation, New York, 1982, Springer-Verlag.

Mayer, D.J., Price, D.D., and Becker, D.P.: Neurophysiological characterization of the anterolateral spinal cord neurons contributing to pain perception in man, Pain **1:**59, 1975.

Melzack, R.: The puzzle of pain, New York, 1973, Basic Books.

Melzack, R.: The McGill Pain Questionnaire: major properties and scoring methods, Pain **1:**277, 1975.

Melzack, R., Stillwell, D., and Fox, E.: Trigger points and acupuncture points for pain: correlations and implications, Pain **3:**3-23, 1977.

Melzack, R., and Törgerson, W.S.: On the language of pain, Anesthesiology **34:**50, 1971.

Melzack, R., and Wall, P.D.: Pain mechanisms: a new theory, Science **150:**971, 1965.

Melzack, R., and Wall, P.: The challenge of pain, New York, 1982, Penguin Books.

Mense, S.: Effects of temperature on the discharges of muscle spindles and tendon organs, Pflugers Arch. **374:**159, 1978.

Mense, S., and Schmidt, R.F.: Muscle pain: which receptors are responsible for the transmission of noxious stimuli? In Rose, F.C. editor: Psychological aspects of clinical neurology, Oxford, 1977, Blackwell Scientific Publications.

Merskey, H., and Able-Fessard, D.G.: Pain terms: a list with definitions and notes on usage, Pain **6:**249, 1979.

Nathan, P.W.: The gate-control theory of pain: a critical review, Brain **99:**123, 1976.

Nyquist, J.K.: Somatosensory properties of neurons of thalamic nucleus ventralis lateralis, Exp. Neurol. **48:**123, 1975.

Ohnhaus, E.E., and Adler, R.: Methodological problems in the measurement of pain: a comparison between the verbal rating scale and the visual analogue scale, Pain **1:**379, 1975.

Parsons, C.M., and Goetzl, F.R.: Effect of induced pain on pain threshold, Proc. Soc. Exp. Bio. Med. **60:**327, 1945.

Pelletier, G., Steinbusch, H.W.M., et al.: Immunoreactive substance P and serotonin present in the same dense-core vesicles, Nature **293:**71, 1981.

Pert, C.: Opiate receptors and pain pathways, Neurosci. Res. Program Bull. **16:**133, 1978.

Price, D.D., and Dubner, R.: Neurons that subserve the sensory-discriminative aspects of pain, Pain 3:307, 1977.

Price, D.D., Hayes, R.L., Ruda, M., et al.: Spatial and temporal transformation of input to spinothalamic tract neurons and their relation to somatic sensation, J. Neurophysiol. **41**:933, 1978.

Price, D.D., Hu, J.W., Dubner, R., et al.: Peripheral suppression of first pain and central summation of second pain evoked by noxious heat pulses, Pain 3:57, 1977.

Procacci, P., and Zoppi, M.: Pathophysiology and clinical aspects of visceral and referred pain. In Bonica, J.J., Lindblom, V., et al.: Advances in pain research and therapy, vol. 5, New York, 1981, Raven Press.

Reading, A.E.: A comparison of MPQ in chronic and acute pain, Pain **13**:185, 1982.

Roeser, W., Meeks, L., Veins, R., and Strickland, G.: The use of transcutaneous stimulation for pain control in athletic medicine: a preliminary report, Am. J. Sports Med.

Simons, D.G., and Travell, J.G.: Myofascial origins of low back pain, Postgrad. Med. J. **73**:66, 1983.

Tait, R.C.: Psychological factors in chronic benign pain: evaluation and treatment, Curr. Concepts Pain 1(1):10-15, 1983.

Torebjörk, H.E., and Hallin, R.G.: Perceptual changes accompanying controlled preferential blocking of A and C fibre responses in intact human skin nerves, Exp. Brain. Res. **16**:321, 1973.

Torebjörk, H.E., and Hallin, R.G.: Excitation failure in thin nerve fiber structure and accompanying hypalgesia during repetitive electrical skin stimulation. In Bonica, J.J., editor: Advances in neurology, vol. 4, New York, 1974, Raven Press.

Travell, J.: Temporomandibular joint dysfunction, J. Prosthet. Dent. **10**:745, 1960.

Travell, J.: Myofascial trigger points: clinical view. In Bonica, J.J., Able-Fessard, D.G., editors: Advances in pain research and therapy, vol. 1, New York, 1976, Raven Press.

Travell, J.G., and Simons, D.G.: Myofascial trigger point manual, Baltimore, 1982, Williams & Wilkins.

Travell, J.G., and Simons, D.G.: Myofascial pain and dysfunction, Baltimore, 1983, Williams & Wilkins, pp. 29-37.

Turk, D.C.: Measuring pain behavior, Aches Pains 35-36, 1983.

Van Hees, J.: Human C-fiber input during painful and nonpainful skin stimulation with radiant heat. In Bonica, J.J., and Able-Fessard, D., editors: Advances in pain research and therapy, vol. 1, New York, 1976, Raven Press.

Wall, P.D.: The gate control theory of pain mechanisms: a re-examination and re-statement, Brain **101**:1, 1978.

Wall, P.D.: The role of substantia gelatinosa as a gate control. In Bonica, J.J., editor: Pain, New York, 1980, Raven Press.

Wall, P.D., and Sweet, W.H.: Temporary abolition of pain in man, Science **155**:108, 1967.

Warfield, C.A., and Stein, J.M.: Chronic pain: contributory factors, Hosp. Pract. 49-56, 1982.

Watson, J.: Pain mechanisms: a review, III, Aust. J. Physiother. **28**(2):38-45, 1982.

Weissmann, G.: The pain mediators, Aust. J. Physiother. **28**(2):17-21, 1982.

Weissmann, G.: Anesthet and analgesic action, Aust. J. Physiother. **28**(2):36-38, 1982.

White, J.C., and Sweet, W.H.: Pain and the neurosurgeon: a forty-year experience. Springfield, 1969, Charles C Thomas.

Wolf, S.L.: Perspectives on central nervous system responsiveness to transcutaneous electrical stimulation, Phys. Ther. **58**:1443-1449, 1978.

Yaksh, T.L., and Hammond, D.L.: Peripheral and central substances involved in rostrad (ascending) transmission of nociceptive information, Pain **13**:1, 1982.

Zimmerman, M: Peripheral and central nervous mechanisms of nociception, pain, and pain therapy: facts and hypotheses. In Bonica, J.J. et al., editors: Advances in pain research and therapy, vol. 3, New York, 1979, Raven Press.

Therapeutic Modalities in Relation to the Electromagnetic and Acoustic Spectra

William E. Prentice

2

OBJECTIVES

Following completion of this chapter, the student will be able to:

- Discuss what radiant energy is and how it is produced.

- Describe the relationship between wavelength and frequency.

- Indicate how the sports therapist can make use of electromagnetic radiations to affect the biologic tissues of the body.

- Discuss the physiologic effects produced by each therapeutic modality.

- Differentiate between the electromagnetic and acoustic spectra.

There is considerable confusion among sports therapists regarding the relationship of the various therapeutic modalities to the **electromagnetic** and **acoustic spectra.** Electrical stimulating currents, shortwave and microwave **diathermy,** the **infrared** modalities, **ultraviolet** therapy, and low-power lasers are all therapeutic agents that emit a type of energy with **wavelengths** and **frequencies** that can be classified as electromagnetic radiations. **Ultrasound** is a form of radiation whose wavelength and frequency of vibration are best classified in the acoustic spectrum rather than in the electromagnetic spectrum. Each of the modalities that make use of these varying types of energy will be discussed in the following chapters.

RADIANT ENERGY

Radiation is a process by which energy in various forms travels through space. Most of us are familiar with the effects of radiation from the sun. Sunlight is a type of radiant energy, and we know that it not only makes objects visible but also produces heat. The sun emits radiant energy as a result of high-intensity chemical reactions. This radiant energy in the form of sunlight travels through space at about 300,000 meters per second and eventually reaches earth where its effects may be felt or seen. But the sun is not the only object capable of producing this radiant energy.[1,7]

All matter produces energy that radiates in the form of heat. The sun produces radiation through chemical reactions. But when a sufficiently intense chemical or electrical force is applied to any object, radiant energy in various forms can be produced by movement of electrons. Many of the therapeutic modalities to be discussed in this text produce radiant energy (i.e., the infrared modalities, the diathermies, lasers, and the electrical stimulating modalities).

If a ray of sunlight is passed through a prism, it will be broken down into various regions of colors (Fig. 2-1). Each of these colors represents a different form of radiant energy. They appear because the various forms of radiant energy are **refracted** or change direction as a result of differences in wavelength and frequency of each color, thus resulting in distinct bands of color called a spectrum. These color variations that we can detect with our eyes are referred to as visible light or luminous radiations. It becomes apparent when looking at this colorful display that there is a region of red at one end of the spectrum and a region of violet at the other end. When passed through a prism, the type of radiant energy refracted the least appears as the color red, whereas that refracted the most is violet.[7]

This beam of sunlight passing through the prism is also propagating forms of radiant energy that are not visible to our eyes. If a thermometer is placed close to the red end of the spectrum, heat will be detected. Likewise, a photographic plate placed close to the violet end of the spectrum will indicate chemical changes. The form of radiant energy that produces heat and is located in the spectrum beyond the visible red portion is referred to as the infrared radiation region. The form of radiant energy that produces chemical changes and is located beyond the violet end of the visible spectrum is called the ultraviolet radiation region (Fig. 2-2). Ultraviolet, infrared, and visible light rays are produced by heat. As the temperature increases in a particular substance, the vibration of molecules tends to increase the activity of the electrons. The movement of electrons produces electromagnetic waves. The higher the temperature, the greater the frequency of electromagnetic waves produced. These elec-

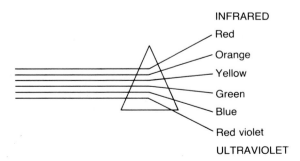

Figure 2-1. When a beam of light is shone through a prism, the various electromagnetic radiations in visible light are refracted and appear as a distinct band of color called a spectrum.

Region	Clinically Used Wavelength	Clinically Used Frequency*	Estimated Effective Depth of Penetration	Physiologic Effects
Electrical stimulating currents	3×10^8 Km to 75,000 Km	1–4000 Hz	Effects may occur anywhere between elect-rodes	Pain modulation, muscle contraction, relaxation, ion movement
Commercial radio and television				
Shortwave diathermy	22 m 11 m	13.56 MHz 27.12 MHz	3 cm	Deep tissue tempera-ture increase, vaso-dilation, increased blood flow
Microwave diathermy	69 cm 33 cm 12 cm	433.9 MHz 915 MHz 2450 MHz	5 cm	Deep tissue tempera-ture increase, vaso-dilation, increased blood flow
Infrared				
Cold packs (8° F)	111,000 A	2.7×10^{12} Hz		Superficial temperature decrease
Cold whirlpool (63° F)	99,514 A	3.01×10^{12} Hz		
Hot whirlpool (99° F)	93,097 A	3.22×10^{12} Hz	1 cm	Vasoconstriction— decreased blood flow
Paraffin bath (117° F)	90,187 A	3.32×10^{12} Hz		Analgesia
Hydrocollar (170° F)	82,457 A	3.63×10^{12} Hz		
Luminous IR (1341° F)	28,860 A	1.04×10^{13} Hz		Superficial temperature increase
Nonluminous IR (3140° F)	14,430 A	2.08×10^{13} Hz		Vasodilation— increased blood flow
Red	**Laser**			
Visible light	GaAs 9100 A HeNe 6328 A	3.3×10^{13} Hz 4.74×10^{13} Hz	5 cm 10–15 mm	Pain modulation and wound healing
Violet				
Ultraviolet				Superficial chemical changes
UV-A	3200–4000 A	9.38×10^{13}–7.5×10^{13} Hz		
UV-B	2900–3200 A	1.03×10^{14}–9.38×10^{13} Hz	2 mm	Tanning effects
UV-C	2000–2900 A	1.50×10^{14} –1.03×10^{14} Hz		Bactericidal
Ionizing radiation (x-ray, gamma rays, cosmic rays)				

*Calculated using C = λ × F, C = velocity (3 × 10 m/sec), λ = wavelength, F = frequency.

Figure 2-2. Electromagnetic spectrum.

tromagnetic waves produced by heat are usually absorbed by many objects and have little penetration.[6]

　　It is known that other forms of radiation beyond the infrared and ultravio-let portions of the spectrum may be produced when an electrical force is ap-plied.[7] Beyond the infrared portion of the spectrum lie several large regions of radiations known as the diathermies; these include radio, television, and nerve-

and muscle-stimulating currents. Beyond the ultraviolet end of the spectrum lie the high-frequency ionizing and penetration radiation region (i.e., x-ray, alpha, beta, and gamma rays).

All of these various classifications of radiations collectively constitute the electromagnetic spectrum (Fig. 2-2).

ELECTRO-MAGNETIC RADIATIONS

All the electromagnetic radiations lying within this spectrum have several theoretical characteristics in common:[2]

1. They may be produced when sufficiently intense electrical or chemical forces are applied to any material.
2. They all travel readily through space at an equal velocity.
3. Their direction of travel is always in a straight line.
4. They may be reflected, refracted, absorbed, or transmitted, depending on the specific medium that they strike.

The luminous, infrared, and ultraviolet rays in sunlight travel in waves through a vacuum or through space at a velocity of about 300 million meters per second and all reach the earth at about the same time. These rays are emitted from chemical reactions taking place on the sun, and each type of radiation processes its own individual physical characteristics. The basis of differentiation between the different regions of the electromagnetic spectrum is defined by analyzing the wavelengths and frequencies of the radiations within this spectrum.

The electromagnetic radiations produced by the different modalities all share the same physical characteristics as any other type of electromagnetic radiation. However, when these radiations come in contact with various biologic tissues, the velocity and direction of travel will be altered within the various types of tissues.

WAVELENGTH AND FREQUENCY

Wavelength is defined as the distance between the peak of one wave and the peak of either the preceding or succeeding wave. Frequency is defined as the number of wave oscillations or vibrations occurring in 1 second and is expressed in hertz (Hz) units.

Each of the various types of radiation in the electromagnetic spectrum has a specific wavelength and frequency of vibrations. Since it is accepted theoretically that all forms of electromagnetic radiation are produced simultaneously, travel at a constant velocity through space, and reach earth at the same time, it follows that longer wavelengths must have shorter frequencies and shorter wavelengths must have higher frequencies.

$$\text{Velocity} = \text{Wavelength} \times \text{Frequency}$$
$$C = \lambda \times F$$

Thus an inverse or reciprocal relationship exists between wavelength and frequency.

Velocity is a constant 3×10^8 km/sec. Therefore, if we know the wavelength, frequency can be calculated.

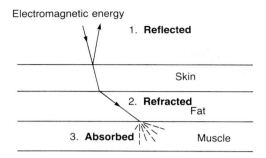

Figure 2-3. When electromagnetic radiations contact human tissues they may be reflected, refracted, or absorbed. Energy that is transmitted through the tissues must be absorbed before any physiologic changes can take place.

When electromagnetic radiations strike or come in contact with various objects several things may happen. Some rays may be **reflected,** while others are transmitted through the tissues where they may be refracted. Still others penetrate to deeper layers where they may be **absorbed** (Fig. 2-3). Generally, those radiations that have the longest wavelengths tend to have the greatest depths of penetration regardless of their frequency. It must be added, however, that a number of other factors, which will be discussed later, can also contribute to the depth of penetration.

　　The purpose of using therapeutic modalities is to stimulate a specific body tissue to perform its normal function. This stimulation will only occur if energy produced by the electrotherapeutic device is absorbed by the tissue. The **Arndt-Schultz principle** states that no reactions or changes can occur in the body tissues if the amount of energy absorbed is insufficient to stimulate the absorbing tissues. The goal of the sports therapist should be to deliver sufficient energy in one form or another to stimulate the tissues to perform their normal function while realizing that too much energy absorbed in a given period of time may seriously impair normal function and, if severe enough, may cause irreparable damage.[2]

　　If the therapeutic energy is not absorbed by the tissues, then according to the **Law of Grotthus-Draper,** it must be transmitted to deeper layers. The greater the amount of energy absorbed, the less transmitted and thus the less penetration.[5] The transmitted energy tends to (1) travel in a straight line, (2) come in contact with a tissue that reflects or turns away the energy, or (3) have its angle of transmission changed or refracted within the tissue. Radiant energy is more easily transmitted to deeper tissues if the source of radiation is at a right angle to the area being radiated. Thus the smaller the angle between the propagating ray and the right angle, the less radiation reflected and the greater the absorption. This principle, known as the **cosine law,** will be extremely important in the chapters dealing with the diathermies, ultraviolet light, and infra-

LAWS GOVERNING THE EFFECTS OF ELECTRO-MAGNETIC RADIATIONS

red heating, since the effectiveness of these modalities is based to a large extent on how they are positioned with regard to the patient (Fig. 2- 4).

The intensity of the radiation striking a particular surface is known to vary inversely with the square of the distance from the source. For example, a source of radiation that is 2 inches away from the surface will have one quarter of the intensity of a source of radiation that is 1 inch from the surface. This principle, known as the **inverse square law,** will obviously be of great consequence when setting up a specific modality to achieve a desired physiologic effect (Fig. 2-5). Regardless of the path this transmitted energy takes, the physiologic effects will only be apparent when the energy is absorbed by a specific tissue.

$$\frac{1}{2^2} = \frac{1}{4}$$

All physical modalities emitting electromagnetic radiations are subject to the relationship between absorption and transmission of energy. The modalities that emit radiations with relatively longer wavelengths have the ability to transmit energy through the superficial tissue layers, thus penetrating to the deeper tissues where it is absorbed.

THE APPLICATION OF THE ELECTRO-MAGNETIC SPECTRUM TO THERAPEUTIC MODALITIES

The therapeutic modalities discussed in detail in later chapters (with the exception of ultrasound and massage) all emit radiations with physical characteristics that may be classified as electromagnetic radiations.

Figure 2-2 represents the electromagnetic spectrum and places all of the modalities in order based on wavelengths and corresponding frequencies. It is apparent, for example, that the electrical stimulating currents have the longest wavelength and the lowest frequency and, all other factors being equal, should therefore have the greatest depth of penetration. As we move down the chart, the wavelengths in each region become progressively shorter and the frequencies progressively higher. Shortwave and microwave diathermy, the various sources of infrared heating, and the ultraviolet regions have progressively less depth of penetration.

It should be mentioned that the regions labeled as radio and television frequencies, visible light, and high-frequency ionizing and penetrating radiations certainly fall under the classification of electromagnetic radiations. However, they do not have application as therapeutic modalities and, while extremely important to our everyday way of life, warrant no further consideration in the context of this discussion.

Electrical Stimulating Currents

The electrical stimulating currents that affect nerve and muscle tissue have the longest wavelengths and the lowest frequencies of any of the modalities. The wavelengths of electrical stimulating units are extremely long, ranging somewhere around 15,000 km. Clinically used frequencies range from 1 to 4000 Hz. Most stimulators have the flexibility to alter the frequency output of the device to elicit a desired physiologic response. The nerve and muscle stimulating currents are capable of (1) pain modulations either through stimulation of cutaneous sensory nerves at high frequencies or through production of β-endorphin at lower frequencies, (2) producing muscle contraction and relaxation or tetany depending on the type of current (alternating or direct) and frequency, and (3)

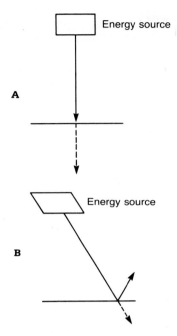

Figure 2-4. The cosine law states that the smaller the angle between the propagating ray and the right angle, the less radiation reflected and the greater absorbed. Thus the energy absorbed in *A* would be greater than in *B*.

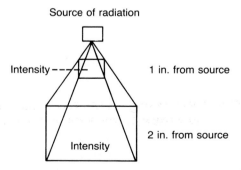

Figure 2-5. The inverse square law states that the intensity of the radiation striking a particular surface varies inversely with the square of the distance from the source.

producing a net movement of ions and thus eliciting a chemical change (direct current only).[8] The electrical stimulating currents and their various physiologic effects will be discussed in detail in Chapter 4.

Shortwave and Microwave Diathermy

The diathermies are considered to be high-frequency currents because they have more than a million cycles per second. When impulses of such a short duration come in contact with human tissue there is not sufficient time for ion movement to take place. Consequently there is no stimulation of either motor or sensory nerves. The energy of this rapidly vibrating electrical current produces heat as it passes through tissue cells, resulting in a temperature increase.

The electrotherapeutic shortwave and microwave devices have preset frequencies and wavelengths that cannot be altered. Shortwave diathermy units are set at either (1) 13.56 MHz (1 MHz = 10 million Hz) with a corresponding wavelength of 22 m or (2) 27.12 MHz with a wavelength of 11 m.[2]

Microwave units have shorter wavelengths than do shortwave diathermy units and are set at wavelengths of 33 or 12 cm with respective frequencies of 915 or 2450 MHz. The depth of penetration with microwave is a bit deeper than with shortwave because the amount of energy when using microwave is concentrated in one spot rather than spread out over a large area.[2] This will be discussed in more detail in Chapter 7.

Infrared Modalities

Perhaps the greatest confusion over this relationship between electromagnetic radiations and therapeutic modalities is associated with the infrared region. We tend to think of the infrared modalities as being the luminous and nonluminous infrared bakers or lamps only, when in fact the largest number of modalities used by sports therapists actually emit radiations with wavelengths and frequencies that clearly fall within this infrared region. Cold packs, hydrocollator packs, whirlpools, paraffin baths, and contrast baths are all infrared modalities.[4]

Earlier it was stated that any object heated (or cooled) to a temperature different than the surrounding environment will dissipate heat through radiation to the other materials with which it comes in contact. The infrared modalities are used to produce a local and occasionally a generalized heating or cooling of the superficial tissues. It is generally accepted that the infrared modalities have a maximum depth of penetration of 1 cm or less. The infrared modalities can elicit either increases or decreases in circulation depending on whether heat or cold is used. They are also known to have some analgesic effects as a result of stimulation of sensory cutaneous nerve endings.

The infrared region of the spectrum is located adjacent to the red end of the visible light region. The wavelengths of the infrared modalities are obviously much shorter than are those of the electrical stimulating currents and the diathermies and are expressed in Angstrom (A) units; 1 A is equal to 10^{-10} meters (m).

Both the infrared and ultraviolet wavelengths are temperature dependent.

Those modalities with the lower temperature have the longer wavelength. This means that an ice pack will have a longer wavelength and thus a greater depth of penetration than will a hydrocollator pack. Temperatures used with the infrared modalities range from $0°$ C with ice to more than $3000°$ C with the infrared lamps. The wavelengths in this temperature range fall between 10,000 and 105,000 A with corresponding frequencies ranging between 2×10^{12} and 4×10^{13} Hz.

It should be pointed out that an Angstrom unit is an extremely small unit of measure and thus the differences in depth of penetration are not great between any of the infrared modalities. The critical factor is the superficial increase or decrease in tissue temperature that elicits the same physiologic response regardless of wavelength.

Laser

Of the modalities discussed in this text, the low-power **laser** is certainly the newest used by the sports therapist. The word *laser* is an acronym for *l*ight application by *s*timulated emission of *r*adiation. Laser is a form of electromagnetic radiation that is classified within both the infrared and visible light portions of the spectrum.

Lasers are either high-power or low-power. High-power lasers are used in surgery for purposes of incision, coagulation of vessels, and thermolysis, owing to their thermal effects. The low-power or cold laser produces little or no thermal effects but seems to have some significant clinical effect on soft tissue and fracture healing as well as pain management through stimulation of acupuncture and trigger points.

Two types of low-power lasers are used by sports therapists: the helium-neon laser (HeNe), and the gallium-arsenide laser (GaAs). The HeNe laser has a wavelength of 632.8 nanometers (nm) and a direct depth of penetration to 0.8 mm, although there may be some indirect effects up to 10 to 15 mm. The GaAs laser has a wavelength of 910 nm and can penetrate indirectly as much as 5 cm. The laser as a therapeutic tool will be discussed in Chapter 9.

Ultraviolet Therapy

The ultraviolet portion of the electromagnetic spectrum is adjacent to the violet end of the visible light region. As stated previously, the radiations in the ultraviolet region are undetectable by the human eye. However, if a photographic plate is placed at the ultraviolet end, chemical changes will be apparent. Although an extremely hot source ($7000°$ to $9000°$ C) is required to produce ultraviolet wavelengths, the physiologic effects of ultraviolet are mainly chemical in nature and occur entirely in the cutaneous layers of skin. The maximum depth of penetration with ultraviolet is about 1 mm. The wavelengths with ultraviolet range between 2000 and 4000 A. The ultraviolet region is subdivided into three different areas; near ultraviolet or UV- A (3200 to 4000 A); middle ultraviolet or UV-B (2900 to 3200 A); and for ultraviolet or UV-C (2000 to 2900 A). Clinically used frequencies with ultraviolet range between 7×10^{13} and 7×10^{14}Hz.[2,5,8] Ultraviolet therapy is used rarely by the sports therapist to treat cutaneous lesions.

THE ACOUSTIC SPECTRUM AND ULTRASOUND

One additional therapeutic modality frequently used by sports therapists is ultrasound. Ultrasound devices produce a type of energy that must be classified as a portion of the acoustic spectrum rather than the electromagnetic spectrum. Ultrasound is frequently classified along with shortwave and microwave diathermy as a deep-heating, conversion-type modality, and it is certainly true that all of these are capable of producing a temperature increase in human tissue to a considerable depth. However, ultrasound is a mechanical vibration, a sound wave, produced and transformed from high-frequency electrical energy.[2] Ultrasound must be considered a type of acoustic vibration rather than a type of electromagnetic radiation.

Acoustic and electromagnetic radiations have very different physical characteristics. When acoustic vibrations are produced, they travel at a velocity that is significantly lower than electromagnetic radiations. Electromagnetic waves travel at approximately 300 million meters (m) per second while sound waves travel at speeds from hundreds to several thousand m per second.

The relationship between velocity, wavelength, and frequency is a bit different with acoustic energy than with electromagnetic energy even though the inverse relationship between wavelength and frequency still exists. The distinction lies in the fact that the velocity of travel is much greater for electromagnetic energy than for acoustic energy. Therefore wavelengths are considerably shorter in acoustic vibrations than in electromagnetic radiations at any given frequency.[2] For example, ultrasound traveling in the atmosphere has a wavelength of approximately 0.3 mm while electromagnetic radiations have wavelengths of 297 m at a similar frequency.

We stated that electromagnetic radiations were capable of traveling through space or through a vacuum. As the density of the transmitting medium is increased, the velocity of travel significantly decreases as a result of refraction, reflection, or absorption by the molecules in the medium. Acoustic vibrations will not be transmitted at all through a vacuum since they depend on conduction through molecular collisions. The more dense the transmitting medium, the greater the velocity of travel. In human tissue ultrasound has a much greater velocity of transmission in bone tissue (3500 m per second), for example, than in fat tissue (1500 m per second).

Frequencies of ultrasound wave production are between 700,000 and 1,000,000 cycles per second. Frequencies up to around 20,000 Hz are detectable by the human ear. Thus the ultrasound portion of the acoustic spectrum is inaudible. Ultrasound generators are generally set at a standard frequency of 1 megacycle (1000 KHz). The depth of penetration with ultrasound is much greater than with any of the electromagnetic radiations. At a frequency of 1 megacycle, 50% of the energy produced will penetrate to a depth of about 5 cm. The reason for this great depth of penetration is that ultrasound travels very well through homogeneous tissue (e.g., fat tissue) while electromagnetic radiations are almost entirely absorbed. Thus when therapeutic penetration to deeper tissues is desired, ultrasound is the modality of choice.[3,6]

Clinical ultrasound is capable of producing a temperature increase in the deeper tissues and thus to some extent pain relief as a result of both mechanical and chemical effects.[3] These physiologic effects will be discussed in greater detail in Chapter 6.

SUMMARY

1. Radiant energy may be produced when a sufficiently intense chemical or electrical force is applied to any object.
2. Electrical stimulating currents, shortwave and microwave diathermy, the infrared modalities, and ultraviolet therapy are all classified as portions of the electromagnetic spectrum according to corresponding wavelengths and frequencies associated with each region.
3. All electromagnetic radiations travel at the same velocity; thus wavelength and frequency are inversely related.
4. Radiations may be reflected, refracted, absorbed, or transmitted in the various tissues.
5. Those radiations with the longer wavelengths tend to have the greatest depth of penetration.
6. The purpose of using any therapeutic modality is to stimulate a specific tissue to perform its normal function.
7. Ultrasound is part of the acoustic spectrum and is best propagated through dense tissue such as biologic tissue; thus it is extremely effective in reaching deep tissues.

GLOSSARY

absorption Energy that stimulates a particular tissue to perform its normal function.

acoustic spectrum The range of frequencies and wavelengths of sound waves.

Arndt-Schultz Principle No reactions or changes can occur in the body if the amount of energy absorbed is not sufficient to stimulate the absorbing tissues.

cosine law Optimal radiation occurs when the source of radiation is at right angles to the center of the area being radiated.

diathermy The application of high-frequency electrical energy that is used to generate heat in body tissue as a result of the resistance of the tissue to the passage of energy.

electromagnetic spectrum The range of frequencies and wavelengths associated with radiant energy.

frequency The number of cycles or pulses per second.

infrared The portion of the electromagnetic spectrum associated with thermal changes located adjacent to the red portion of the visible light spectrum.

inverse square law The intensity of radiation striking a particular surface varies inversely with the square of the distance from the radiating source.

Law of Grotthus-Draper Energy not absorbed by the tissues must be transmitted.

radiation The process of emitting energy from some source in the form of waves. A method of heat transfer through which heat can be either gained or lost.

reflection The bending back of light or sound waves from a surface that they strike.

refraction The change in direction of a soundwave or radiation wave when it passes from one medium or type of tissue to another.

ultrasound A portion of the acoustic spectrum located above audible sound.

ultraviolet The portion of the electromagnetic spectrum associated with chemical changes located adjacent to the violet portion of the visible light spectrum.

wavelength The distance from one point in a propagating wave to the same point in the next wave.

REFERENCES

1 Goldman, L.: Introduction to modern phototherapy, Springfield, Ill., 1978, Charles C Thomas, Publisher.

2 Griffin, J., and Karselis, T.: Physical agents for physical therapists, Springfield, Ill., 1978, Charles C Thomas Publisher.

3 Lehmann, J.F., and Guy, A.W.: Ultrasound therapy. Proc Workshop on Interaction of Ultrasound and Biological Tissues. Washington, D.C., HEW Pub. (FDA 73:8008), Sept., 1972.

4 Lehmann, J., editor: Therapeutic heat and cold, ed. 2, New Haven, 1982, Elizabeth Licht, Publisher.

5 Licht, S.: Therapeutic electricity and ultraviolet radiation, New Haven, 1959, Elizabeth Licht, Publisher.

6 Schriber, W.: A manual of electrotherapy, Philadelphia, 1975, Lea & Febiger.

7 Sears, F., Zemansky, M., and Young, H.: University physics, Reading, Mass., 1976, Addison-Wesley Publishing Co., Inc.

8 Stillwell, K.: Therapeutic electricity and ultraviolet radiation, Baltimore, 1983, Williams & Wilkins.

SUGGESTED READINGS

Goodgold, J., and Eberstein, A.: Electrodiagnosis of neuromuscular diseases, Baltimore, 1972, Williams & Wilkins.

Jehle, H.: Charge fluctuation forces in biological systems, Ann. NY Acad. Sci. **158**:240-255, 1969.

Koracs, R.: Light therapy, Springfield, Ill., 1950, Charles C Thomas, Publisher.

Licht, S., editor: Electrodiagnosis and electromyography, ed. 3, New Haven, 1971, Elizabeth Licht, Publisher.

Scott, P., and Cooksey, F.: Clayton's electrotherapy and actinotherapy, London, 1962, Bailliere, Tindall and Cox.

Basic Principles of Electricity

3

William E. Prentice

OBJECTIVES

Following completion of this chapter, the student will be able to:

- Define potential difference, ampere, volt, ohm, and watt.
- Give Ohm's law and its mathematical expression.
- Differentiate between alternating and direct currents.
- Discuss various waveforms.
- Discuss waveform modulation and frequency.
- Differentiate between series and parallel circuit arrangement.
- Discuss current flow through various types of biologic tissue.
- Discuss safety in the use of electrical equipment by the sports therapist.

Many of the modalities discussed in this text may be classified as electrical modalities. These pieces of equipment have the capabilities of taking the electrical current flowing from a wall outlet and modifying that current to produce a specific, desired physiologic effect in human biologic tissue.

Understanding the basic principles of electricity is usually difficult even for the sports therapist who is accustomed to using electrical modalities on a daily basis. To understand how current flow effects biologic tissue it is first necessary to become familiar with some of the principles that describe how electricity is produced and how it behaves in an electrical circuit.

These principles can be applied to all of the electrical modalities to be discussed in later chapters but are particularly applicable to Chapter 4, Electrical Stimulating Currents.

All matter is composed of atoms that contain positively and negatively charged particles called **ions.** These charged particles possess electrical energy and thus have the ability to move about. They tend to move from an area of higher concentration toward an area of lower concentration. An electrical force is capable of propelling these particles from higher to lower energy levels, thus

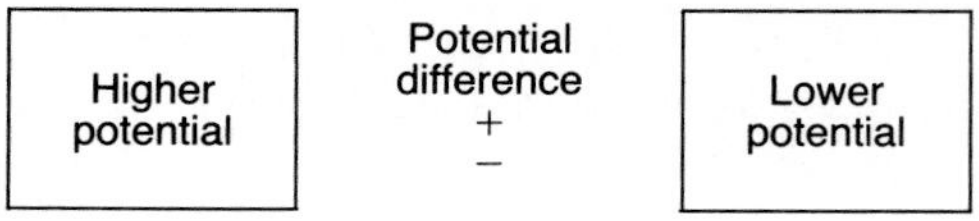

Higher potential	Potential difference + −	Lower potential

Figure 3-1. The difference between high potential and low potential is potential difference. Electrons tend to flow from areas of higher concentration to areas of lower concentration. A potential difference must exist if there is to be any movement of electrons.

establishing **electrical potentials.** The more ions an object has, the higher its potential electrical energy. Particles with a positive charge tend to move toward negatively charged particles, and those that are negatively charged tend to move toward the positively charged particles (Fig. 3-1).[9]

Electrons are particles of matter possessing a negative charge and very small mass. The net movement of electrons is referred to as an electrical **current.** The movement or flow of these electrons will always go from a higher potential to a lower potential.[13] An electrical force is oriented in one direction of the applied force. This flow of electrons may be likened to a domino reaction.

The unit of measurement that indicates the rate at which electrical current flows is the **ampere** (amp); 1 amp is defined as the movement of 1 **coulomb** or 6.25×10^{18} electrons per second. Amperes indicate the rate of electron flow while coulombs indicate the number of electrons. In the case of therapeutic modalities, current flow is generally described in **milliamperes** (1/1000 of an amp, denoted as **mamp**) or in microamperes (1/1,000,000 of an amp, denoted as µamp).

The electrons will not move unless an electrical potential difference in the concentration of these charged particles exists between two points. The electromotive force, which must be applied to produce a flow of electrons, is called a **volt** (V) and is defined as the difference in electron population (potential difference) between two points.[3]

Voltage is the force resulting from an accumulation of electrons at one point in an electrical circuit, usually corresponding to a deficit of electrons at another point in the circuit. If the two points are connected by a suitable conductor, the potential difference (difference in electron population) will cause electrons to move from the area of higher population to the area of lower population.

Commercial current flowing from wall outlets produces an electromotive force of either 115 V or 220 V. The electrotherapeutic devices used in injury rehabilitation modify voltages. Devices that use up to about 150 V are called **low-voltage** or low-tension currents. Those using from several hundred to several thousand volts are referred to as **high-voltage** or high-tension currents.[3]

Electrons can move in a current only if there is a relatively easy pathway to move along. Materials that permit this free movement of electrons are referred to as conductors. **Conductance** is a term that defines the ease with which current flows along a conducting medium. Metals (copper, gold, silver, aluminum) are good conductors of electricity, as are electrolyte solutions, because both are composed of large numbers of free electrons that are given up readily. Thus materials that offer little opposition to current flow are good conductors. Materials that resist current flow are called insulators. Insulators contain relatively fewer free electrons and thus offer greater resistance to electron flow. Air, wood, and glass are all considered insulators. The number of amps flowing in a given conductor is dependent both on the voltage applied and on the conduction characteristics of the material.[12]

The opposition to electron flow in a conducting material is referred to as resistance or electrical impedance and is measured in a unit known as an ohm. Thus, an electrical circuit that has high resistance (ohms) will have less flow (amps) than a circuit with less resistance and the same voltage.[2]

The mathematical relationship between current flow, voltage, and resistance is demonstrated in the formula:

$$\text{Current flow} = \frac{\text{Voltage}}{\text{Resistance}}$$

This formula is the mathematical expression of **Ohm's law,** which states that the current in an electrical circuit is directly proportional to the voltage and inversely proportional to the resistance.

An analogy comparing the movement of water with the movement of electricity may help to clarify this relationship between current flow, voltage, and resistance (Table 3-1). In order for water to flow, some type of pump must create a force to produce movement. Likewise, the volt is the pump that produces the electron flow. The resistance to water flow is dependent on the length, diameter, and smoothness of the water pipe. The resistance to electrical flow depends on the characteristics of the conductor. The amount of water flowing is measured in gallons while the amount of electricity flowing is measured in amperes.

The amount of energy produced by flowing water is determined by two factors: (1) the number of gallons flowing per unit of time and (2) the pressure created in the pipe. Electrical energy or power is a product of the voltage or electromotive force and the amount of current flowing. Electrical power is measured in a unit called a **watt.**

$$\text{Watts} = \text{Volts} \times \text{Amperes}$$

Simply, the watt indicates the rate at which electrical power is being used. A watt is defined as the electrical power needed to produce a current flow of 1 amp at a pressure of 1 volt.

TABLE 3-1   Electron Flow as Analogous to Water Flow

Electron Flow		Water Flow
Volt	=	Pump
Amperes	=	Gallons
Ohm (properties of conductor)	=	Resistance (length and distance of pipe)

**ELECTRO-
THERAPEUTIC
CURRENTS**

Electrotherapeutic devices generate two different types of current, which when introduced into biologic tissue are capable of producing specific physiologic changes. These two types of current are referred to as **alternating** (AC) and **direct** (DC).

In an alternating current, the flow of electrons constantly changes direction, or stated differently, reverses its polarity. Electrons flowing in an alternating current always move from the negative to positive pole reversing direction when polarity is reversed (Fig. 3-2, *A*). The direct current, also referred to as galvanic current, has a unidirectional flow of electrons toward the positive pole (Fig. 3-2, *B*). On most modern direct current devices the polarity and thus the direction of current flow can be reversed.[13]

The therapeutic physiologic effects of alternating and direct currents when applied to biologic tissues are different from and should not be confused with electrical generators, which are classified as either alternating or direct current generators. The therapeutic effects of nerve and muscle stimulating currents, which may be either alternating or direct, will be discussed in detail in Chapter 4.

Electrotherapeutic devices are usually classified as being either high-

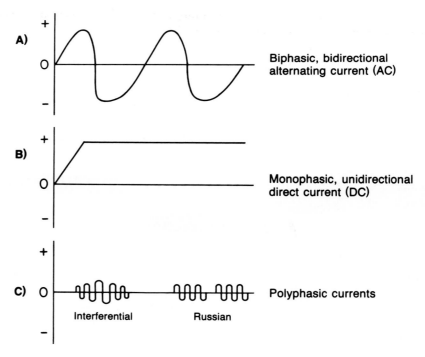

Figure 3-2. A, Alternating current periodically changes its polarity or direction of flow. **B,** Direct current always flows in the same direction and may flow in either a positive or negative direction. **C,** Polyphasic currents are usually referred to as interferential or "Russian" currents.

voltage generators or low-voltage generators. High-voltage devices produce waveforms with an amplitude of 150 V or greater and a relatively short pulse duration of less than 100 msec. Most high-voltage devices produce direct current, but some alternating current generators are also available. The amplitude of high-voltage currents is greater than that of low-voltage currents, and this factor combined with a short pulse duration enables high-voltage currents to produce a muscle contraction, as well as selectively stimulating sensory nerves. Most modern high-voltage generators produce twin pulses of high amplitude and short pulse width, thus allowing for nonirritating stimulation of nerve and muscle tissue.[14]

Low-voltage generators produce voltages lower than 150 V and are capable of generating from one to several thousand pulses per second. These devices seem to be more effective when thermal or chemical effects are desired; however, they are also used for producing muscular contractions. A direct current generator that produces only a one-pulse continuous current causes only chemical effects.

Generators that produce electrotherapeutic currents may be driven by either alternating or direct currents. Devices that plug into the standard electrical wall outlet use alternating current. The commercially produced alternating current changes its direction of flow 120 times per second. In other words, there are 60 complete cycles per second. The number of cycles occurring in 1 second is called **frequency** and is indicated in Hertz (Hz), pulses per second, or cycles per second. The voltage of electromotive force producing this alternating directional flow of electrons is set at a standard 115 V or 220 V. Thus, commercial alternating current is produced at 60 Hz with a corresponding voltage of either 115 or 220.

Other electrotherapeutic devices are driven by batteries that always produce direct current, ranging between 1.5 and 9 V, although the devices driven by batteries may in turn produce modified types of current.

There is no relationship between the type of current being delivered by the power source (i.e., a wall outlet or battery) and the type of current being output to the patient by the generator. For example, a stimulating unit that plugs into a wall outlet is being driven by an AC power source, but that same unit may very well output DC current to the patient. This "conversion" from an AC power source to a DC output is accomplished by a series of electrical components within the stimulating unit: a transformer, a rectifier, a filter, a regulator, an amplifier, and an oscillator.[6] A transformer "steps down" or reduces the amount of voltage from the power supply. The rectifier converts AC current to pulsating DC current. The filter changes the pulsating DC current to smooth DC. The regulator produces a specific controlled voltage output. An output amplifier within the stimulating unit is used to magnify or increase the amplitude of the voltage output of the generator and control it at a specific level, regardless of the electrical impedance of the remainder of the circuit (including the electrodes and patient). The oscillator is used to produce and output a specific waveform, which again may be different from that used to power or drive the stimulating unit.

WAVEFORMS   Once the electrotherapeutic device receives power, the components within the electrical circuit of the machine have the ability to alter the current flow and produce a specific **waveform** or pulse of variable intensity that can elicit a desired physiologic response. The term *waveform* indicates a graphic representation of the shape, direction, amplitude, and duration of the electrical current being produced by the electrotherapeutic device, as displayed by an instrument called an oscilloscope.

Both alternating and direct currents may take on a sine, square, or triangular waveform configuration depending on the capabilities of the machine producing the current. The basic difference between the two is that in each instance, the alternating current flow reverses direction one time in each cycle. Conversely, the direct current flow does not reverse direction. If the electrical modality has the capability of automatically reversing polarity (i.e., the direction of flow), a direct current will elicit the same physiologic responses as an alternating current.[11]

Waveforms may be either unidirectional or bidirectional, meaning that electrons flow either in one direction or in both directions. Unidirectional waveforms also may be called monopolar or monophasic and are associated with direct or galvanic current. Bidirectional waveforms may be referred to as bipolar or biphasic and are associated with alternating current. Polyphasic currents contain three or more grouped phases in a single pulse and are used in interferential and so-called "Russian" currents.[1]

The **amplitude** of each waveform reflects the intensity of the current, the maximum amplitude being the tip or highest point of each peak. The term *amplitude* is synonymous with the terms *voltage* and *current intensity*. The higher the amplitude, the greater the voltage and thus the amount of current being delivered to the tissues.

The **rate of rise** in amplitude or the rise time refers to how quickly the waveform reaches its maximum amplitude. Conversely, **decay time** refers to the time in which a waveform goes from peak amplitude to 0 V. The rate of rise is important physiologically because of the accommodation phenomenon, in which a fiber that has been subjected to a constant level of depolarization will become unexcitable at that same intensity or amplitude. Rate of rise and decay times are generally short, ranging from nanoseconds (billionths of a second) to milliseconds (thousandths of a second).

By observing the three different waveforms it is apparent that the sine wave has a gradual increase and decrease in amplitude for both alternating and direct currents (Fig. 3-3, *A* and *B*). The square wave has an almost instantaneous increase in amplitude, which plateaus for a period of time and then abruptly falls off (Fig. 3-3, *C* and *D*). The triangular wave has a rapid increase and decrease in amplitude (Fig. 3-3, *E* and *F*). The shape of these waveforms as they reach their maximum amplitude or intensity is directly related to the excitability of nervous tissue. The more rapid the increase in amplitude or the rate of rise, the greater the current's ability to excite nervous tissue. The effects of the various waveforms on biologic tissue will be discussed in Chapter 4.

The **duration** of each waveform indicates the length of time current is

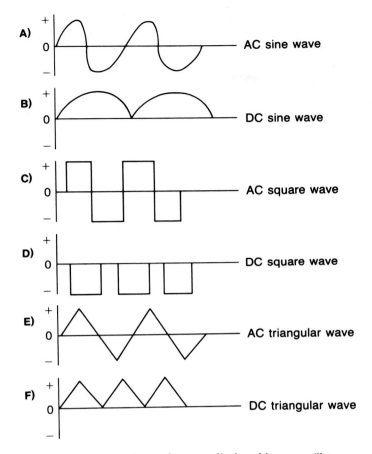

Figure 3-3. Theoretical waveforms as displayed by an oscilloscope.

flowing in one cycle. In some electrotherapeutic devices the duration or pulse width is preset by the manufacturer. Other devices have the capability of changing duration. The pulse width may be as short as a few microseconds or may be a long-duration uninterrupted direct current (Fig. 3-2, *B*). Most high-voltage generators make use of a twin peak pulse of very short duration (1 to 70 microseconds) and peak amplitudes as high as 500 V (Fig. 3-4). Combining a high peak intensity with a short pulse duration produces a very comfortable type of current as well as an effective means of stimulating sensory, motor, and pain fibers.

There are two additional waveforms that are seldom available on electro-therapeutic devices used by sports therapists but which for informational purposes must be mentioned. Both these currents have asymmetric waveforms.

Occasionally, manufacturers will indicate that their equipment is producing faradic current. However, the true faradic waveform is no longer used. The so-called faradic current is most likely a high-frequency (greater than 100 Hz)

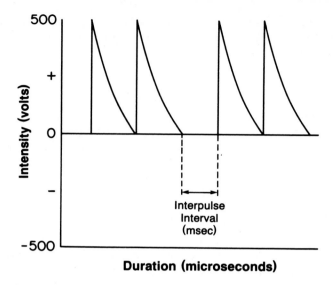

Figure 3-4. Most high-voltage generators produce a twin peak pulsed wave of short duration and high amplitude.

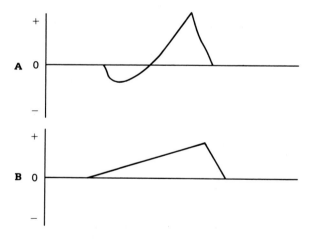

Figure 3-5. A, Original faradic waveform, which is no longer used. **B,** Sawtooth or exponential waveform.

pulsed wave. The original faradic waveform (Fig. 3-5, *A*) could only have used alternating current because there was always a reversal of direction. The amplitude of the portion of the wave in the negative direction was not great enough to produce any physiologic response. Thus the effects of this faradic wave would be similar to those of a direct current pulsed wave.[8]

The sawtooth or exponential waveform (Fig. 3-5, *B*) always uses direct current. The amplitude rises very gradually and then falls abruptly. The sawtooth current is used to stimulate denervated muscle without affecting normally innervated muscle, since the gradual rise in amplitude allows accommodation of the normal muscle.[8]

The physiologic responses to the various waveforms depend primarily on two factors: current **modulation** and frequency.

Modulation refers to any alteration in the magnitude or any variation in duration of these pulses. Modulation may be *continuous, interrupted,* or *surged.*[8] The parameters of this modulation must be established according to various treatment goals.

Continuous modulation means that the amplitude of current flow remains the same for several seconds or perhaps minutes. Continuous modulation is usually associated with uninterrupted direct current (Fig. 3-6, *A*). With direct current, flow is always in a uniform direction. In the discussion of physiologic responses to electrical currents, it was indicated that positive and negative ions are attracted toward poles or, in this case, electrodes of opposite polarity. This accumulation of charged ions over a period of time results in an acidic or alkaline environment, either of which may cause considerable discomfort to the pa-

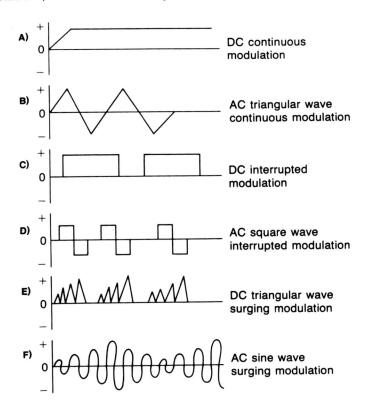

Figure 3-6. Modulated current using various waveforms as displayed by an oscilloscope.

tient. If the amplitude is great enough to produce a muscle contraction, the contraction will occur only when the current flow is turned on or off. Thus with direct current continuous modulation, there will be a muscle contraction both when the current is turned on and when it is turned off.

With interrupted modulation, current flow or groups of pulses are turned off periodically. The pulses are generated for one second or more and then turned off for one second or longer. Interrupted currents are sometimes referred to as pulsatile currents. These pulses may be either monophasic (DC), biphasic (AC), or polyphasic and again may take on sine, square, or triangular shapes (Fig. 3-6, *C* and *D*). The majority of modern stimulators used in a sports medicine setting output short duration pulses (<65 microseconds) with relatively long interruptions (up to 1 microsecond) between the pulses. These interruptions between pulses are called **interpulse intervals.**

With polyphasic currents, sets of three or more pulses are combined. These combined pulses are referred to in the literature as packets, envelopes, or beats. They may also be called **bursts,** although this term may be used with monophasic and biphasic currents as well. The time between each pulse in a burst is called an interburst interval. The interburst interval is much too short to have any effect on a muscle contraction. Thus the physiologic effects of a burst of pulses will be the same as with a single pulse.[1]

Muscle will respond with individual twitch contractions to frequencies of less than 50 pulses per second. At 50 pulses per second or greater a tetanic contraction will result, regardless of whether the current is biphasic, monophasic, or polyphasic.

In surging modulation, also called **ramping** modulation, current amplitude will increase or ramp up gradually to some preset maximum and may also decrease or ramp down in intensity (Fig. 3-6, *E* and *F*). Ramp up time is usually preset at about one third of the on time. The ramp down option is not available on all machines. Most modern stimulators allow the sports therapist to set the on time and the off time between 1 and 10 seconds. Surging modulation is generally considered to be a very comfortable type of current since it allows for a gradual increase in sensory stimulation or muscle contraction.

Frequency indicates the number of cycles or pulses per second. Physiologically, as the frequency of any waveform is increased, the amplitude tends to increase and decrease more rapidly, thus more closely resembling a pulsed current. Each individual pulse represents a rise and fall in amplitude. The muscular and nervous system responses depend on the length of time between pulses and on how the pulses or waveforms are modulated.[12]

Stimulators have been clinically labeled as either low-, medium-, or high-frequency generators, and a great deal of misunderstanding exists over how these frequency ranges are classified.[1] Generally, all stimulating units are low-frequency electrical generators that deliver between one and several hundred pulses per second. Recently a number of so-called medium-frequency generators have been developed that are claimed to have frequencies of 2500 to as high as 10,000 pulses per second. However, these high-frequency pulses are in reality groups of pulses combined as bursts that range in frequency from 1 to

200 pulses per second. These modulated bursts are capable of producing a physiologically effective frequency of stimulation only in this 1 to 200 pulse-per-second range owing to the limitations of the absolute refractory period of nerve cell membranes. Therefore, many of the claims of equipment manufacturers relative to medium-frequency generators are inaccurate.[1]

ELECTRICAL CIRCUITS

The path of current from a generating power source through various components back to the generating source is called an electrical **circuit.** A closed circuit is one in which electrons are flowing, and in an open circuit the current flow ceases. Electronic circuits are not ordinarily composed of single elements; they often encompass several branches or components with different resistances. The current in each branch may be easily calculated if the individual resistances are known and if the amount of voltage applied to the circuit is also known.[5]

With the development of the microelectronics industry, we all know that electrical circuits can be extremely complex. However, all electrical circuits have several basic components. There is a power source, which is capable of producing voltage. There is some type of conducting medium or pathway, which current travels along and which carries the flowing electrons. Finally, there is some component or group of components that are driven by this flowing current. These driven elements provide resistance to electrical flow.[5]

SERIES AND PARALLEL CIRCUITS

The components that provide resistance to current flow may be connected to one another in one of two different patterns, (1) a series circuit or (2) a parallel circuit. The main difference between these two is that in a series circuit there is only one path for current to get from one terminal to another. In a parallel circuit two or more routes exist for current to pass between the two terminals.

In a series circuit the components are placed end to end (Fig. 3-7). The number of amperes of an electrical current flowing through a series circuit is exactly the same at any point in that circuit. The resistance to current flow in

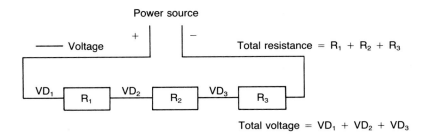

Figure 3-7. In a series circuit the component resistors are placed end to end. The total resistance to current flow is equal to the resistance of all the components added together. There is a voltage decrease at each component such that the sum of the voltage decrease is equal to the total voltage.

this total circuit is equal to the resistance of all the components in the circuit added together.

$$R_T = R_1 + R_2 + R_3$$

Electrical energy is required to force the current through the resistor, and this energy is dissipated in the form of heat. Consequently, there is a decrease in voltage at each component such that the total voltage at the beginning of the circuit is equal to the sum of the voltage decreases at each component.

$$V_T = VD_1 + VD_2 + VD_3$$

In a parallel circuit, the component resistors are placed side by side and the ends are connected (Fig. 3-8). Each of the resistors in a parallel circuit receives the same voltage. The current passing through each component depends on its resistance. So the total voltage will be exactly the same as the voltage at each component.

$$V_T = V_1 = V_2 = V_3$$

Each additional resistance added to a parallel circuit in effect decreases the total resistance. Adding an alternative pathway regardless of its resistance to current flow improves the ability of the current to get from one point to another. The current will, in general, choose the pathway that offers the least resistance. The formula for determining total resistance in a parallel circuit according to Ohm's law is

$$\frac{1}{R_T} = \frac{1}{R_1} + \frac{1}{R_2} + \frac{1}{R_3}$$

Thus component resistors connected in a series circuit have a higher resistance and lower current flow, and resistors in a parallel circuit have a lower resistance and a higher current flow.

The electrical modalities in general make use of some combination of both series and parallel circuits.[8] For example, to elicit a muscle contraction, the elec-

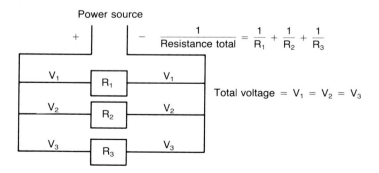

Figure 3-8. In a parallel circuit the component resistors are placed side by side and the ends are connected. The current flow in each of the pathways is inversely proportional to the resistance of the pathway. The total voltage is the sum of the voltages at each component.

trodes from an electrical stimulating unit are placed on the skin (Fig. 3-9). The current from those electrodes must pass directly through the skin and fat. The total resistance to current flow seen by the electrical stimulating unit is equal to the combined resistances at each electrode. This passage of current through the skin is basically a series circuit.

After the current passes through the skin and fat, it comes in contact with a number of different types of biologic tissue (i.e., bone, connective tissue, blood, muscle). The current has several different pathways through which it may reach the muscle to be stimulated. The total current traveling through these tissues is the sum of the currents in each different type of tissue, and since there are additional tissues through which current may travel, the total resistance is effectively reduced. Thus in this typical application of a therapeutic modality, both parallel and series circuits are used to produce the desired physiologic effect.

As stated previously, electrical current tends to choose the path that offers the least resistance to flow or, stated differently, the material that is the best conductor.[14] The conductivity of the different types of tissue in the body is variable. Typically tissue that is highest in water content and consequently highest in ion content is the best conductor of electricity.

CURRENT FLOW THROUGH BIOLOGIC TISSUES

The skin has different layers that vary in water content, but generally the skin offers the primary resistance to current flow and is considered an insulator. Skin preparation for the purpose of reducing electrical impedance is of primary concern with electrodiagnostic apparatus, but it is also important with electrotherapeutic devices. The greater the impedance of the skin, the higher the voltage of the electrical current must be to stimulate underlying nerve and muscle.

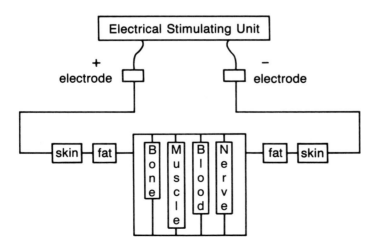

Figure 3-9. The electrical circuit that exists when electrons flow through human tissue is in reality a combination of a series and a parallel circuit.

Chemical changes in the skin can make it more resistant to certain types of current. Thus skin impedance is generally higher with direct current than with alternating current.

Blood is a biologic tissue that is composed largely of water and ions and is consequently the best electrical conductor of all of the tissues. Muscle is composed of about 75% water and depends on the movement of ions for contraction. Muscle tends to propagate an electrical impulse much more effectively in a longitudinal direction than transversely. Muscle tendons are considerably more dense than muscle, contain relatively little water, and are considered poor conductors. Fat contains only about 14% water and is thought to be a poor conductor. Peripheral nerve conductivity is approximately 6 times that of muscle. However, the nerve is generally surrounded by fat and a fibrous sheath, both of which are considered to be poor conductors. Bone is extremely dense, contains only about 5% water, and is considered to be the poorest biologic conductor of electrical current. It is essential for the sports therapist to understand that many biologic tissues will be stimulated by an electrical current. Selecting the appropriate treatment parameters is critical if the desired tissue response is to be attained.

PHYSIOLOGIC RESPONSES TO ELECTRICAL CURRENT

The effects of electrical current passing through the various tissues of the body may be thermal, chemical, or physiologic.[11]

All electrical currents cause a rise in temperature in a conductor (tissue). The tissues of the body possess varying degrees of resistance, and those of higher resistance should heat up more when electrical current passes through. As indicated in previous chapters, the diathermies generate a continuous high-frequency current that is designed to produce a tissue temperature increase. The electrical currents used for stimulation of nerve and muscle have a relatively low average current flow that produces minimal thermal effects.

Most biologic tissue contains negatively and positively charged ions. A direct current flow will cause migration of these charged particles toward the pole of opposite polarity. At the positive pole the negatively charged particles cause an acid reaction in which there is coagulation of protein and hardening of the tissues. At the negative pole the positively charged particles produce an alkaline reaction, liquefying protein and causing softening of the tissues.

Basically, electrical currents are used to produce either muscle contractions or modification of pain impulses through effects on the motor and sensory nerves. This function is dependent to some extent on the intensity or voltage of current and on the frequency of the impulses.

SAFETY IN THE USE OF ELECTRICAL EQUIPMENT

Electrical safety in the sports medicine setting should be of maximal concern to the professional sports therapist. Too often there are reports of athletes being electrocuted as a result of faulty electrical circuits in whirlpools. This type of accident can be avoided by taking some basic precautions and acquiring some understanding of the power distribution system and electrical grounds.

The typical electrical circuit consists of a source producing electrical power, a conductor that carries the power to a resistor or series of driven elements, and a conductor that carries the power back to the power source.

Electrical power is carried from generating plants through high-tension powerlines carrying 2200 V. The power is decreased by a transformer and is supplied in the wall outlet at 220 V or 120 V with a frequency of 60 Hz. The voltage at the outlet is alternating current, which means that one of the poles, the "hot" or "live" wire, is either positive or negative with respect to other neutral lines. Theoretically the voltage of the neutral pole should be zero. Actually the voltage of the neutral line is about 10 V. Thus both hot and neutral lines carry some voltage with respect to the earth, which has zero voltage. The voltage from either of these two leads may be sufficient to cause physiologic damage.

The two-pronged plug has only two leads, both of which carry some voltage. Consequently the electrical device has no true **ground.**

The term *true ground* literally means the electrical circuit is connected to the earth or the ground, which has the ability to accept large electrical charges without becoming charged itself. The ground will continually accept these charges until the electrical potential has been neutralized. Therefore any electrical charge that may be potentially hazardous (i.e., any electricity escaping from the circuit) is almost immediately neutralized by the ground. If an individual were to come in contact with a short-circuited instrument that was not grounded, the electrical current would flow through that individual to reach the ground.

Electrical devices that have two-pronged plugs generally rely on the chassis or casing of the power source to act as a ground. The danger with the two-pronged plug devices is that there is no true ground. So if an individual were to touch the casing of the instrument while in contact with some object or instrument that has a true ground, an electrical shock may result. With three-pronged plugs, the third prong is grounded directly to the earth and all excess electrical energy should theoretically be neutralized through this.

By far the most common mechanism of injury from therapeutic devices results when there is some damage, breakdown, or short circuit to the power cord. When this happens, the casing of the machine becomes electrically charged. In other words, there is a voltage leak and in a device that is not properly grounded electrical shock may occur (Fig. 3-10).

The magnitude of the electrical shock is a critical factor in terms of potential health danger (Table 3-2). Shock from electrical currents flowing at one or less mamps will not be felt and is referred to as **microshock.** Shock from a current flow greater than 1 mamp is called **macroshock.** Currents that range between 1 and 15 mamps produce a tingling sensation or perhaps some muscle contraction. Currents flowing at 15 to 100 mamps cause a painful electrical shock. Currents between 100 and 200 mamps may result in fibrillation of cardiac muscle or respiratory arrest. When current flow is above 200 mamps, there is rapid burning and destruction of tissue.

Most electrotherapeutic devices (e.g., muscle stimulators, ultrasound, and

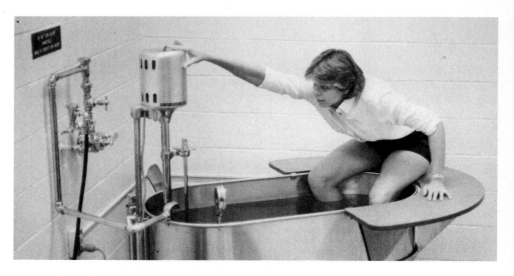

Figure 3-10. There is danger of electrical shock when a therapeutic device is not properly grounded. This is a major problem in a whirlpool.

TABLE 3-2   **Physiologic Effects of Electrical Shock at Varying Magnitudes**

Intensity	Physiologic Effects
0-1 mamps	Imperceptible
1-15 mamps	Tingling sensation and muscle contraction
15-100 mamps	Painful electrical shock
100-200 mamps	Cardiac or respiratory arrest
>200 mamps	Instant tissue burning and destruction

the diathermies) are generally used in dry environments. All new electrotherapeutic equipment being produced has three-pronged plugs and is thus grounded to the earth. However, in a wet or damp area the three-pronged plug may not provide sufficient protection from electrical shock.

We know that the body will readily conduct electricity because of its high water content. If the body is wet or if an individual is standing in water, the resistance to electrical flow is reduced even more. Thus if a short should occur, the shock could be as much as 5 times greater in this damp or wet environment. The potential danger that exists with whirlpools or tubs is obvious. The ground on the whirlpool will supposedly conduct all current leakage from a faulty motor or power cord to the earth. However, an individual in a whirlpool is actually a part of that circuit and is subject to the same current levels as any other component of the circuit. Small amounts of current can therefore be potentially harmful no matter how well the apparatus is grounded. For this reason in 1981 the National Electrical Code required that all health care facilities using whirlpools and tubs install ground-fault circuit breakers (Fig. 3-11). These de-

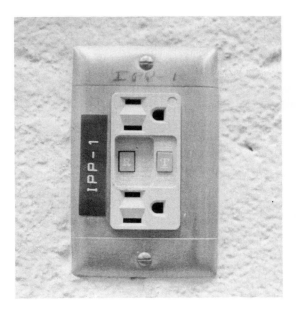

Figure 3-11. A typical ground-fault circuit breaker.

vices constantly compare the amount of electricity flowing from the wall outlet to the whirlpool turbine with the amount returning to the outlet. If there is any leakage in current flow detected, the ground-fault circuit breaker will automatically interrupt current flow in as little as one fortieth of a second, thus shuting off current flow and reducing the chances of electrical shock.[10] These devices may be installed either in the electrical outlet or in the circuit-breaker box.

Regardless of the type of electrotherapeutic device being used and the type of environment, the following safety practices should be considered:

1. The entire electrical system of the building or training room should be designed or evaluated by a qualified electrician. Problems with the electrical system may exist in older buildings or in situations where rooms have been modified to accommodate therapeutic devices (e.g., putting a whirlpool in a locker room where the concrete floor is always wet or damp).
2. It should not be assumed that all three-pronged wall outlets are automatically grounded to the earth. The ground must be checked.
3. The sports therapist should become very familiar with the equipment being used and with any potential problems that may exist or develop.
4. The plug should not be jerked out of the wall by pulling on the cable.
5. Extension cords or multiple adaptors should not be used.
6. Equipment should be reevaluated on a yearly basis and should conform to National Electrical Code guidelines. If a training room is not in compliance with this code, then there is no legal protection in a lawsuit.
7. Common sense should always be exercised when using electrotherapeutic devices. A situation that appears to be potentially dangerous may in fact result in injury or death.

SUMMARY

1. The movement or flow of electrons from a higher electrical potential to a lower potential is referred to as an electrical current.
2. A volt is the electromotive force that produces this net movement of electrons; an ampere is a unit of measurement that indicates the rate at which electrical current is flowing.
3. Ohm's law expresses the relationship between current flow voltage and resistance. The current flow is directly proportional to the voltage and inversely proportional to the resistance.
4. Electrical energy or power is a product of the voltage or electromotive force and the amount of current flowing; it is expressed in watts.
5. The main difference between a series and a parallel circuit is that in a series circuit there is a single pathway for current to get from one terminal to another, and in a parallel circuit two or more routes exist for current to pass.
6. The electrical circuit that exists when electron flow is through human tissue is in reality a combination of both a series and a parallel circuit.
7. The effects of electrical current moving through biologic tissue may be chemical, thermal, or physiologic.
8. Alternating current periodically changes the direction of electron flow while direct current has a unidirectional flow of electrons.
9. The term *waveform* indicates a graphic representation of the shape, direction, amplitude, and duration of the electrical current being produced by the electrotherapeutic device. Alteration of any of these four factors can produce an altered physiological response.
10. Alternating current has a biphasic waveform while direct current has a monophasic waveform. Interferential current has a polyphasic waveform.
11. Current modulation refers to any alteration in magnitude or variation in the duration of the waveforms. Modulation may be continuous, interrupted, or surged.
12. High-voltage generators have amplitudes greater than 150 V while low-voltage generators produce less than 150 V.
13. Electrical safety is critical when using electrotherapeutic devices. It is the responsibility of the sports therapist to make sure that all electrical modalities conform to the National Electrical Code.

GLOSSARY

accommodation Adaptation by the sensory receptors to various stimuli over an extended period of time.

alternating current Current that periodically changes its polarity or direction of flow.

ampere Unit of measure that indicates the rate at which electrical current is flowing.

amplitude The intensity of current flow as indicated by the height of the waveform from baseline.

biphasic current Another name for alternating current, in which the direction of current flow reverses direction.

bursts A combined set of three or more pulses; also referred to as *packets* or *envelopes*.

circuit The path of current from a generating source through the various components back to the generating source.

conductance The ease with which a current flows along a conducting medium.

coulomb Indicates the number of electrons flowing in a current.

current The flow of electrons.

decay time The time required for a waveform to go from peak amplitude to 0 V.

direct current Galvanic current that always flows in the same direction and may flow in either a positive or a negative direction.

duration Sometimes also referred to as pulse width. Indicates the length of time the current is flowing.

electrical potential The difference between charged particles at a higher and lower potential.

electron Fundamental particles of matter possessing a negative electrical charge and very small mass.

frequency The number of cycles or pulses per second.

ground A wire that makes an electrical connection with the earth.

high-voltage current Current in which the waveform has an amplitude of greater than 150 V with a relatively short pulse duration of less than .100 μsec.

interpulse interval The interruptions between individual pulses or groups of pulses.

ion A positively or negatively charged particle.

low-voltage current Current in which the waveform has an amplitude of less than 150 V.

macroshock An electrical shock that can be felt and has a leakage of electrical current of greater than 1 mamp.

microshock An electrical shock that is imperceptible because of a leakage of current of less than 1 mamp.

modulation Refers to any alteration in the magnitude or any variation in the duration of an electrical current.

monophasic current Another name for direct current, in which the direction of current flow remains the same.

Ohm's law The current in an electrical circuit is directly proportional to the voltage and inversely proportional to the resistance.

polyphasic current Current that contains three or more grouped phases in a single pulse and that is used in interferential and "Russian" currents.

ramping Another name for surging modulation, in which the current builds gradually to some maximum amplitude.

rate of rise How quickly a waveform reaches its maximum amplitude.

tetany Muscle condition that is caused by hyperexcitation and results in cramps and spasms.

volt The electromotive force that must be applied to produce a movement of electrons.

watt A measure of electrical power. Mathematically Watts = Volts × Amperes.

waveform The shape of an electrical current as displayed on an oscilloscope.

REFERENCES

1 Alon, G.: Principles of electrical stimulation. In Nelson, R., and Currier, D., editors: Clinical electrotherapy, Norwalk, Conn., 1987, Appleton-Lange.

2 Bergueld, P.: Electromedical instrumentation: a guide for medical personnel, Cambridge, 1980, Cambridge University Press.

3 Chamishion, R.: Basic medical electronics, Boston, 1964, Little, Brown & Co., Inc.

4 Cromwell, L., Arditti, M., Weibell, F., et al: Medical instrumentation for health care, Englewood Cliffs, N.J., 1976, Prentice-Hall, Inc.

5 Cohen, H.L., and Brumlik, J.: Manual of electroneuromyography, ed. 2, New York, Harper & Row, Publishers, Inc.

6 Cook, T.: Instrumentation. In Nelson, R., and Currier, D., editors: Clinical electrotherapy, Norwalk, Conn., 1987, Appleton-Lange.

7 DeDomenico, G.: Basic guidelines for interferential therapy, Sydney, Australia, 1981, Theramed.

8 Griffin, J., and Karselis, T.: Physical agents for physical therapists, Springfield, Ill., 1978, Charles C Thomas, Publisher.

9 Licht, S.: Therapeutic electricity and ultraviolet radiation, vol. IV, ed. 2, Baltimore, 1969, Waverly.

10 Porter, M., and Porter, J.: Electrical safety in the training room, Athletic Training 16(4):263-264, 1981.

11 Shriber, W.: A manual of electrotherapy, ed. 4, Philadelphia, 1975, Lea & Febiger.

12 Stillwell, G.K.: Therapeutic electricity and ultraviolet radiation, ed. 3, Baltimore, 1983, Williams & Wilkins.

13 Watkins, A.L.: A manual of electrotherapy, ed. 3, Philadelphia, 1968, Lea & Febiger.

14 Wolf, S.L.: Electrotherapy: clinics in physical therapy, vol. 2, New York, 1981, Churchill Livingstone, Inc.

SUGGESTED READINGS

Alon, G.: High voltage stimulation: a monograph, Chattanooga, Tenn., 1984, Chattanooga Corporation.

Alon, G.: Electrical stimulators, Chattanooga, Tenn., 1985, Chattanooga Corporation. (Video presentation).

Alon, G., Allin, J., and Inbar, G.: Optimization of pulse duration and pulse charge during TENS, Aust. J. Physiother. 29:195, 1983.

Benton, L., Baker, L., Bowman, B., et al.: Functional electrical stimulation: a practical clinical guide, Downey, Calif., 1980, Rancho Los Amigos Hospital.

Binder, S.: In Wolf, S., editor: Electrotherapy, New York, 1981, Churchill Livingstone, Inc.

Brown, I.: Fundamentals of electrotherapy, course guide, Madison, Wis., 1963, University of Wisconsin Press.

Campbell, J.: A critical appraisal of the electrical output characteristics of ten TENS units, Clin. Phys. Physiol. Meas. **3:**141, 1982.

Geddes, L., and Baker, L.: Applied biomedical instrumentation, New York, 1975, John Wiley.

Geddes, L.: A short history of electrical stimulation of excitable tissue, Physiologist **27:**1, 1984.

Kottke, F.: Handbook of physical medicine and rehabilitation, ed. 3, Philadelphia, 1982, W.B. Saunders Co.

Lane, J.: Electrical impedances of superficial limb tissues, epidermis, dermis, and muscle sheath, Ann. N.Y. Acad. Sci. **238:**812, 1974.

Licht, S.: Electrodiagnosis and electromyography, vol. 1, ed. 3, Baltimore, 1971, Waverly.

Mannheimer, J., and Lampe, G.: Clinical transcutaneous electrical nerve stimulation, Philadelphia, 1984, F.A. Davis.

Nelson, R., and Currier, D.: Clinical electrotherapy, Norwalk, Conn., 1987, Appleton-Lange.

Newton, R.A.: Electrotherapeutic treatment: selecting appropriate wave form characteristics. Clinton, N.J., 1984, Preston.

Newton, R.A.: Electrotherapy: selecting wave form parameters, paper presented at the American Physical Therapy Association Conference, Washington, D.C., 1981.

Reismann, M.: A comparison of electrical stimulators eliciting muscle contraction, Phys. Ther. **64:**751, 1984.

Scott, P.: Clayton's electrotherapy and actinotherapy, eds. 5 and 7, Baltimore, 1965 and 1975, Williams & Wilkins.

Sunderland, S.: Nerves and nerve injuries, Baltimore, 1968, Williams & Wilkins.

Wadsworth, H., and Chanmugan, A.: Electrophysical agents in physical therapy, Marickville, Australia, 1983, Science Press.

Ward, A.: Electricity waves and fields in therapy, Marickville, Australia, 1980, Science Press.

Electrical Stimulating Currents

4

Daniel N. Hooker

OBJECTIVES

Following completion of this chapter, the student will be able to:

- Describe muscle and nerve responses to electrical stimulation.

- Describe the modulation of pain through the use of electrical stimulating currents.

- Describe two methods of electrode placement for pain relief.

- Describe electromyographic biofeedback.

- Identify problems that might respond to electrical stimulation.

Often the sports therapist uses electrical currents for treatment in an effort to create a quick cure for the physical problems suffered by his or her patients or athletes. Although electrical treatments can provide dramatic results at times, this is the exception rather than the rule. The use of electricity in treating an injury can be beneficial, but the sports therapist must base the use of electricity on facts about the effects of electricity on biologic tissues. The treatment program must be tailored toward influencing the problems identified in the evaluation. Electrical therapy should not be used in a "shotgun" approach if we are to maximize the effectiveness of this modality.

All biologic tissue will have some response when an electrical current is passed through it.[40] The type and extent of this response are dependent on (1) the type of tissue and its response characteristics (for example, how it normally functions and how it grows or changes under normal stress); and (2) the nature of the current applied (that is, direct or alternating, intensity, duration, voltage, and density). The tissue should respond to electrical energy in a manner similar to that in which it normally functions or grows. These statements are true within a certain range of current parameters, but current density above critical levels can cause coagulation and tissue destruction.

PHYSIOLOGIC RESPONSE TO ELECTRICAL CURRENTS

Clinically, sports therapists use electrical currents for the following:
1. Creating muscle contraction through nerve or muscle stimulations.
2. Stimulating sensory nerves to help in treating pain.
3. Creating an electrical field in biologic tissues to stimulate or alter the healing process.
4. Creating an electrical field on the skin surface to drive ions beneficial to the healing process into or through the skin.

Muscle and Nerve Responses to Electrical Currents

The major therapeutic uses of electricity center on muscle contraction or sensory stimulation or both. Let us look in a general way at the physiologic effects of electricity on nerve and muscle tissue. Specific currents or frequencies will be discussed later in the chapter.

Nerves and muscles are both excitable tissues. This excitability is dependent on the cell membrane's **voltage sensitive permeability.** The nerve or muscle cell membrane regulates the interchange of substances between the inside of the cell and the environment outside the cell. This voltage sensitive permeability produces an unequal distribution of charged ions on each side of the membrane, which in turn creates a potential difference between the charge of the interior of the cell and that of the exterior of the cell. The membrane then is considered to be *polarized.* The potential difference between the inside and outside is known as the **resting potential,** because the cell tries to maintain this difference in electrical charge as its normal homeostatic environment.[15]

Both electrical and chemical gradients are established along the cell membrane, with a greater concentration of diffusable positive ions on the outside of the membrane than on the inside. Using its active transport mechanism, the cell continually moves Na^+ from inside the cell to outside and balances this positive charge movement by moving K^+ to the inside. K^+ will have a larger concentration on the inside of the cell, but the overall charge difference produces an electrical gradient with + charges outside and − charges inside (Fig. 4-1). As explained by Guyton, "The potential is proportional to the difference in tendency of the ions to diffuse in one direction versus the other direction. Two conditions are necessary for the membrane potential to develop: (1) The membrane must be semipermeable, allowing ions of one charge to diffuse through the pores more readily than ions of the opposite charge. (2) The concentration of the diffusable ions must be greater on one side of the membrane than on

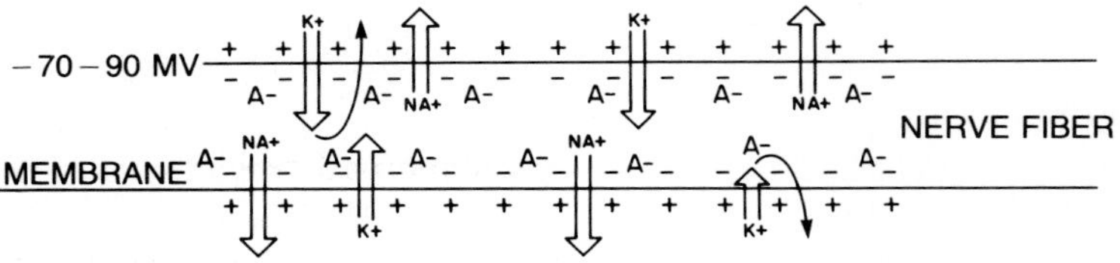

Figure 4-1. Nerve cell membrane with active transport mechanisms maintaining the resting membrane potential.

the other side."[15] In addition to the ability of the nerve and muscle cell membranes to develop and maintain the resting potential, the membranes are excitable.[15]

To create transmission of an impulse in the nerve tissue, this resting membrane potential must be reduced to below a threshold level. Changes in the membrane's permeability then occur. These changes create an **action potential** that will propagate the impulse down the nerve in both directions from the location of the stimulus. An action potential created by a stimulus from chemical, electrical, thermal, or mechanical means always creates the same result, membrane **depolarization.**

Not all stimuli are effective in causing action potential and depolarization. To be an effective agent, the stimulus must have an adequate intensity and last long enough to equal or exceed the membrane's basic threshold for excitation. The stimulus must alter the membrane so that a number of ions are pushed across the membrane, exceeding the ability of the active transport pumps to maintain the resting potentials. A stimulus of this magnitude forces the membrane to depolarize and results in an action potential.[15,44]

CLINICAL RESPONSE TO ELECTRICAL CURRENTS

When an electrical system is applied to the soft tissues of an extremity, the system provides the force to induce ion movement in the tissues and create an action potential. At the positive electrode (also called the **anode**), positive ions are repelled and negative ions are attracted. At the negative electrode (also called the **cathode**), the negative ions are repelled and the positive ions are attracted.[44]

DEPOLARIZATION

As the charged ions move across the nerve fiber membranes beneath the anode and cathode, membrane depolarization occurs. The cathode usually is the site of depolarization (Fig. 4-2, *A*). As the concentration of negatively charged ions increases, the membrane's voltage potential becomes low and is brought toward its threshold for depolarization (Fig. 4-2, *B*). The anode makes the nerve cell membrane potential more positive, increasing the threshold necessary for depolarization (Fig. 4-2, *C*). The cathode in this example becomes the **active electrode;** the anode becomes the **indifferent electrode.** The anode and cathode may switch active and indifferent roles under other circumstances.[3,44] The number of ions needed to exceed the membrane pump's ability to maintain the normal membrane resting potential is tissue dependent.

Depolarization Propagation

Once the threshold has been reached, the depolarization is propagated along the nerve in both directions from the site of excitation. Following this excitement and propagation of the impulse along the nerve fiber, there is a brief period during which the nerve fiber is incapable of reacting to a second stimulus. This is the **absolute refractory period,** which lasts about 0.5 μsec. Excitability is restored gradually as the nerve cell membrane repolarizes itself. The nerve then is capable of being stimulated again. The maximum number of possible

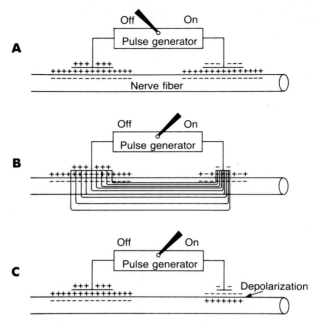

Figure 4-2. Depolarization of nerve cell membranes.

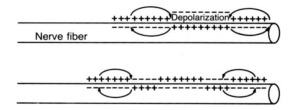

Figure 4-3. Propagation of the nerve impulse.

discharges of a nerve is approximately 1000 per second, depending on fiber type.[2,3,15,44]

The difference in electrical potential between the depolarized region and the neighboring inactive regions causes the current to flow from the depolarized region through the intracellular material to the inactive membrane. The current also flows through the extracellular materials, back to the depolarized area, and finally into the cell again. This forms a complete local circuit and makes the depolarization self propagating as the process is repeated all along the fiber in each direction from the depolarization site. Energy released by the cell keeps the intensity of the impulse uniform as it travels down the cell.[2,3,15,44] This process is illustrated in Fig. 4-3.

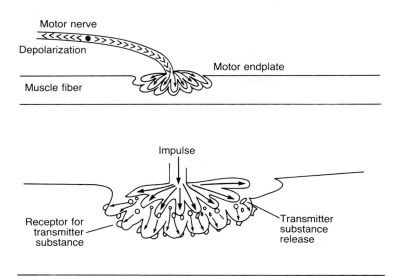

Figure 4-4. Change of electrical impulse to transmitter substance at the motor end plate. When activated, the muscle cell membrane will depolarize and contraction will occur.

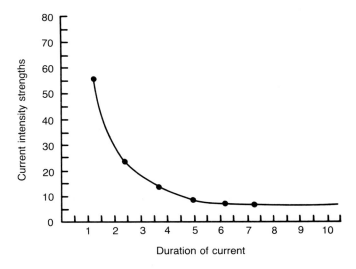

Figure 4-5. Strength-duration curve.

As the nerve impulse reaches its effector organ or another nerve cell, the impulse is transferred between the two at a motor end plate or a synapse. At this junction, a transmitter substance is released from the nerve, rather than the impulse jumping from one to another. This transmitter substance causes the other excitable tissue to discharge (Fig. 4-4).[3,44]

In terms of muscle excitation, a **twitch muscle contraction** results. This

Depolarization Effects

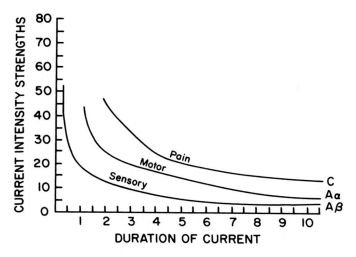

Figure 4-6. Strength-duration curves for motor, sensor, and pain nerve fibers.

contraction, initiated by an electrical stimulus, is the same as a twitch contraction coming from voluntary activity. Voluntary muscular activity is different only in the rate and synchrony (simultaneous response) of the muscle fiber contractions.[3,32] A graphic illustration of this threshold and propagation and contraction is the **strength-duration curve** (Fig. 4-5).

As illustrated, there is a nonlinear relationship between current duration and current intensity, in which shorter duration stimuli require increasing intensities in order to reach the threshold of the nerve or muscle. Nerve and muscle membrane thresholds differ significantly. Different sizes and types of nerve

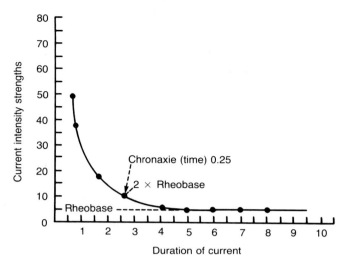

Figure 4-7. Excitation time of nerve cell membranes.

fibers also have different thresholds. The strength-duration curves for different classes of nerve and muscle tissue illustrate the different thresholds of excitability of these tissues. The curves are basically symmetric, but the intensity of current necessary to reach the membrane's threshold for excitation differs for each tissue (Fig. 4-6).[15,32,44,46]

STRENGTH-DURATION CURVE

Three important concepts are represented in the strength-duration curve. These terms and ideas are used frequently in discussions on the biologic effects of electrical currents.[17,44]

1. The shape of the curve relates the intensity of the electrical stimulus and the length of time (duration) necessary to cause the tissue to depolarize.
2. The **rheobase** describes the minimum intensity of current necessary to cause tissue excitation when applied for a maximum duration (Fig. 4-7).
3. **Chronaxie** describes the length of time (duration) required for a current of twice the intensity of the rheobase current to produce tissue excitation (Fig. 4-7).

MUSCULAR RESPONSES TO ELECTRICAL CURRENT

Stimulation of the motor nerve is the method used in most clinical applications of electrical muscular contractions. In the absence of innervation, muscle contraction can be stimulated by an electrical current that causes the muscle membrane to depolarize. This will create the same muscle contraction as a natural stimulus.

The **all-or-none response** is another important concept in applying electrical current to nerve or muscle tissue. Once a stimulus reaches a depolarizing threshold, the nerve or muscle membrane depolarizes, and propagation of the impulse or muscle contraction occurs. This reaction remains the same regardless of increases in the strength of the stimulus used. Either the stimulus causes depolarization—the all—or it does not cause depolarization—the none. There is no gradation of response; the response of the single nerve or muscle fiber is maximal or nonexistent.[3,32,44]

This all-or-none phenomenon does not mean that muscle fiber shortening and overall muscle activity cannot be influenced by changing the intensity, pulses per second, or duration of the stimulating current. Adjustments in current parameters can cause changes in the shortening of the muscle fiber and in the overall muscle activity.

ELECTRICAL CONCEPTS: EFFECTS OF CHANGES IN CURRENT PARAMETERS AND THEIR EFFECT ON TREATMENT PROTOCOLS

When using any of the treatment protocols aimed at the electrical stimulation of muscle or nerve tissue, several concepts must be understood for sports therapists to accomplish their goals:
1. Alternating versus direct current
2. Tissue impedance
3. Current density
4. Frequency of wave or pulse
5. Intensity of wave or pulse
6. Duration of wave or pulse
7. Polarity of electrodes
8. Motor point location stimulation

Changes in these parameters affect how the electrical current changes the physiology of the body part being treated. The wave form used gives us a graphic way to measure and quantify these parameters.[47]

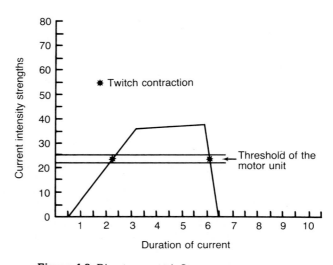

Figure 4-8. Direct current influence on a motor unit.

To further understand electrically stimulated muscle contractions, we must think in terms of multiple stimuli rather than a simple direct current response. The motor nerves are not stimulated by a steady flow of direct current. The nerve repolarizes under the influence of the current and will not depolarize until a sudden change in current intensity occurs.

Alternating Versus Direct Current

If continuous direct current were the only current mode available, we would get a muscle contraction only when the current intensity rose to a stimulus threshold. Once the membrane repolarized, another change in the current intensity would be needed to force another depolarization and contraction (Fig. 4-8).

The biggest difference in the effects of alternating and direct currents is the ability of direct current to cause chemical changes. Chemical effects from using direct current will occur only when the stimulus is continuous and is applied over a period of time. These chemical changes become measurable when the duration of the stimulus reaches the 1-minute mark, but the effect is cumulative over the total treatment time. This type of current is available in most low-voltage equipment. The duration of the current in most high-voltage stimulators is nonadjustable and is too short to create any chemical effect.[33,44]

Tissue Impedance

Impedance is the resistance of the tissue to the passage of electrical current. Bone and fat are high-impedance tissues; nerve and muscle are low-impedance tissues. If a low-impedance tissue is located under a large amount of high-impedance tissue, the current will never become high enough to cause a depolarization.[3,44]

Current Density

The **current density** (amount of current flow per cubic volume) at the nerve or muscle must be high enough to cause depolarization. The current density is highest where the electrodes meet the skin and diminishes as the electricity penetrates into the deeper tissues (Fig. 4-9).[3,44] If there is a large fat layer between the electrodes and the nerve, the electrical energy may not have a high enough density to cause depolarization (Fig. 4-10).

If the electrodes are spaced closely together, the area of highest current density is relatively superficial (Fig. 4-11, *A*). If the electrodes are spaced farther apart, the current density will be higher in the deeper tissues, including nerve and muscle (Fig. 4-11, *B*).

Electrode size will also change current density. As the size of one elec-

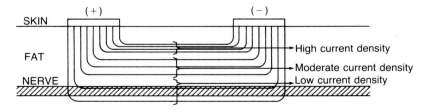

Figure 4-9. Current density using equal size electrodes spaced close together.

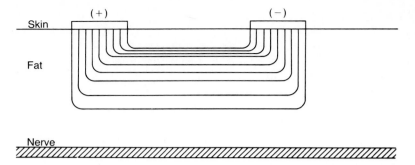

Figure 4-10. Equal size electrodes spaced close together on body part with thick fat layer. Thus, the electrical current does not reach the nerve.

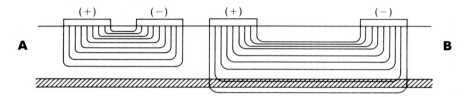

Figure 4-11. A, Electrodes very close together, producing a high-density current in the superficial tissues. **B,** Increasing the distance between the electrodes increases the current density in the deeper tissues.

trode relative to another is decreased, the current density beneath the smaller electrode is increased. The larger the electrode, the larger the area over which the current is spread, decreasing the current density (Fig. 4-12).[1,3,32,44]

Using a large electrode (dispersive) remote from the treatment area while placing a small electrode (active) as close as possible to the nerve or muscle motor point will give the greatest effect at the small electrode. The large electrode disperses the current over a large area; the small electrode concentrates the current in the area of the motor point (Fig. 4-12).

Frequency

The amount of shortening of the muscle fiber and the amount of recovery allowed the muscle fiber is a function of the frequency. The mechanical shortening of the single muscle fiber response can be influenced by stimulating again as soon as the tissue membrane repolarizes. Only the membrane has the absolute refractory period; the contractile mechanism operates on a different timing sequence and is just beginning to contract. When the second stimulus is received by the muscle membrane, the myofilaments are already overlapping, and the second stimulus causes an increased mechanical shortening of the muscle fiber. This process of superimposing one twitch contraction on another is called **summation of contractions.** As the number of twitch contractions per second increases, single twitch responses cannot be distinguished, and **tetanization** of the muscle fiber is reached (Fig. 4-13). The tension developed by a muscle fiber

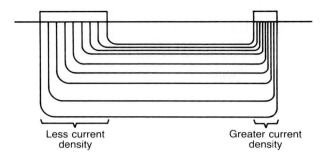

Figure 4-12. Unequal size electrodes increase the current density under the smaller electrode.

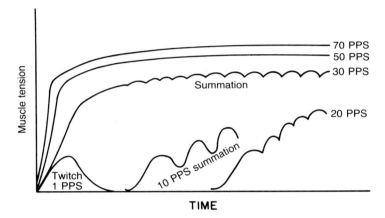

Figure 4-13. Summation of contractions and tetanization.

in tetany is much greater than the tension from a twitch contraction. This muscle fiber tetany is strictly a function of the frequency of the stimulating current; it is not dependent on the intensity of the current.[3,32]

The primary difference between electrically induced muscle contraction and voluntary muscle contraction is the asynchrony of firing of motor units under voluntary control versus the synchronous firing of electrically stimulated motor units. Each time the electrical stimulus is applied, the same motor units respond. This may lead to greater fatigue in the electrically stimulated muscles. Normal firing in voluntary muscle contraction varies from one movement to the next, because some motor units are contracting while others are inactive. Voluntary contractions do not lead to muscular fatigue as early in the exercise period as do electrical contractions. This synchrony of contraction may also be important in training the muscle to use more synchronous contractions to improve muscular strength.[3,32]

In cases that need strengthening, muscle reeducation, retardation of atro-

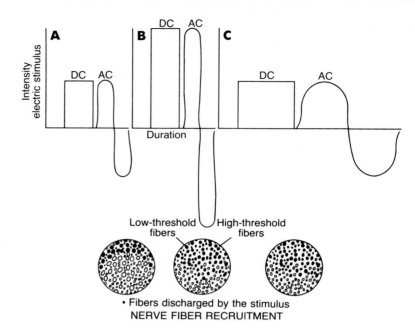

Figure 4-14. Recruitment of nerve fibers. **A,** A stimulus pulse at a duration-intensity just above threshold will excite the closest and largest fibers. Each electrical pulse of the same intensity at the same location will cause the same fibers to contract. **B,** Increasing the intensity will excite smaller fibers and fibers farther away. **C,** Increasing the duration will also excite smaller fibers and fibers farther away.

phy, and frequency in the range needed for tetany are required (30 to 40 pulses per second). In cases that need a prolonged contraction or many contractions during a treatment time, frequencies at the beginnings of tetany (15 to 20 pulses per second) may allow greater muscle recovery and less fatigue.

Intensity

Increasing the intensity of the electrical stimulus in Fig. 4-14, *A* to that in Fig. 4-14, *B* causes the current to reach deeper into the tissue. Depolarization of more fibers then is accomplished by two methods: (1) higher threshold fibers within the range of the first stimulus (Fig. 4-14, *A*) are depolarized by the higher intensity stimulus; and (2) fibers with the same threshold but deeper in the structure are depolarized by the deeper spread of the current. High-voltage stimulators are capable of deeper penetration into the tissue than low-voltage stimulators and may be desirable when stimulating deep muscle tissue. This is the most significant difference between high-voltage and low-voltage generators.[32]

Duration

We also can stimulate more nerve fibers with the same intensity current by increasing the length of time (duration) that an adequate stimulation is available to depolarize the membranes (Fig. 4-14, *C*). Greater numbers of nerve fibers then would react to the same intensity stimulus, because the current would be available for a longer period of time.[3,17,44] This method requires the use of a stimulator with an adjustable duration. The low-voltage stimulators usually are available with this parameter, whereas the high-voltage stimulators usually have a preset pulse duration.

During the use of any stimulator, an electrode that has a greater level of electrons is called the *negative electrode* or the *cathode.* The other electrode in this system has a lower level of electrons and is called the *positive electrode* or the *anode.* The negative electrode attracts positive ions and the positive electrode attracts negative ions and electrons. With AC waves, these electrodes change polarity with each current cycle.

Polarity

    With a direct current generator, the sports therapist can designate one electrode the negative and one the positive, and for the duration of the treatment the electrodes will provide that polar effect.

    The polar effect can be thought of in terms of three characteristics: (1) chemical effects, (2) ease of excitation, and (3) direction of current flow.[2,3,26,32,37,44]

    CHEMICAL EFFECTS. Changes in pH under each electrode, a reflex vasodilation, and the ability to drive oppositely charged ions through the skin into the tissue (iontophoresis) are all thought of as chemical effects. A tissue-stimulating effect is ascribed to the negative electrode and a bacteriostatic effect to the positive electrode. To create these effects, longer pulse durations (greater than 1 minute) are required.[2,13,33,37]

    EASE OF EXCITATION OF EXCITABLE TISSUE. The polarity of the active electrode usually should be negative when the desired result is a muscle contraction, because of the greater facility for membrane depolarization at the negative pole. However, current density under the positive pole can be increased rapidly enough to create a depolarizing effect. Using the positive electrode as the active electrode is not as efficient, because it will require more current intensity to create an action potential; this may cause the patient to be less comfortable with the treatment. In treatment programs requiring muscle contraction or sensory nerve stimulation, patient comfort should dictate the choice of positive or negative polarity. Negative polarity usually is the most comfortable in this instance.[3,32,44]

    DIRECTION OF CURRENT FLOW. In some treatment schemes, the direction of current flow is also considered important. Generally speaking, the negative electrode is positioned distally and the positive electrode proximally. This arrangement tries to replicate the naturally occurring pattern of electrical flow in the body.[2,26]

    The direction of current flow could also influence shifting of the water content of the tissues and movement of colloids (fluid suspension of the intracellular fluid). Neither of these phenomena is well documented or understood, and further study is needed before clinical treatments are designed around these concepts.[31,44]

    True polar effects can be substantiated when they occur close to the electrodes through which the current is entering the tissue. In laboratory situations in physics and physical therapy, polar effects occur in very close proximity to the electrode. To cause these effects, the current must flow through a medium. If the tissue to be treated is centrally located between the two electrodes and the current flowing through the area causes changes, the changes are caused by the current flow and cannot be assigned to polar effects.[2] Clinically, polar effects are an important consideration in iontophoresis and stimulating motor points or peripheral nerves, but for other treatment protocols, they probably have little impact.

Motor Point Location Stimulation

To find the motor point of a muscle, a probe electrode should be used to stimulate the muscle. Stimulation should be started in the approximate location of the desired motor point. (See Appendix A for motor point chart.) The intensity should be increased until contraction is visible, and the current intensity should be maintained at that level. The probe should be moved around until the best visible contraction for that current intensity is found; this is the motor point.[3,35,44] By stimulating this location, the current density is increased in an area where numerous fibers can be affected, maximizing the muscular response from the stimulation.

THERAPEUTIC USES OF ELECTRICALLY INDUCED MUSCLE CONTRACTION

A variety of therapeutic gains can be made by electrically stimulating a muscle contraction:
1. Muscle reeducation
2. Muscle pump contractions
3. Retardation of atrophy
4. Muscle strengthening
5. Increasing range of motion

Any electrical stimulator—high voltage, low voltage, alternating current, **hybrid current,** or transcutaneous electrical nerve stimulating (TENS) units—may be used to cause muscle contraction. The efficiency and effectiveness of treatment can be increased by following the protocols as closely as possible with the available equipment.

Muscle Reeducation

Muscular inhibition after surgery or injury is the primary indication for muscle reeducation. If the neuromuscular mechanisms of a muscle have not been damaged, then central nervous system inhibition of this muscle usually is a factor in loss of control. A muscle contraction usually can be forced by electrically stimulating the muscle. Forcing the muscle to contract causes an increase in the sensory input from that muscle. The patient feels the muscle contract, sees the muscle contract, and can attempt to duplicate this muscular response.[3,9,12,16,32]

Protocols for muscle reeducation do not list specific parameters to make this treatment more efficient, but the following criteria are essential for effective electrical stimulation:
1. Current intensity must be adequate for muscle contraction but comfortable for the athlete.

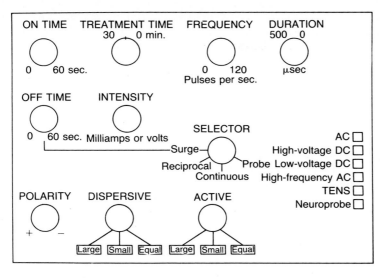

Figure 4-15. Electrical stimulator control panel.

2. Pulse duration must be set as close as possible to the duration needed for chronaxie of the tissue to be stimulated. This is preset on most of the new therapeutic generators.
3. Pulses per second should be high enough to give a tetanic contraction (30 to 40 pulses per second).
4. Interrupted or surged current must be used.
5. On time should be 1 to 2 seconds.
6. Off time should be 2 to 4 seconds.
7. The patient should be instructed to allow just the electricity to make the muscle contract, allowing the patient to feel and see the response desired. Next, the patient should alternate voluntary muscle contractions with current-induced contractions.
8. Total treatment time should be about 15 minutes, but this can be repeated several times daily.
9. High-voltage galvanic or high-frequency alternating current may be most effective (Fig. 4-15).[3,9,12,16]

Muscle Pump Contractions

Electrically induced muscle contraction can be used to duplicate the regular muscle contractions that help stimulate circulation by pumping fluid and blood through venous and lymphatic channels back into the heart. In most traumatic injuries and surgical interventions, one of the major problems is excessive accumulation of fluid. This edema is the result of damage to the vascular structures, loss of normal muscular activity, and dependency of the extremity. Electrical stimulation of muscle contractions in the affected extremity can help in reestablishing the proper circulatory pattern while keeping the injured part protected.

The following criteria must be satisfied for the electrical treatment to be successful in helping to reduce swelling:
1. Current intensity must be high enough to provide a strong, comfortable muscle contraction.
2. Pulse duration is preset on most of the new therapeutic generators. If adjustable, it should be set as close as possible to the duration needed for chronaxie of the tissue to be stimulated.
3. Pulses per second should be in the beginnings of tetany range (20 pulses per second).
4. Interrupted or surged current must be used.
5. On time should be 2 to 5 seconds.
6. Off time should be 5 to 8 seconds.
7. The part to be treated should be elevated.
8. The patient should be instructed to allow the electricity to make the muscles contract. Active range of motion may be encouraged at the same time if it is not contraindicated.
9. Total treatment time should be between 20 and 30 minutes; treatment should be repeated two to five times daily.
10. High-voltage galvanic or high-frequency alternating current may be most effective.[9,12,37,38,41] (See Fig. 4-15.)

Retardation of Atrophy

Prevention or retardation of atrophy has traditionally been a reason for treating patients with electrically stimulated muscle contraction. The maintenance of muscle tissue, after an injury that prevents normal muscular exercise, can be accomplished by substituting an electrically stimulated muscle contraction. The electrical stimulation reproduces many of the physical and chemical events associated with normal voluntary muscle contraction and helps to maintain normal muscle function.

Again, no specific protocols exist. In designing a program, the practitioner should try to duplicate muscle contractions associated with normal exercise routines. The following criteria can be used as guidelines in developing effective treatment protocols:
1. Current intensity should be as high as can be tolerated by the patient. This can be increased during the treatment as some sensory accommodation takes place. The contraction should be capable of moving the limb through the antigravity range or of achieving 60% of the normal isometric contraction torque for the muscle.
2. Pulse duration is preset on most of the new therapeutic generators. If it is adjustable, it should be set as close as possible to the duration needed for chronaxie of the tissue to be stimulated.
3. Pulses per second should be well into the tetany range (30 to 60 pulses per second).
4. Interrupted or surge type current should be used.
5. On time should be between 6 and 15 seconds.
6. Off time should be at least double on time.
7. The muscle should be given some resistance, either gravity or external re-

sistance provided by addition weights or by fixing the joint so that the contraction becomes isometric.

8. The patient can be instructed to work with the electrically induced contraction, but voluntary effort is not necessary for the success of this treatment.
9. Total treatment time should be 15 to 20 minutes, or enough time to allow a minimum of 10 contractions; the treatment time can be repeated two times daily.
10. A high-frequency alternating current stimulator is the machine of choice.* (See Fig. 4-15.)

Muscle Strengthening

Muscle strengthening from electrical muscle stimulation has been used with some good results in patients with weakness or denervation of a muscle group. Several studies also indicate that strength gain can be achieved. The protocol is better established for this use, but more research is needed to clarify the procedures and allow us to generalize the results to other electrical stimulators. The following are the protocols used successfully:

1. Current intensity should be high enough to make the muscle develop 60% of the torque developed in a maximum voluntary contraction.
2. Pulse duration is preset on most of the new therapeutic generators. If adjustable, it should be set as close as possible to the duration needed for chronaxie of the tissue to be stimulated.
3. Pulses per second should be near the top of the tolerable range (approximately 50 to 60 pulses per second).
4. Surged interrupted current should be used with a 10 msec on-off cycle of 2,500 cps and gradual current rise.
5. On time should be 15 seconds.
6. Off time should be 50 seconds.
7. Resistance usually is applied by immobilizing the limb. The muscle is then given an isometric contraction torque equal to or greater than 60% of the maximum voluntary contraction torque.
8. The patient can be instructed to work with the electrically induced contraction, but voluntary effort is not necessary for the success of the treatment.
9. Total treatment time should include 10 repetitions three times weekly. Some protocols recommend stimulation 1 to 6 hours per day in 30- to 60-minute treatment sessions. Generally, strength gains begin after 2 weeks and continue for 5 to 6 weeks.
10. A high-frequency alternating current stimulator is the machine of choice.† (See Fig. 4-15.)

Increasing Range of Motion

Increasing the range of motion in contracted joints is also a possible and documented use of electrical muscle stimulation. Electrically stimulating a muscle pulls the joint through the limited range. The continued contraction of this muscle group over an extended time appears to make the contracted joint and mus-

---

*11, 18, 19, 27, 32, 35, 44
†References 3, 9, 10, 12, 18, 19, 23, 32, 38, 44.

cle tissue modify and lengthen. Reduction of contractures in patients with hemiplegia has been reported, although no studies have reported this type of use in contracted joints from athletic injuries or surgery. The protocol needed to affect joint contracture is the following:

1. Current intensity must be high enough to make a muscle contract strongly enough to move the body part through its antigravity range. Intensity should be increased gradually during treatment if possible.
2. Pulse duration is preset on most of the new therapeutic generators. If it is adjustable, it should be set as close as possible to the duration needed for chronaxie of the tissue to be stimulated.
3. Pulses per second should be at the beginning of the tetany range (20 to 30 pulses per second).
4. Interrupted or surged current should be used.
5. On time should be between 15 and 20 seconds.
6. Off time should be equal to or greater than on time.
7. The stimulated muscle group should be antagonistic to the joint contracture and should be forced to work at the limits of the available range.
8. The patient is passive in this treatment and does not work with the electrical contraction.
9. Total treatment time should be 90 minutes daily. This can be broken into three 30-minute treatments.
10. High-voltage galvanic or high-frequency alternating current stimulators are the best choices.[3] (See Fig. 4-15.)

THERAPEUTIC USES OF ELECTRICAL STIMULATION OF SENSORY NERVES

Clinically, efforts are made to stimulate the sensory nerves to change the patient's perception of a painful stimulus coming from an injured area. To understand how to maximally affect the perception of pain through electrical stimulation, it is necessary to understand pain perception. The gate control theory, the central biasing theory, and the opiate pain control theory are the theoretical bases for pain reduction phenomena. The information in this area is rapidly expanding, and current knowledge will be obsolete quickly. These theories are covered in depth in Chapter 1.

Gate Control Theory

Electrically stimulating the large sensory fibers when there is pain in a certain area will force the central nervous system to make the brain's recognition area aware of the electrical stimuli. As long as the stimuli are applied, the perception of pain is diminished. Electrical stimulation of sensory nerves will evoke the gate control mechanism and diminish awareness of painful stimuli. As long as the stimulation is causing firing of the sensory nerves, the gate to pain should be closed. If accommodation to the electrical stimulus occurs or if the stimulus stops, the gate is then open, and pain returns to perception.[4,5,19,21,22,28,29,45]

Central Biasing Theory

Intense electrical stimulation of the smaller fibers (C fibers or pain fibers) at peripheral sites (trigger and acupoint) for short time periods causes stimulation of descending neurons, which then affect transmission of pain information by closing the gate at the spinal cord level.[6] (See Fig. 1-3.)

Opiate Pain Control Theory

Electrical stimulation of sensory nerves may stimulate the release of enkephalin from local sites throughout the central nervous system and the release of β-endorphin from the pituitary gland into the cerebral spinal fluid. The mechanism that causes the release and then the binding of enkephalin and β-endorphin to some nerve cells is still unclear. It is certain that a diminution or elimination of pain perception is caused by applying an electrical current to areas close to the site of pain or to acupuncture or trigger points, both local and distant to the pain area.[6,29,30,39,45]

Physical Dominance and Enkephalin Release

The techniques for stimulation of sensory nerves based on the physical dominance theory and enkephalin release should be aimed at maximum depolarization of the sensory nerve. This depolarization is best accomplished by an electrical current that matches the sensory nerve strength-duration curve. The following criteria can be used as guidelines in developing effective treatment protocols:

1. Current intensity should be adjusted to tolerance but should not cause a muscular contraction—the higher the better.
2. Pulse duration (pulse width) should be 75 to 150 msec.
3. Pulses per second should be 80 to 125.
4. A transcutaneous electrical stimulator waveform should be used.
5. On time should be continuous mode.
6. Total treatment time should correspond to fluctuations in pain; the unit should be left on until pain is no longer perceived, turned off, then restarted when pain begins again.
7. Any stimulator that can deliver this current is acceptable. Portable units are better for 24-hour pain control.[21,22,25] (See Fig. 4-15.)

    CENTRAL BIASING. Changing the bias of the central nervous system and increasing the descending influences on the transmission of pain are best accomplished with the following protocols:

1. Current intensity should be very high, approaching a noxious level; muscular contraction is not desirable.
2. Pulse duration should be 10 msec.
3. Pulses per second should be 80.
4. On time should be 30 seconds to 1 minute.
5. Stimulation should be applied over trigger or acupuncture points.
6. Selection and number of points used varies according to the part treated.
7. A low-frequency, high-intensity generator is the stimulator of choice for central biasing.[6] (See Fig. 4-16.)

    β-ENDORPHIN. β-Endorphin production may be stimulated using the following protocols:

1. Current intensity should be high, approaching a noxious level; muscular contraction is acceptable.

2. Pulse duration should be 200 to 500 μsec.
3. Pulses per second should be between 1 and 5.
4. High-voltage galvanic waveform should be used.
5. On time should be 30 to 45 seconds.
6. Stimulation should be applied over trigger or acupuncture points.
7. Selection and number of points used varies according to the part and condition being treated.
8. A high-voltage galvanic or a low-frequency, high-intensity machine is best for this effect.[6,29,30] (See Fig. 4-15.)

ELECTRODE PLACEMENT

When using any of the treatment protocols aimed at the electrical stimulation of sensory nerves for pain suppression, there are several guidelines that will help the practitioner select the appropriate sites for electrode placement. Transcutaneous electrical nerve stimulation (TENS) uses similar-sized electrodes placed according to a pattern and moved in a trial-and-error pattern until pain is decreased. The following patterns may be used:

1. Electrodes may be placed on or around the painful area.
2. Electrodes may be placed over specific dermatomes, myotomes, or sclerotomes that correspond to the painful area.
3. Electrodes may be placed close to the spinal cord segment that **innervates** an area that is painful.
4. Peripheral nerves that innervate the painful area may be stimulated by placing electrodes over sites where the nerve becomes superficial and can be stimulated easily.
5. Both acupuncture and trigger points have been conveniently mapped out and illustrated. A reference on acupuncture and trigger areas is included in Appendix A. The sports therapist should systematically attempt to stimulate the points listed as successful for certain areas and types of pain. If they are effective, the patient will have decreased pain. These points also can be identified using an ohm meter point locator to determine areas of decreased skin resistance.
6. Combinations of any of the above systems and bilateral electrode placement can also be successful.[21,22,25,47]
7. Crossing patterns, also referred to as an *interferential technique,* involve electrode application such that the electrical signals from each set of electrodes add together at some point in the body and the intensity accumulates. The electrodes are usually arranged in a criss-cross pattern around the point to be stimulated (Fig. 4-16).

The practitioner should not be limited to any one system but should evaluate electrode placement for each patient. The effectiveness of this treatment is closely tied in with proper electrode placement. As in all trial-and-error treatment approaches, a systematic, organized search is always better than a "shotgun," hit-and-miss approach. Numerous articles have identified some of the best locations for common pain problems, and these may be used as a start-

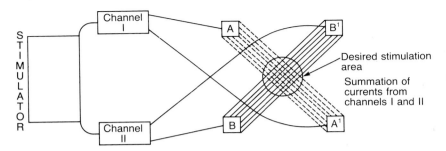

Figure 4-16. Current flow would be from A to A and B to B. As the currents cross the area of stimulation, they summate in intensity.

ing point for the first approach.[21] If the treatment is not achieving the desired results, the electrode placement should be reconsidered.

PROTOCOL FOR ELECTRICAL HYPER-STIMULATION AND β-ENDORPHIN RELEASE

To use the influence of hyperstimulation analgesia and β-endorphin release, a point stimulation setup must be used. A large dispersive pad and a small pad or handheld probe point electrode are utilized in this approach. The point electrode is applied to the chosen site, and the intensity is increased until it is perceived by the patient. The probe is then moved around the area and the patient is asked to report relative changes in perception of intensity. When a location of maximum-intensity perception is found, the current intensity is increased to maximum tolerable levels. This is much the same as finding a motor point, as described earlier.[6,35]

A combination of intense point stimulation and transcutaneous electrical nerve stimulation may be used. The transcutaneous electrical nerve stimulation applications should be used as much as needed to make the patient comfortable, and the intense point stimulation should be used on a periodic basis. Periodic use of intense point stimulation gives maximal pain relief for a period of time and allows some gains in overall pain suppression. Daily intense point stimulation may eventually bias the central nervous system and decrease the effectiveness of this type of stimulation.

CLINICAL USES OF LOW-VOLTAGE UNINTERRUPTED DIRECT CURRENT

The application of uninterrupted low-voltage direct current causes several physiologic changes that can be used therapeutically. The therapeutic benefits are related to the polar and vasomotor effects and to the acid reaction around the positive pole and the alkaline reaction at the negative pole. The sports therapist must be concerned with the damaging effects of this variety of current. Acidic or alkaline changes can cause severe skin reactions.[44] These reactions occur only with low-voltage uninterrupted direct current and are not possible with the high-voltage galvanic machines. The pulse duration of the high-voltage galvanic machines is too short to cause these chemical changes.[33]

There is also a vasomotor effect on the skin, increasing blood flow between the electrodes. The benefits from this type of direct current are usually attributed to the increased blood flow through the treatment area.[44]

The following protocols for uninterrupted low-voltage direct current can be used to give the greatest vasomotor effects:

1. Current intensity should be to the patient's tolerance; it should be increased as accommodation takes place.
2. Continuous uninterrupted direct current should be used.
3. Pulses per second should be 0.
4. A low-voltage direct current stimulator is the machine of choice.
5. Treatment time should be between a 15-minute minimum and a 50-minute maximum.
6. Equal-sized electrodes are used over gauze that has been soaked in saline solution and lightly squeezed.
7. Skin should be unbroken.[35] (See Fig. 4-15.)

Promotion of Wound Healing

Similar direct current has been used to treat skin ulcers that have poor blood flow. The treated ulcers show accelerated healing rates when compared with untreated skin ulcers. The wound areas should be treated for the first 3 days with the negative electrode at the wound site and the positive electrode positioned 25 cm from the wound. The negative electrode and its alkaline reaction seem to inhibit the growth of bacteria. In cases in which infection was present, the negative electrode was used until the infection cleared and for 3 days thereafter.

After the initial negative pole treatment, the electrodes were reversed, and the positive pole was placed in the wound. The positive pole promotes the migration of skin cells toward the center of the wound and decreases healing time in these ulcers.[13]

Promotion of Fracture Healing

The use of uninterrupted low-voltage direct current may be an adjunctive modality in the treatment of fractures, especially fractures prone to nonunion. Fracture healing may be accelerated by passing a direct current through the fracture site. Getting the current into the bony area without an invasive technique is difficult.[2,5,8,26,46]

Using a standard transcutaneous electrical nerve stimulation unit, Kahn reported favorable results in the electrical stimulation of callus formation in fractures that had nonunions after 6 months. This information is based on a case study. Results of a more extensive population of nonunions have not been documented. Kahn used the following protocol:

1. Current intensity was just perceptible to the patient.
2. Pulse duration was the longest duration allowed on the unit (100 to 200 msec).
3. Pulses per second were set at the lowest frequency allowed on the unit (5 to 10 pps).
4. Standard monophasic or biphasic direct current transcutaneous electrical stimulating units were used.

5. Treatment time was from 30 minutes to 1 hour, three to four times daily.
6. A negative electrode was placed close to but distal to the fracture site. A positive electrode was placed proximal to the immobilizing device.
7. If four pads were used, the interferential placement described earlier was used.
8. Results were reassessed at monthly intervals.[20] (See Fig. 4-15.)

Iontophoresis

Direct current has been used for many years to drive ions from the heavy metals into and through the skin for treatment of skin infections or for a counterirritating effect. There are three techniques of application: (1) an active pad is applied over gauze that is saturated with a solution containing the ions (this is positioned as close as possible to the involved tissue); (2) the active electrode is suspended in a container of the ion solution, then the part to be treated is immersed in the container; and (3) special stimulators with a specially adapted electrode containing the treatment ions is positioned as close to the involved tissue as possible. In all cases, a large dispersive pad is applied to the patient and the proper polarity of the active electrode is selected based on the polarity of the ions in the solution.

Positive ions require an active electrode that is positive; negative ions require an active electrode that is negative. Treatment time will vary. A more comprehensive source dealing with iontophoresis should be consulted before using this technique.[20,44]

CONTRAINDICATION TO UNINTERRUPTED DIRECT CURRENTS

Skin burns are the greatest hazard of any uninterrupted direct current technique. These burns result from excessive density in any area, usually from direct metal contact with skin or from setting the intensity too high for the size of the active electrode. Both these problems cause a very high density of current in the area of contact.[11]

"RUSSIAN CURRENT"

"Russian current" is associated with the class of stimulators developed in Canada and the United States after the Russian scientist Yadou M. Kots presented his research at a seminar in Canada in 1977. The stimulators developed out of this presentation deliver a polyphasic AC wave form with frequency ranging from 2000 to 10,000 Hz. Earlier models had nonadjustable frequencies fixed at 2500 Hz. The pulse width can be varied from 50 to 250 μsec; the phase duration will be 0.5 pulse width. Earlier models had a fixed pulse duration of 400 μsec. As the pulse frequency increases, the pulse duration decreases.[18,32,38]

According to strength-duration curve data, to obtain the same effect as the duration decreases, the intensity must be increased. To make this intensity of current tolerable, it is generated in 50-burst-per-second envelopes with an interburst interval of 10 MS. This slightly reduces the total current but allows enough of a peak current intensity to stimulate muscle very well (Fig. 4-17). If the current continued without the burst effect, the total current delivered would equal the lightly shaded area in Fig. 4-18. When generated with the

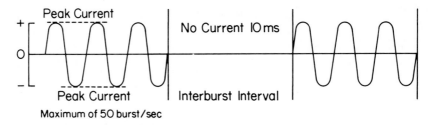

Figure 4-17. "Russian" current with polyphasic AC wave form and 10 MS interburst interval.

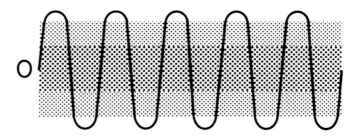

Figure 4-18. "Russian" current (without an interburst interval). The light shaded area is equal to the total current.

burst effect, the total current is decreased. Here the total current would equal the darkly shaded area in Fig. 4-19. This allows tolerance of greater current intensity by the patient. As the intensity increases, more muscle fibers are stimulated, increasing the magnitude of the contraction. Because it is a fast oscillating AC current, as soon as the nerve repolarizes it is stimulated again, producing a current that will maximally summate muscle contraction.

The frequency (pulses per second or, in this case, bursts per second) is also a variable that can be controlled. This would make the muscle respond with a twitch rather than a gradually increasing mechanical contraction. Gradually increasing the numbers of bursts interrupts the mechanical relaxation cycle of the muscle and causes more shortening to take place.[32] (See Fig. 4-13.)

Recent changes in this type of stimulator have added greater flexibility to changes in waveform. The waveform can be switched from a sine wave to a symmetric biphasic pulse wave. This makes the current more efficient, and less total current is required to obtain the same stimulation effect.[18]

INTERFERENTIAL CURRENTS

The research and use of interferential currents (IFC) has taken place primarily in Europe. An Austrian scientist, Ho Nemec, introduced the concept and suggested its therapeutic use. Nemec's concept resulted in the creation of a type of electrical generator that is difficult to understand, not because the theory is so complex, but because the electrical engineers added so many options to the

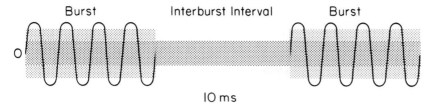

Figure 4-19. "Russian" current (with an interburst interval). Dark shaded area represents total current, and light shading indicates total current without the interburst interval.

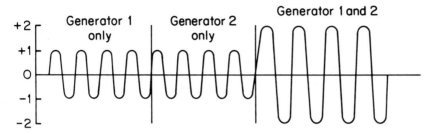

Figure 4-20. Sine wave from Generator 1 and sine wave from Generator 2 showing a constructive interference pattern.

generator that the current can be modified substantially while still maintaining its basic waveform.

The theories and behavior of electrical waves are part of basic physics. This behavior is easiest to understand when continuous sine waves are used as an example.

With only one circuit the current behaves as described earlier; if put on an oscilloscope, it looks like Generator 1 in Fig. 4-20. If a second generator is brought into the same location, the currents may interfere with each other. This interference can be summative—that is, the amplitudes of the electric wave are combined and increase (Fig. 4-20). Both waves are exactly the same; if they are produced in phase or originate at the same time, they combine. This is called **constructive interference.**

If these waves are generated out of sync, Generator 1 starts in a positive direction at the same time that Generator 2 starts in a negative direction; the waves then will cancel each other out. This is called **destructive interference;** in the summation the waves end up with an amplitude of 0. (Fig. 4-21).

To make this a bit more complex, assume that one generator has a slightly slower or faster frequency and that the generators begin producing current simultaneously. Initially, the electric waves will be constructively summated; however, because the frequencies of the two waves differ, they gradually will get out of phase and become destructively summated. When dealing with sound waves, we hear distinct beats as this phenomenon occurs. We borrow

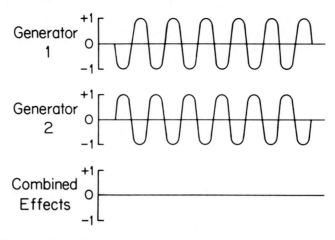

Figure 4-21. Sine wave from Generator 1 and sine wave from Generator 2 showing destructive interference.

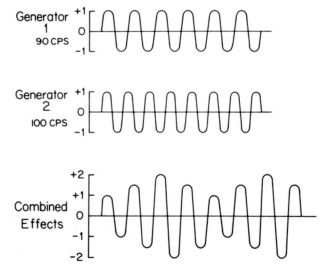

Figure 4-22. Sine wave from Generator 1 at 90 CPS and sine wave from Generator 2 at 100 CPS showing the heterodyne, or beating behavior, of wave interference.

the term *beat* when describing this behavior. When any waveforms are out of phase but are combined in the same location, the waves will cause a beat effect. The blending of the waves is caused by the constructive and destructive interference patterns of the waves and is called *heterodyne.* (Fig. 4-22).[32,34]

The heterodyne effect is seen on an oscilloscope as a cyclic, rising and falling waveform. The peaks or beat frequency in this heterodyne wave behavior occur regularly, according to the difference of each current; for example, 100 cps − 90 cps = 10 cps beat frequency. In electric currents, this beat frequency

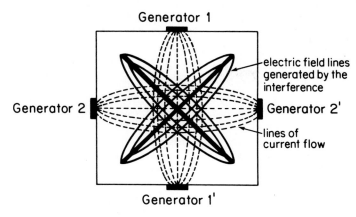

Figure 4-23. Square electrode alignment and interference pattern of current in a homogeneous medium.

is, in effect, the stimulation frequency of the waveform, because the destructive interference negates the effects of the other part of the wave. The intensity (amplitude) will be set according to sensations created by this peak.[32] When using an interference current for therapy, the sports therapist should select the frequencies to create a beat frequency corresponding to his or her choices of frequency when using other stimulators—20 to 50 pps for muscle contraction, 50 to 120 pps for pain management, 1 pps for acustim pain relief.

When the electrodes are arranged in a square alignment and interferential currents are passed through a homogeneous medium, a predictable pattern of interference will occur. In these patterns, an electric field is created that resembles a four-petaled flower, with the center of the flower located where the two currents cross and the petals falling between the electric current force lines. The maximum interference effect takes place near the center, with the field gradually decreasing in strength as it moves toward the points of the petal. (Fig. 4-23).[32]

Because the body is not a homogeneous medium, we cannot predict the exact location of this interference pattern; we must rely on the patient's perception. If the patient has a localized structure that is painful, locating the stimulation in the correct location is relatively easy. The therapist moves the electrode placement until the patient centers the feeling of the stimulus in the problem area.[32,34] When a patient has poorly localized pain, the task becomes more difficult. The engineers added features to the generators and created a scanning interferential current that moves the flower petals of force around while the treatment is taking place. This enlarges the effective treatment area. Additional technology and another set of electrodes create a three-dimensional flower effect when one looks at the electrical field. This is called a *stereodynamic interference current.*[32,34]

All these alterations and modifications are designed to spread the heterodyne effect throughout the tissue. Because it is controlled by a cyclic electrical pattern, however, we actually may be decreasing the current passed through the structures we are trying to treat. The machines seem complex but lack the versatility to do much more than the conventional TENS treatment.[32,38]

Nikolova[34] has used IFC for a variety of clinical problems and found them effective in dealing with pain problems, (e.g., joint sprains with swelling, restricted mobility and pain; neuritis; retarded callus formation following fractures; and pseudarthrosis). These claims are supported by other researchers. Each of these researchers used slightly different protocols in treating the different clinical problems. To be successful in achieving the desired results with interferential currents, the sports therapist must thoroughly review existing protocols and acquire a good working knowledge of the application techniques.

Microcurrent Electrical Neuromuscular Stimulation

Generators that use microcurrent electrical neuromuscular stimulation (MENS) are among the newer electrical therapy units available to today's sports therapist. The currents generated by these devices are not substantially different from the currents discussed previously. These currents still have a direction, and both AC and DC waveforms are available. The currents also have amplitude (intensity), pulse duration, and frequency.

This equipment apparently is being developed around the research into the normal electrical charges at work in cellular function and maintenance, as well as on the effects of electrical currents on single cell behavior.[2] Although electrical fields and electromagnetic forces have always been present in the natural world, they are just beginning to be researched, and good supporting studies are not available. The scientific community has just begun the process of testing and research that is required to begin to understand the effects of electrical forces on cellular behavior.

Most of the literature on microcurrents has been generated by researchers interested in stimulating the healing process in fractures and skin wounds. Subsequent research aims at identifying why and how microcurrents work. The best-researched area of application of MENS-type currents is in the stimulation of bone formation in delayed union or nonunion of fractures of the long bones. Most of this research was done using implanted rather than surface electrodes, and most have used DC with the negative pole placed at the fracture site.[2,7,26] We are in danger of generalizing treatments for all problems based on success in this one area. These applications were intended to mimic the normal electrical field created during the injury and healing process.[2,32] At present these electrical changes are poorly understood, and the effects of adding additional electric current to the normal electrical activity created by the injury and healing process are still being investigated. There is only scant evidence to back up protocols; the efficacy of using this type of current is still under scrutiny, with only one study supporting its use for sports therapy patients.[42,43]

For the purposes of our discussion, MENS currents will be defined as those with a very low frequency (1 Hz or less) and low intensity or amplitude (1 to 1000 microamps). They are considered subsensory, because they will not stimulate an action potential from the excitable tissues (nerves and muscles). Conventional stimulators (TENS, low-volt, HVPGS) may be capable of delivering this type of current if the controls of the device allow the necessary adjustments. The frequency should be set as low as possible, and the intensity should be at a subsensory level. The pulse duration is reported to be 1 to 500 msec. This either varies as the frequency changes or is preset, as is the case when using pulsed currents.[36]

If the current generator can be adjusted to allow increases of current above 1000 microamps and frequencies higher than 1 Hz, the current becomes like those previously described in this text. If the current provokes an action potential in a sensory or motor nerve, the results on that tissue will be the same as previously described for other currents—sensation or muscle contraction.

When using MENS to stimulate the healing process, there is some research on which to base the clinical protocols; it is contradictory, however, and its lack of consensus gives the sports therapist limited security in devising protocols.

Direct currents have been used most often, although alternating currents also have had a positive effect. The frequency should be kept under 1 cycle per second, and the intensity can vary from 1 to 150 microamps. The treatment time varies from 12 to 15 minutes to 8 to 24 hours.[2,26] One study[42,43] investigated the use of microcurrents in treating shoulder impingement problems by using a treatment time of 5 to 20 minutes on a daily basis. The majority (70%) of patients responded in 6 treatment days, with most (84%) becoming pain-free in 10 treatment days.

Some studies indicate that there is a polar effect and that healing is stimulated to the greatest levels under the negative pole.[2] Positive polarity has been used in the presence of infection for the first treatment day because of its bacteriostatic effect. In a study on skin wounds in rats by Harrington,[48] the greatest healing activity occurred under the positive electrode. This study did not follow the complete course of healing; the results came from studying the progress made during the first 48 hours postincision. Other studies did not discuss the polar effects, because the tissue undergoing treatment was located centrally in an area of current flow and away from areas where polar effects could be substantiated. The positive electrode in most of the bone healing studies was moved frequently to keep the skin irritation at a minimum and to promote the current flow in a variety of directions along the axis of the bone.

Microamp currents may be a valuable addition to the electrical therapies, but they are untested clinically, and the practitioner is certainly entitled to be very skeptical of the manufacturers' claims until more research is reported. Existing protocols for use are not well established; this, again, leaves the practitioner with an insecure feeling about this modality.

The world of electrical therapy is constantly changing, owing to the advances in research, engineering, and technology and because of the competitive pressures of the marketplace. Equipment manufacturers will develop a different machine and try to market it on the basis of a single feature of their product. The old adage "let the buyer beware" is certainly good advice. The more understanding of electrical currents the sports therapist has, the less likely he or she is to be "snowed" or confused by the salesman's spiel. Even more important, the greater the understanding, the easier it becomes to manipulate the treatment protocols for each patient to optimize the results.

BIOFEEDBACK   In the previous sections we have been concerned with adding electrical energy to the body tissues to achieve a therapeutic result. Using the natural electrical activity generated by a contracting muscle to selectively train that muscle to relax or contract is called **electromyographic biofeedback.**[16,27]

The term *biofeedback* should be familiar, because all sports therapists are instruments of biofeedback in teaching a therapeutic exercise or in coaching a particular movement pattern. The sports therapist acts as the knowledge-of-results loop in a motor-learning sequence in this situation.

In all motor learning sequences, the athlete has some expectation of what is to be accomplished in any exercise session. The athlete then produces a motor output from brain-originated commands. Internal sensors and external stimuli tell the athlete how a movement was performed and what the movement accomplished in the environment, relative to the original expectations. Through practice, the athlete can adjust motor outputs to reach expected goals. The sports therapist adds to the external stimuli, giving the athlete the knowledge of results and cues for improving performance (Fig. 4-24).

Electromyographic signals, which graphically display electrical muscle activity, can provide a useful external stimulus from the internal functioning of the muscle; this can lead to better training of a given muscular response. As each motor unit contracts, electrical currents are generated as the membranes of the nerve and muscle discharge. These electrical signals are picked up by sensing electrodes. The signals are then amplified and converted to visual or auditory displays.[27]

This display is useful in two ways in a therapeutic exercise program: (1)

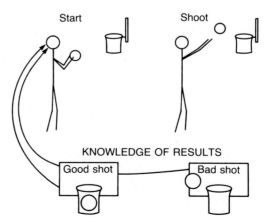

Figure 4-24. Through practice the student can learn to adjust motor outputs to reach the expected goals.

muscle contraction can be trained to provide any desired effect, and (2) the muscle also can be trained not to contract in situations in which muscle tension or muscular contractions from particular muscle groups are not desirable.[16,24,27]

Protocol

1. The motor point of the muscle under treatment must be found, using the method described earlier.
2. The electrodes should be placed as close to this motor point as possible, and the **electromyography** unit should be turned on.
3. The patient then can be instructed to maximize or minimize the contraction of the involved muscle.

    The information gained from the electromyographic signals gives the athlete augmented feedback on his or her muscular activity and allows greater control to be gained through repetition, practice, and increased knowledge of results.[16,27]

SUMMARY

1. When an electrical system is applied to muscle or nerve tissue, the result will be tissue membrane depolarization, provided that the current has the appropriate intensity, duration, and waveform to reach the tissue's excitability threshold.
2. Nerve function and muscle contraction are the same regardless of the stimulation mechanism (i.e., natural or electrical).
3. Muscle and nerve tissue respond in an all-or-none fashion; there is no gradation of response.
4. Muscle contraction will change according to changes in current. As the frequency of the electrical stimulus increases, the muscle will develop more tension as a result of the summation of the contraction of the muscle fiber through progressive mechanical shortening. Increases in intensity spread the current over a larger area and increase the number of motor units activated by the current. Increases in the duration of the current also will cause more motor units to be activated.
5. Electrically stimulated muscle contractions are used clinically to help with muscle reeducation, muscle contraction for muscle pumping action, reduction of swelling, prevention or retardation of atrophy, muscle strengthening, and increasing range of motion in tight joints.
6. To stimulate a given muscle, location of the muscle's motor point, size and spacing of electrodes, and impedance of the tissue between the electrodes and the motor points must be selected and adjusted to provide the most effective therapy. This also must be taken into account when selecting a stimulation site.
7. Electrically stimulated discharges of sensory nerves help decrease pain perceptions.
8. The pain gating effect of electrical stimulation may occur at different levels

in the central nervous system, depending on the type of electrical current used. Types of current similar to that used in transcutaneous electrical nerve stimulation will be gated at the spinal cord level. Hyperstimulation analgesia will stimulate central biasing with inhibitory influences descending from the brain and brain stem levels. Noxious stimuli to acupuncture or trigger areas will cause production of β-endorphin in the spinal cord and brain, with a resultant analgesic effect.

9. Constant direct current has several major influences. The primary uses involve polar effects (acid or alkaline), increased blood flow, **bacteriostatic** effects (negative electrode), and migration and alignment of cellular building blocks in the healing processes.

10. Specialized current waveforms ("Russian," interferential, microamp, and so on) all have physiologic responses that can be attributed to the characteristics of their waveforms. The differences in the waveforms and the physiologic response of each have particular effects that can be used therapeutically.

11. Electromyographic biofeedback can enhance exercise by increasing knowledge of results during the exercise. This type of feedback can be used to increase or decrease the activity of any muscle.

GLOSSARY

absolute refractory period Brief time period (.5 μsec) following membrane depolarization during which the membrane is incapable of depolarizing again.

action potential A recorded change in electrical potential between the inside and outside of a nerve cell, resulting in muscular contraction.

active electrode Electrode at which greatest current density occurs.

all or none response The depolarization of nerve or muscle membrane is the same once a depolarizing intensity threshold is reached; further increases in intensity do not increase the response. Stimuli at intensities less than threshold do not create a depolarizing effect.

anode Positively charged electrode in a direct current system.

cathode Negatively charged electrode in a direct current system.

central biasing The use of hyperstimulation analgesia to bias the central nervous system against transmitting painful stimuli to the sensory recognition area. This occurs through hormonal influences created by brain stem stimulation.

chronaxie The duration of time necessary to cause observable tissue excitation, given a current intensity of 2 times rheobasic current.

current density Amount of current flow per cubic area.

depolarization Process or act of neutralizing the cell membrane's resting potential.

electromyography The pickup and amplification of electrical signals generated by the muscle as it contracts.

hybrid currents Currents that have wave forms containing parameters that are not classically alternating or direct.

impedance Resistance of the tissue to the passage of electrical current.

indifferent or dispersive electrode Large electrode used to spread out electrical charge and decrease current density at that electrode site.

iontophoresis The use of constant direct current to drive heavy metal ions into and through the skin.

rheobase The intensity of current necessary to cause observable tissue excitation, given a long current duration.

strength-duration curve A graphic illustration of the relationship between current intensity and current duration in causing depolarization of a nerve or muscle membrane.

summation of contractions Shortening of muscle myofilaments caused by increasing the frequency of muscle membrane depolarization.

twitch muscle contraction A single muscle contraction caused by one depolarization phenomenon.

voltage sensitive permeability The quality of some

cell membranes that makes them permeable to different ions based on the electric charge of the ions. Nerve and muscle cell membranes allow negatively charged ions into the cell while actively transporting some positively charged ions outside the cell membrane.

REFERENCES

1 Alon, G.: High voltage stimulation: effects of electrode size on basic excitatory responses, Phys. Ther. **65**:890, 1985.

2 Becker, R.O., and Selden, G.: The body electric, New York, 1985, William Morrow & Co., Inc.

3 Benton, L.A., Baker, L.L., Bowman, B.R., et al.: Functional electrical stimulation: a practical clinical guide, Downey, Calif., 1980, Rancho Los Amigos Hospital.

4 Bishop, B.: Pain: its physiology and rationale for management, Phys. Ther. **60**:13-37, 1980.

5 Brighton, C.T.: Bioelectric effects on bone and cartilage, Clin. Orthop. **124**:2-4, 1977.

6 Castel, J.C.: Pain management with acupuncture and transcutaneous electrical nerve stimulation techniques and photo simulation (laser), Symposium on Pain Management, Walter Reed Army Medical Center, Nov. 13, 1982.

7 Chen, N., Van Houf, H., Bockx, E., et al.: The effects of electric current on ATP Generation, protein synthesis, and membrane transport in rat skin, Clin. Orthop. Relat. Res. **171**:264-272, 1982.

8 Connolly, J.F., Hahn, H., and Jardon, O.M.: The electrical enhancement of periosteal proliferation in normal and delayed fracture healing, Clin. Orthop. **124**:97-105, 1977.

9 Currier, D.P., Lehman, J., and Lightfoot, P.: Electrical stimulation in exercise of the quadriceps femoris muscle, Phys. Ther. **59**:1508-1512, 1979.

10 Currier, D.P., and Mann, R.: Muscular strength development by electrical stimulation in healthy individuals, Phys. Ther. **63**:915-921, 1983.

11 Electrotherapy safety rules and general principles of treatment, Course Handout, Medical College of Virginia Physical Therapy School, 1966.

12 Eriksson, E., and Haggmark, T.: Comparison of isometric muscle training and electrical stimulation supplement, isometric muscle training in the recovery after major knee ligament surgery, Am. J. Sports Med. **7**:169-171, 1979.

13 Gault, W.R., and Gatens, P.F., Jr.: Use of low intensity direct current in management of ischemic skin ulcers, Phys. Ther. **56**:265-269, 1976.

14 Goodgold, J., and Eberstein, A.: Electrodiagnosis of neuromuscular diseases, Baltimore, 1972, Williams & Wilkins.

15 Guyton, A.C.: Textbook of medical physiology, ed. 2, Philadelphia, 1961, W.B. Saunders Co.

16 Howson, D.: Report on neuromuscular re-education, Minneapolis, 1978, Medical General.

17 Howson, D.C.: Peripheral neural excitability, Phys. Ther. **58**:1467-1473, 1978.

18 Instruction manual for Electrostim 180-2, Promatek, Canada.

19 Johnson, D.H., Thurston, P., and Ashcroft, P.J.: The Russian technique of faradism in the treatment of chondromalacia patellae, Physiotherapy (Can.) **29**:266-268, 1977.

20 Kahn, J.: Low voltage technique, ed. 4, Syossett, N.Y., 1983, Joseph Kahn.

21 Lampe, G.N.: A clinical approach to transcutaneous electrical nerve stimulation in the treatment of chronic and acute pain, Minneapolis, July, 1978, Med. General.

22 Lampe, G.N.: Introduction to the use of transcutaneous electrical nerve stimulation devices, Phys. Ther. **58**:1450-1454, 1978.

23 Laughman, R.K., Youdss, J., Garrett, T., et al: Strength changes in the normal quadriceps femoris muscle as a result of electrical stimulation, Phys. Ther. **63**:494-499, 1983.

24 LeVeau, B.F., and Rogers, C: Selective training of the vastus medialis muscle using EMG biofeedback, Phys. Ther. **60**:1410-1415, 1980.

25 Mannheimer, J., and Lampe, G.: Clinical transcutaneous electrical nerve stimulation, Philadelphia, 1984, F.A. Davis Co.

26 Marino, A., and Becker, R.O.: Biologic effects of extremely low frequency electric and magnetic fields: a review, Phys. Chem. Physics **9**:131-143, 1977.

27 McDermott, J.F., Modaff, W.L., and Boyle, R.W.: Electromyography, GP **27**(1):103-108, 1963.

28 Melzack, R.: The puzzle of pain, New York, 1973, Basic Books, Inc.

29 Melzack, R.: Prolonged relief of pain by brief, intense transcutaneous electrical stimulation, Pain **1**(4):357-373, 1975.

30 Melzack, R., Stillwell, D.M., and Fox, E.J.: Trigger points and acupuncture points for pain: correlations and implications, Pain **3**(1):3-23, 1977.

31 Mohr, T., Akers, T., and Landry, R.: Effect of high voltage stimulation on edema reduction in the rat hind limb, Phys. Ther. **67**:1703-1707, 1987.

32 Nelson, R.L., and Currier, D.P.: Clinical electrotherapy, Norwalk, CT, 1987, Appleton and Lange.

33 Newton, R.A., and Karselis, T.C.: Skin pH following high voltage pulsed galvanic stimulation, Phys. Ther. **63**:1593-1596, 1983.

34 Nikolova, L.: Treatment with interferential current, New York, 1987, Churchill Livingstone.

35 Notes on low volt therapy, White Plains, NY, 1966, TECA Corporation.

36 Protocol for monad instruments, Pomona, CA, 1988, Monad Corporation.

37 Randall, B.F., Imig, C.J., and Hines, H.M.: Effect of electrical stimulation upon blood flow and temperature of skeletal muscles, Arch. Phys. Med. **33**:73-78, 1952.

38 Synder-Mackler, L., Garrett, M., and Roberts, M.: A comparison of torque generating capabilities of three different electrical stimulating currents, JOSPT **10**:297-301, 1989.

39 Snyder, S.H.: Opiate receptors and internal opiates, Sci. Am. **236**:44-56, 1977.

40 Stillwell, G.K.: Therapeutic electricity and ultraviolet radiation, Baltimore, 1983, Williams & Wilkins.

41 Svacina, L.: Modified interferential technique, Pain Control, April 1978, pp. 1-2, Staodynamics, Inc.

42 Wallace, L.: Microcurrent electrical neuromuscular stimulation therapy and the shoulder impingement syndrome, unpublished report, 1988, Lyndhurst, Ohio.

43 Wallace, L.: Personal communication, January 12, 1989.

44 Watkins, A.L.: A manual of electrotherapy, ed. 3, Philadelphia, 1968, Lea & Febiger.

45 Wolf, S.L.: Perspectives on central nervous system responsiveness to transcutaneous electrical nerve stimulation, Phys. Ther. **58**:1443-1449, 1978.

46 Wolf, S.L.: Electrotherapy, New York, 1981, Churchill Livingstone.

47 Wolf, S.L., Gersh, M.R., and Kutner, M.: Relationship of selected clinical variables to current delivered during transcutaneous electrical nerve stimulation, Phys. Ther. **58**:1478-1483, 1978.

48 Harrington, D., Meyer, R., Jr., and Klein, R.: Effects of small amounts of electric current at the cellular level, Ann. N. Y. Acad. Sci. **238**:300-306, 1974.

SUGGESTED READINGS

Abramowitsch, D., and Neoussikine, B.: Treatment by ion transfer, New York, 1946, Grune & Stratton, p 124.

Adams, J.A.: The effects on frequency of high voltage pulsed galvanic stimulation on the results of treatment for pain in chronic low back pain patients, PhD thesis, Richmond, Va, Medical College of Virginia, Virginia Commonwealth University, 1983.

Akers, T.K., and Gabrielson, A.L.: The effect of high voltage galvanic stimulation on the rate of healing of decubitus ulcers, Biomed. Sci. Instrum. **20**:99, 1984.

Alon, G.: High voltage stimulation: effects of electrode size on basic excitatory responses, Phys. Ther. **65**:890, 1985.

Alon, G., Allin, J., and Inbar, G.E.: Optimization of pulse duration and pulse charge during transcutaneous electrical stimulation, Aust. J. Physiother. **29**:195, 1983.

Alon, G., Bainbridge, J., Croson, G., et al.: High-voltage pulsed direct current effects on peripheral blood flow, Phys. Ther. **61**:678, 1981.

Andersson, S.A.: Pain control by sensory stimulation. In Bonica, J.J., et al., editors: Advances in pain research and therapy, New York, 1979, Raven, vol. 3, pp. 569-584.

Andersson, S.A., Hansson, G., Holmgren, E., et al.: Evaluation of the pain suppression effect of different frequencies of peripheral electrical stimulation in chronic pain conditions, Acta Orthop. Scand. **47**:149, 1979.

Augustinsson, L.E., Bohlin, P., Bundsen, P., et al.: Pain relief during delivery by transcutaneous electrical nerve stimulation, Pain **4**:59, 1977.

Baker, L.L.: Neuromuscular electrical stimulation in the restoration of purposeful limb movements. In Wolf, S.L., editor: Electrotherapy—clinics in physical therapy, New York, 1981, Churchill Livingstone, pp 25-48.

Barranco, S.D., Spadero, J.A., Berger, T.J., et al.: In vitro effect of weak direct current on staphylococcus aureus, Clin. Orthop. Relat. Res. **100**:250, 1974.

Benton, L.A., Baker, L.L., Bowman, B.R., et al.: Functional electrical stimulation. Downey, CA, 1980, Rancho Los Amigos Rehabilitation Engineering Center.

Benton, L.A., Baker, L.L., Bowman, B.R., and Waters, R.L.: Functional electrical stimulation—a practical clinical guide, ed. 2, Downey, CA, 1981, Professional Staff Association of Rancho Los Amigos Medical Center.

Berlandt, S.R.: Method of determining optimal stimulation sites for transcutaneous nerve stimulation, Phys. Ther. **64**:924, 1984.

Bertolucci, L.E.: Introduction of antiinflammatory drugs by iontophoresis: double-blind study, J. Orthop. Sports Phys. Ther. **4**:103, 1982.

Bigland, B., and Lippold, O.C.J.: The relation between force, velocity, and integrated electrical activity in human muscles, J. Physiol. **123**:214, 1954.

Brandell, B.R.: Development of a universal control unit for functional electrical stimulation (FES), Am. J. Phys. Med. **61**:279, 1982.

Brown, M.D., Cotter, M., Hudlicka, O., et al.: The effects of long-term stimulation of fast muscles on their ability to withstand fatigue, J. Physiol. (London) **238**:47, 1974.

Brown, M.D., Cotter, M., Hudlicka, O., et al.: Metabolic changes in long-term stimulated fast muscles. In Howland, H., and Poortmans, J.R., editors: Metabolic adaptation to prolonged physical exercise, Basel, 1975, Birkhauser, pp. 471-475.

Burr, H.S., Harvey, S.C.: Bio-electric correlates of wound healing, Yale J. Biol. Med. **11**:103, 1938-1939.

Burr, H.A., Taffel, M., and Harvey, S.C.: An electrometric study of the healing wound in man. Yale J. Biol. Med. **12**:483, 1940.

Campbell, J.A.: A critical appraisal of the electrical output characteristics of ten transcutaneous nerve stimulators, Clin. Phys. Physiol. Meas. **3**:141, 1982.

Carey, I.C., and Lepley, D.: Effect of continuous direct electric current on healing wounds, Surg. Forum **13**:33, 1955.

Carley, P.J., and Wainapel, S.F.: Electrotherapy for acceleration of wound healing: low intensity direct current, Arch. Phys. Med. Rehab. **66**:443, 1985.

Chan, C.S., and Chow, S.P.: Electroacupuncture in the treatment of post-traumatic sympathetic dystrophy (Sudek's atrophy), Br. J. Anesth. **53**:899, 1981.

Chase, J.: Elicitation of periods of inhibition in human muscle by stimulation of cutaneous nerves, J. Bone Joint Surg. (Am.) **54**:1737, 1972.

Cooperman, A.M.: Use of transcutaneous electrical stimulation in the control of post-operative pain: results of a prospective, randomized, controlled study, Am. J. Surg. **133**:185, 1977.

Curico, F., and Berweger, R.: A clinical evaluation of the pain supressor TENS, Fairleigh Dickenson University School of Dentistry, 1983.

Currier, D.P., Lehman, J., and Lightfoot, P.: Electrical stimulation in exercise of the quadriceps femoris muscle, Phys. Ther. **59**:1508, 1979.

Currier, D.P., and Mann, R.: Muscular strength development by electrical stimulation in healthy individuals, Phys. Ther. **63**:915, 1983.

Currier, D.P., and Mann, R.: Pain complaint: comparison of electrical stimulation with conventional isometric exercise, J. Orthop. Sports Phys. Ther. **5**:318, 1984.

Currier, D.P., Petrilli, C.R., and Threlkeld, A.J.: Effect of medium frequency electrical stimulation on local blood circulation to healthy muscle, Phys. Ther. **66**:937, 1986.

DeDomenico, G.: Basic guidelines for interferential therapy, Sydney, Australia, 1981, Theramed.

DeDomenico, G.: Pain relief with interferential therapy, Aust. J. Physiother. **28**:14, 1982.

DeGirardi, C.Q., Seaborne, D., Goulet, F.S., et al: The analgesic effect of high voltage galvanic stimulation combined with ultrasound in the treatment of low back pain: a one-group pre-test/post-test study, Physiother. Can. **36**:327, 1984.

Dougherty, R.: TENS: an alternative to drugs in the treatment of acute and chronic pain, presented at American Academy of Family Physicians, San Francisco, October 1982.

DuBois-Reymond, E.: Untersuchungen fiber thierische elektrizitat, Virchow's Arch **2**:258.1, 1845.

Ebersold, M.J., Laws, Jr., E.R., and Albers, J.W.: Measurements of autonomic function before, during, and after transcutaneous stimulation in patients with chronic pain and in control subjects, Mayo Clin. Proc. **52**:228, 1977.

Ebersold, M., Laws, E., Stonnington, H., et al.: Transcutaneous electrical stimulation for treatment of chronic pain: a preliminary report, Surg. Neurol. **4**:96, 1976.

Eigler, E.: Success achieved by treatment with interferential current on patients with epicondylitis humeri. Presented at the 84th Congress of the German Society of Physical Medicine and Rehabilitation, Hannover, 1979.

(Editorial) Iontophoresis—a major advancement, Eye, Ear, Nose, Throat **55**:13, 1976.

Eisenberg, B.R., and Gilai, A.: Structural changes in single muscle fibers after stimulation at a low frequency, J. Gen. Physiol. **74**:1, 1979.

Eriksson, E., and Haggmark, T.: Comparison of isometric muscle training and electrical stimulation supplementing isometric muscle training in the recovery after major knee ligament surgery, Am. J. Sports Med. **7**:169, 1979.

Eriksson, E., Haggmark, T., Kiessling, K.H., et al.: Effect of electrical stimulation on human skeletal muscle, Int. J. Sports Med. **2**:18, 1981.

Eriksson, M., Schuller, H., et al.: Hazard from transcutaneous nerve stimulation in patients with pacemakers (letter), Lancet **1**:1219, 1978.

Ersek, R.: Transcutaneous electrical neurostimulation—a new modality for controlling pain. Clin. Orthop. Relat. Res. **128**:314, 1977.

Ersek, R.A.: Relief of acute musculoskeletal pain using transcutaneous electrical neurostimulation, J. Am. Coll. Emerg. Phys. **6**:300, 1977.

Evaluation—transcutaneous electrical nerve stimulators (TENS) units. Health Dev. **10**:179, 1981.

Feedar, J.A., and Kloth, L.C.: Acceleration of wound helping with high voltage pulsating direct current, Phys. Ther. **65**:741, 1985 (abstr).

Fields, S.A.: High voltage galvanic stimulation: effect on peripheral blood flow. Unpublished study, University of Kentucky, 1982.

Fox, F.J., and Melzach, R.: Transcutaneous electrical stimulation and acupuncture: comparison of treatment for low back pain, Pain **2**:141, 1976.

Frank, C., Schachar, N., Dittrich, D., et al: Electromagnetic stimulation of ligament healing in rabbits, Clin. Orthop. Relat. Res. **175**:263, 1983.

Gadsby, P.D.: Visualization of the barrier layer through iontophoresis of ferric ions, Med. Instrum. **13**:281, 1979.

Gangarosa, L.P.: Iontophoresis for surface local anesthesia, J. Am. Dent. Assoc. **88**:125, 1974.

Ganne, J.M., Speculand, B., Mayne, L.H., et al.: Inferential therapy to promote union of mandibular fractures, Aust. N.Z. J. Surg. **49**:81, 1979.

Geddes, L.A.: A short history of the electrical stimulation of excitable tissue, Physiologist **27**(suppl):1, 1984.

Geddes, L.A., and Baker, L.E.: Applied biomedical instrumentation, New York, 1975, Wiley.

Godfrey, C.M., Jayawardena, H., Quance, T.A., et al.: Comparison of electro-stimulation and isometric exercise in strengthening the quadriceps muscle, Physiother. Can. **31**:265, 1979.

Gould, M., Donnermeyer, D., Gammon, G.G., et al.: Transcutaneous muscle stimulation to retard disuse atrophy after open meniscectomy, Clin. Orthop. Rel. Res. **178**: 190, 1983.

Greathouse, D.G., Nitz, A.J., Matulionis, D., et al.: Effects of electrical stimulation on ultrastructure of rat skeletal muscles, Phys. Ther. **64**:755, 1984.

Halback, J.W., and Straus, D.: Comparison of electromyostimulation to isokinetic training in increasing power of the knee extensor mechanism, J. Orthop. Sports Phys. Ther. **2**:20, 1980.

Harris, R.: Iontophoresis. In Licht, S., editor: Therapeutic electricity and ultraviolet radiation, Baltimore, 1967, Waverly.

Harris, P.R.: Iontophoresis: clinical research in musculoskeletal inflammatory conditions. J. Orthop. Sports Phys. Ther. **4**:109, 1982.

Hay, K.M.: Control of head pain in migraine using TENS, Practitioner **226** (1366):771, 773-775, 1982.

Houston, M.E., Farrance, B.W., and Wight, R.I.: Metabolic effects of two frequencies of short-term surface electrical stimulation on human muscle, Can. J. Physiol. Pharmacol. **60**:727, 1982.

Howson, D.C.: Peripheral neural excitability: implications for transcutaneous electrical nerve stimulation, Phys. Ther. **58**:1467, 1978.

Hymes, A.C.: The use of karaya electrodes with transcutaneous electrical nerve stimulation. A preliminary report. Unpublished paper, 1978.

Hymes, A.C., Raab, D.E., Yonehiro, E.G., et al.: Acute pain control by electrostimulation: a preliminary report, Adv. Neurol. **4**: 761, 1974.

Ignelzi, R.J., Nyquist, J.K.: Excitability changes in peripheral nerve fibers after repetitive electrical stimulation: implications in pain modulation, J. Neurosurg. **51**:824, 1979.

Ignelzi, R.J., Sternbach, R.A., and Callaghan, M.: Somatosensory changes during transcutaneous electrical analgesia. In Bonica, J.J., et al., editors: Advances in pain research and therapy, New York, 1976, Raven Press, pp. 121-125.

Jehle, H.: Charge fluctuation forces in biological systems, Ann. N.Y. Acad. Sci. **158**:240, 1969.

Johnson, D.H., Thurston, P., and Ashcroft, P.J.: The Russian technique of faradism in the treatment of chrondromalacia patellae, Physiother. Can. **29**:1, 1977.

Jones, D.A., Bigland-Ritchie, B., and Edwards, R.H.T.: Excitation and frequency and muscle fatigue: mechanical responses during voluntary and stimulated contractions, Exper. Neurol. **64**:401, 1979.

Kahn, J.: Low-volt technique, Syosset, N.Y., 1973, Joseph Kahn.

Kirsch, W.M., Lewis, J.A., and Simon, R.H.: Experiences with electrical stimulation devices for the control of chronic pain, Med. Instrum. **9**(5):217, 1975.

Kramer, J.F., and Mendryk, S.W.: Electrical stimulation as a strength improvement technique: a review, J. Orthop. Sports Phys. Ther. **4**:91, 1982.

Kramer, J.F., and Semple, J.E.: Comparison of selected strengthening techniques for normal quadriceps, Physiother. Can. **35**:300, 1983.

Lainey, C.G., Walmsley, R.P., and Andrew, G.M.: Effectiveness of exercise alone versus exercise plus electrical stimulation in strengthening the quadriceps muscle, Physiother. Can. **35**:5, 1983.

Lampe, G.N.: Introduction to the use of transcutaneous electrical nerve stimulation devices, Phys. Ther. **58**:1450, 1978.

Lane, J.F.: Electrical impedances of superficial limb tissue, epidermis, dermis and muscle sheath. Ann. N.Y. Acad. Sci. **238**:812, 1974.

Laughman, R.K., Youdas, J.W., Garrett, T.F., et al.: Strength changes in the normal quadriceps femoris muscle as a result of electrical stimulation, Phys. Ther. **63**:494, 1983.

LeDoux, J., Quinones, M.A.: An investigation of the use of percutaneous electrical stimulation in muscle reeducation, Phys. Ther. **61**:678, 1981.

Leo, K.: Perceived comfort levels of modulated versus conventional TENS current, Phys. Ther. **64**:745, 1984 (abstr).

Licht, S.: History of electrotherapy. In Stillwell, G.K., editor: Therapeutic electricity and ultraviolet radiation, ed. 3, Baltimore, MD, 1983, Williams & Wilkins.

Light, K.E., Nuzik, S., Personius, W., and Barstrom, A.: Low-load prolonged stretch vs. high-load brief stretch in treating knee contractures, Phys. Ther. **64**:330, 1984.

Linzer, M., and Long, D.M.: Transcutaneous neural stimulation for relief of pain, IEEE Trans. Biomed. Eng. **23**:341, 1976.

Liu, H.I.: Optimum repetitions for the development of strength and muscle hypertrophy by electrical stimulation, Master's thesis, University of Kentucky, Lexington, KY, 1984.

Loeser, J.D.: Nonpharmacologic approaches to pain relief. In Ng, L.K.Y., and Bonica, J.J., editors: Pain, discomfort and humanitarian care, New York, 1980, Elsevier, vol. 4, pp. 275-292.

Loesor, J.D., Black, R.G., and Christman, A.: A relief of pain by transcutaneous stimulation, J. Neurosurg. **42**:308, 1975.

Long, D.: Cutaneous afferent stimulation for relief of chronic pain, Clin. Neurosurg. **21**:257, 1974.

Long, D.: The comparative efficacy of drugs vs electrical modulation in the management of chronic pain, unpublished paper.

Loze, G.: Pulsed, high voltage galvanic stimulation: effect on localized blood flow. Unpublished study, University of Kentucky, 1981.

Magistro, C.M.: Hyaluronidase by iontophoresis, Phys. Ther. **44**:169, 1964. Schwartz, M.S.: The use of hyaluronidase by iontophoresis in the treatment of lymphedema.

Mannheimer, J.S.: Electrode placements for transcutaneous electrical nerve stimulation, Phys. Ther. **58**:1455, 1978.

Mannheimer, C., and Carlsson, C.A.: The analgesic effect of transcutaneous electrical nerve stimulation (TNS) in patients with rheumatoid arthritis. A comparative study of different pulse patterns, Pain **6**:329, 1979.

Mannheimer, C., Lund, S., and Carlsson, C.A.: The effect of transcutaneous electrical nerve stimulation (TENS) on joint pain in patients with rheumatoid arthritis, Scand. J. Rheumatol. **7**:13, 1978.

Mannheimer, J., and Russek, A.: How TENS works. Rx Home Care **4**(11):22, 1982.

Mao, W., Ghia, J.N., Scott, D.S., et al.: High versus low intensity acupuncture analgesic for treatment of chronic pain: effects on platelet serotonin, Pain **8**:331, 1980.

Marvie, K.W.: A major advance in the control of post-operative knee pain, Orthopedics **2**:129, 1979.

Massey, B.H., Nelson, R.C., Sharkey, B.C., et al.: Effects of high frequency electrical stimulation on the size and strength of skeletal muscle, J. Sports Med. Phys. Fit. **5**:136, 1965.

McMiken, D.F., Todd-Smith, M., and Thompson, C.: Strengthening of human quadriceps muscles by cutaneous electrical stimulation, Scand. J. Rehab. Med. **15**:25, 1983.

McNeal, D.R.: 2000 years of electrical stimulation. In Hambrecht, F.T., and Reswick, J.B., editors: Functional electrical stimulation: applications in neural prosthesis, New York, 1977, Marcel Dekker, pp. 3-35.

McNeal, D.R., and Bowman, B.R.: Peripheral neuromuscular stimulation. In Myklebust, J.B., et al., editors: Neural stimulation, Boca Raton, FL, 1985, CRC Press, vol. II, pp 95-118.

Melzack, R.: Prolonged relief of pain by brief intense transcutaneous somatic stimulation, Pain **1**:357, 1975.

Melzack, R., Stillwell, D.M., and Fox, E.J.: Trigger points and acupuncture points for pain: correlations and implications, Pain **3**: 3, 1977.

Meyer, G.A., and Fields, H.L.: Causalgia treated by selective large fibre stimulation of peripheral nerve, Brain **95**:163, 1972.

Miles, J.: Electrical stimulation for the relief of pain, Ann. R. Coll. Surg. Engl. **66**(2):108, 1984.

Millard, J.B.: The use of electrical stimulation in the rehabilitation of knee injuries, Proc. Int. Congr. Phys. Med. (Lond.) **317**, 1952.

Miller, B.A., Smith, K.B., Reale, J.L., et al.: A comparison of modulated rate and conventional TENS, Phys. Ther. **64**:744, 1984 (abstr).

Milner-Brown, H.S., and Stein, R.B.: The relation between the surface electro-myogram and muscular force, J. Physiol. **246**:549, 1975.

Mohr, T., Carlson, B., Sulentic, C., et al.: Comparison of isometric exercise and high volt galvanic stimulation on quadriceps, femoris muscle strength, Phys. Ther. **65**:606, 1985.

Mueller, E.E., et al.: Skin impedance in relation to pain threshold testing by electrical means, J. Appl. Physiol. **5**:746, 1952.

Munsat, T.L., McNeal, D.R., and Waters, R.L.: Preliminary observations on prolonged stimulation of peripheral nerve in man, Arch. Neurol. **33**:608, 1976.

Murray, W., Levine, L.S., Seifter, E.: The iontophoresis of C_2, esterified glucocorticoids: preliminary report, Phys. Ther. **43**:579, 1963.

Myers, R.A., Woolf, C.J., and Mitchell, D.: Management of acute traumatic pain by peripheral transcutaneous electrical nerve stimulation, S. Afr. Med. J. **52**:309, 1977.

Myer-Waarden, K., Hansjuergens, A., and Friedman, B.: New research results—demonstration of interferential current in deep biological structures, Biomed. Tech. **25**:295, 1980.

Naess, K., and Storm-Mathison, A.: Fatigue of sustained tetanic contractions, Acta Physiol. Scand. **34**:351, 1955.

Newton, R.A., and Karselis, T.C.: Skin pH following high voltage pulsed galvanic stimulation, Phys. Ther. **63**:1593, 1983.

Nightingale, A.: Physics and electronics in physical medicine, London, 1959, F. Bell, p 178.

Nikolova, L.: Physiotherapeutic rehabilitation in the presence of fracture complications, Med. Wochenschr. (Munich) **111**:592, 1969.

Nikolova-Trocva, L.: Interference current therapy in distortions, contusions and luxations of the joints, Med. Wochenschr. (Munich) **109**:579, 1967.

O'Malley, E., and Oester, Y.: Influence of some physical chemical factors on iontophoresis using radio-isotopes, Arch. Phys. Med. Rehabil. **36**:310, 1955.

Owens, J., and Malone, T.: Treatment parameters of high frequency electrical stimulation as established on the electrostim 180, J. Orthop. Sports Phys. Ther. **4**:162, 1983.

Peking Acupuncture Anesthesia Coordinating Group: Acupuncture anaesthesia. Peking, 1972, Foreign Language Press, Cited in Liu, Y.K., Varela, M., and Oswald, R.: The correspondence between some motor points and acupuncture loci, Ann. J. Chin. Med. **3**:347, 1975.

Pette, D., Smith, M.E., Staudte, H.W., et al.: Effects of long-term electrical stimulation on some contractile and metabolic characteristics of fast rabbit muscles, Pfluegers Arch. **338**:257, 1973.

Picaza, J.A., Cannon, B.W., Hunter, S.E., et al.: Pain suppression by peripheral stimulation, Part I. Observations with transcutaneous stimuli, Surg. Neurol. **4**:105, 1975.

Procacci, P., Corte, D., Zoppi, M., et al.: Pain threshold measurements in man. In Bonica, J.J., editors: Recent advances in pain therapy, Springfield, IL, 1974, Thomas, pp. 105-147.

Procacci, P., Zoppi, M., and Maresca, M.: Transcutaneous electrical stimulation in low back pain: a critical evaluation, Acupunct. Electro-ther. Res. **7**:1, 1982.

Protas, E.G., Dupny, T., and Gardea, R.: Electrical stimulation for strength training, Phys. Ther. **64**:751, 1984 (abstr).

Rack, P.M.H., and Westbury, D.R.: The effects of length and stimulus rate on tension in the isometric cat soleus muscle, J. Physiol. **204**:443, 1969.

Ray, C.D., and Maurer, D.D.: A review of neural stimulation system components useful in pain alleviation, Med. Prog. Technol. **2**:121, 1974.

Reddana, P., Moortly, C.V., and Govidappa, S.: Pattern of skeletal muscle chemical composition during in vivo electrical stimulations, Ind. J. Physiol. Pharmacol. **25**:33, 1981.

Reismann, M.A.: A comparison of electric stimulators eliciting muscle contraction, Phys. Ther. **64**:751, 1984 (abst).

Reswick, J.B.: A brief history of functional electrical stimulation. In Fields, W.S., and Leavitt, L.A., editors: Neural organization and its relevance to prosthetics, New York, 1973, Intercontinental, pp 3-13.

Roeser, W., Meeks, L., Venis, R., and Strideland, G.: The use of transcutaneous nerve stimulation for pain control in athletic medicine. A preliminary report, Am. J. Sports Med. **4**(5):210, 1976.

Romero, J.A., Sanford, T.L., Schroeder, R.V., et al.: The effects of electrical stimulation of normal quadriceps on strength and girth, Med. Sci. Sports Exerc. **14**:194, 1982.

Rose, S.J., and Rothstein, J.M.: Muscle mutability: Part I. General concepts and adaptations to altered patterns of use, Phys. Ther. **62**:1773, 1982.

Rosenberg, M., Vutyid, L., and Bourbe, D.: Transcutaneous electrical nerve stimulation for the relief of post-operative pain, Pain **5**:129, 1978.

Ross, C.R., and Segal, D.: High voltage galvanic stimulation—an aid to post-operative healing, Curr. Podiatry May 1981, 19-25.

Rowley, B.A., McKenna, J.M., Chase, G.R., et al.: The influence of electrical current on an infecting microorganism in wounds, Ann. N.Y. Acad. Sci. **238**:543, 1974.

Arch. Intern. Med. **95**:662, 1955.

Selkowitz, D.M.: Improvement in isometric strength of the quadriceps femoris muscle after training with electrical stimulation, Phys. Ther. **65**:186, 1985.

Shealey, C.N., and Maurer, D.: Transcutaneous nerve stimulation for control of pain, Surg. Neurol. **2**:45, 1974.

Shriber, W.: A manual of electrotherapy, ed. 4, Philadelphia, 1975, Lea & Febiger.

Sjolund, B.H., and Eriksson, M.B.E.: The influence of naloxone or analgesia produced by peripheral conditioning stimulation, Brain. Res. **173**:295, 1979.

Sjolund, B.H., Terenius, L., and Eriksson, M.B.E.: Increased cerebrospinal fluid levels of endorphin after electro acupuncture, Acta Physiol. Scand. **100**:382, 1977.

Smith, W., Michlovitz, S.L., and Watkins, M.P.: A comparative study of ice and high voltage stimulation for ankle sprain, Phys. Ther. **65**:684, 1985 (abstr).

Sorenson, N.K.: Pulsed galvanic (DC) muscle stimulation for post-op edema in the hand, Stimulus, Section on Clinical Electrophysiology, APTA **9**:8, 1984.

Standish, W.D., Valiant, G.A., Bonen, A., et al.: The effects of immobilization and of electrical stimulation on muscle glycogen and myofibrillar ATPase, Can. J. Appl. Sports Sci. **7**:267, 1982.

Steig, R.L.: New methods for achieving pain control with transcutaneous nerve stimulation, paper presented at the annual meeting of the American Academy of Neurology, Toronto, April, 1976.

Stillwell, G.K.: Electrotherapy. In Kottke, F., Stillwell, G., and Lehman, J., editors: Handbook of physical medicine and rehabilitation, Philadelphia, 1982, W.B. Saunders Co., p 370.

Sweet, W.H., Wepsic, J.G.: Treatment of chronic pain by stimulation of primary afferent neuron, Trans. Am. Neurol. Assoc. **93**:103, 1968.

Szehi, E., and David, E.: The stereodynamic interferential current—a new electrotherapeutic technique, Electromedica **48**:13, 1980.

Szeto, A.Y.J., and Nyquist, J.K.: Transcutaneous electrical nerve stimulation for pain control, IEEE Eng. Med. Bio. Mag. **2**:14, 1983.

Tannenbaum, M.: Iodine iontophoresis in reducing scar tissue, Phys. Ther. **60**:792, 1980.

Taub, A.: Percutaneous local electrical analgesia: origin, mechanism, and clinical potential, Minn. Med. **57**:172, 1974.

Taylor, P., Hallet, M., and Flaherty, L.: Treatment of osteoarthritis of the knee with transcutaneous electrical nerve stimulation, Pain **11**:233, 1981.

Taylor, M.K., Newton, R.A., Personius, W.J., et al.: The effects of interferential current stimulation for the treatment of subjects with recurrent jaw pain, Abstract. Phys. Ther. **66**:774, 1986.

Terezhalmy, G.T., Ross, G.R., and Holmes-Johnson, E.: Transcutaneous electrical nerve stimulation treatment of TMJ-MPDS patients, Ear Nose Throat J. **61**:664, 1982.

Thorsteinsson, G., and Stonnington, H.H., et al.: The placebo effect of transcutaneous electrical stimulation, Pain **5**:31, 1978.

Treffene, R.J.: Interferential fields in a fluid medium, Aust. J. Physiother. **29**:209, 1983.

Trubatch, J., Van Harreveld, A.: Spread of iontophoretically injected ions in a tissue, J. Theor. Biol. **36**:355, 1972.

Vander Ark, G.D., and McGrath, K.A.: Transcutaneous electrical stimulation in treatment of post-operative pain, Am. J. Surg. **130**:338, 1975.

Vodovnik, L.: Therapeutic effects of functional electrical stimulation of extremities, Med. Biol. Eng. Comput. **19**: 470, 1981.

Wadsworth, H., and Chanmugan, A.P.P.: Electrophysical agents in physiotherapy, ed. 2, Marrickville, Australia, 1983, Science Press, pp. 276-280.

Ward, A.R.: Electricity fields and waves in therapy, Marickville, 1980, Australia Science Press, p 17.

Waters, R.L., and Bowman, B.R.: Multicenter functional electrical stimulation evaluation for contracture prevention and correction. Final report to the Veterans Administration No. V790p-1441, Washington, D.C., 1981.

Wheeler, P., Wolcott, L., Morris, J., et al.: Neural considerations in the healing of ulcerated tissue by clinical electrotherapeutic application of weak direct current: findings and theory. In Reynolds, D.V., and Sjoberg, A.E., editors: Neuroelectric research, Springfield, IL, 1971, Thomas, pp 83-96.

Williams, J.G.P., and Street, M.: Sequential faradism in quadriceps rehabilitation, Physiotherapy **62**:252, 1976.

Wolf, S.L., Gersh, M.R., and Rao, V.R.: Examination of electrode placements and stimulating parameters in treating chronic pain with conventional transcutaneous nerve stimulation (TENS), Pain **11**:37, 1981.

Wong, R.A., and Jette, D.V.: Changes in sympathetic tone associated with different forms of transcutaneous electrical nerve stimulation in healthy subjects, Phys. Ther. **64**:478, 1984.

Zecca, L., Ferrario, P., Furia, G., et al.: Effects of pulsed electromagnetic field on acute and chronic inflammation, Trans. Biol. Repair Growth Soc. **3**:72, 1983.

Infrared Modalities

5

Gerald W. Bell

OBJECTIVES

Following completion of this chapter, the student will be able to:

- Understand how the infrared modalities are classified in the electromagnetic spectrum.

- Differentiate between the physiologic effects of therapeutic heat and cold.

- Describe the contemporary modalities of the infrared spectrum in thermotherapy and cryotherapy.

- Describe the indications and contraindications for each infrared modality discussed.

- Given a clinical diagnosis, select the most effective infrared modalities.

- Explain how the sports therapist can use the infrared modalities to reduce pain.

Of the therapeutic modalities discussed in this text, perhaps none are more commonly used than those that are classified as infrared modalities. As indicated in Chapter 2, the infrared region of the electromagnetic spectrum falls between the microwave diathermy and the visible light portions of the spectrum in terms of wave length and frequency. There is a great deal of misunderstanding among sports therapists regarding which of the modalities used in a sports medicine setting are actually classified as infrared modalities. Traditionally, the term infrared heating conjures up visions only of infrared lamps and bakers. However, it must be reemphasized that most of the heat and cold modalities, such as hydrocollator packs, paraffin baths, hot and cold whirlpools, and ice packs, as well as infrared lamps, produce forms of radiant energy that have wave lengths and frequencies that fall under the classification of infrared modalities (see Fig. 2-2). This chapter will include a discussion of all the modalities that fall into the infrared portion of the electromagnetic spectrum.

MECHANISMS OF HEAT TRANSFER

Easy application and convenience of use of hot and cold modalities provide the sports therapist with the necessary tools for primary sports injury care. Heat is defined as the internal vibration of the molecules within a body. The transmission of heat occurs by three mechanisms: **conduction, convection,** and **radiation.** A fourth mechanism of heat transfer, **conversion,** is discussed in Chapter 6.

Conduction occurs when the body is in direct contact with the heat or cold source. Convection occurs when particles (air or water) move across the body, thus creating a temperature variation. The final mechanism is radiation or the transfer of heat from a warmer source to a cooler source through a conducting medium such as air (e.g., infrared lamps). It must also be pointed out that the body may either gain or lose heat through any of these three processes of heat transfer. The infrared modalities discussed in this chapter use these three methods of heat transfer to effect a tissue temperature increase or decrease.

APPROPRIATE USE OF THE INFRARED MODALITIES

Infrared modalities are often abused on the basis of random usage by the sports therapist who uses a modality without reviewing its benefits. Placing the athlete in the whirlpool or a slush bucket of ice simply because these two modalities are available is not an acceptable technique of treatment.

Heat modalities are referred to as **thermotherapy.** Thermotherapy is used when a tissue temperature rise is the goal of treatment. The use of cold, or cryotherapy, is most effective in the acute stages of the healing process immediately following injury when tissue temperature loss is the goal of therapy. Cold applications can be continued into the reconditioning stage of athletic injury management. Thermotherapy and cryotherapy are included in this section on the basis of their classification in the electromagnetic spectrum. The term **hydrotherapy** can be applied to any cryotherapy or thermotherapy technique that uses water as the medium for tissue temperature exchange.

The electromagnetic spectrum has a relatively large region of radiations designated as infrared. The infrared wavelength provides the radiant energy that is used therapeutically (see Fig. 2-2). Penetration of the energy is dependent on the source, but is generally considered to be a superficial form of treatment.

While this chapter is concerned primarily with application of the infrared modalities and their physiologic effects, several of the other modalities discussed in this text (e.g., the diathermies and ultrasound) also cause a tissue temperature increase. The effects of heat and cold therapy discussed in this chapter may be applied to any modality that alters tissue temperature.

Heating and cooling agents can be used successfully to treat athletic injuries and trauma. The sports therapist must know the injury mechanism and specific pathology, as well as the physiologic effects of the heating and cooling agents, to establish a consistent treatment schedule.

PHYSIOLOGIC EFFECTS OF HEAT

Local superficial heating (infrared heat) is recommended in subacute conditions for reducing pain and inflammation through **analgesic** effects. Superficial heating produces lower tissue temperatures at the site of the pathology (injury) relative to the higher temperatures in the superficial tissues, resulting in analgesia. During the later stages of injury healing, a deeper heating effect is usually desirable; it can be achieved by using the diathermies or ultrasound.

Heat dilates blood vessels, causing the resting capillaries (patent small blood vessels) to open up and increase circulation. The skin is supplied with sympathetic **vasoconstrictor** fibers that secrete norepinephrine at their endings (especially evident in feet, hands, lips, nose, and ears). At normal body temperature the sympathetic vasoconstrictor nerves keep vascular anastomoses (blood vessel junctions) almost totally closed, but when the superficial tissue is heated, the number of sympathetic impulses is greatly reduced so that the anastomoses dilate and allow large quantities of warm blood to flow into the venous plexuses (a group of veins). This promotes heat loss from the body, which can increase blood flow about twofold.[19]

The hyperemia (increased blood flow) created by heat has a beneficial effect on athletic injury. This is based on increases of blood flow and pooling of blood during the metabolic processes. Recent hematomas (blood clots) should never be treated with heat until resolution of bleeding is completed. Some sports therapists have advocated never using heat during any therapeutic modality application.[22,24,25,27]

The rate of metabolism of tissues is dependent in part on temperature. The metabolic rate has been shown to increase approximately 13% for each 1° C increase in temperature.[22] A similar decrease in metabolism has been demonstrated when temperatures are lowered.

A primary effect of local heating is an increase in the local metabolic rate with a resulting increase in the production of metabolites and additional heat. These two factors lead to an increased intravascular hydrostatic pressure, causing arteriolar **vasodilation** and increased capillary blood flow.[47] However, with increased hydrostatic pressure, there is a tendency toward formation of edema, which may increase the time required for rehabilitation of a particular injury. Increased capillary blood flow is important with many types of injury in which there is mild or moderate inflammation, because it causes an increase in the supply of oxygen, antibodies, leukocytes, and other necessary nutrients and enzymes, along with an increased clearing of metabolites. With higher heat intensities, vasodilation and increased blood flow will spread to remote areas, causing increased metabolism in the unheated area. This is known as consensual heat vasodilation and may be useful in many conditions where local heating is contraindicated.[16]

The application of heat can produce an analgesic effect, resulting in a reduction in the intensity of pain. The analgesic effect is the most frequent **indication** for the use of heat.[47] Although the mechanisms underlying this phenomenon are not well understood, current thinking is that it is in some way related to the gate control theory of pain modulation.

Heat is applied in musculoskeletal and neuromuscular disorders, such as sprains, strains, articular (joint-related) problems, and muscle spasms, which all describe various types of muscle pain.[16] Heat generally is considered to produce a relaxation effect and a reduction in guarding in skeletal muscle. It also increases the elasticity and decreases the viscosity of connective tissue, which is an important consideration in postacute joint injuries or following long periods of immobilization.

Many sports therapists empirically (through observation and experience) believe that in these types of disorders heat has little effect on the disease itself but serves merely to facilitate further treatment by producing relaxation.[16] This is accomplished by relieving pain, lessening hypertonicity (excessive tension) of muscles, producing sedation (which decreases spasticity, tenderness, and spasm), and decreasing tightness in muscles and related structures. The following physiologic effects of heat have been documented:

Increased local temperature superfically
Increased local metabolism
Vasodilation of arterioles and capillaries
Increased blood flow to part heated
Increased leukocytes and phagocytosis
Increased capillary permeability
Increased lymphatic and venous drainage
Increased metabolic wastes
Increased axon reflex activity
Increased elasticity of muscles, ligaments, and capsule fibers
Analgesia
Increased formation of edema
Decreased muscle tone
Decreased muscle spasm

Heat (handwritten margin note)

EFFECTS OF COOLING

The physiologic effects of cold are for the most part opposite those of heat, the primary effect being a local decrease in temperature. Local cooling is strongly indicated in the acute stage of the healing process to decrease pain, muscle spasm, and inflammation. Cold is also known to reduce the metabolic rate, with a corresponding decrease in production of metabolites and metabolic heat.

In acute injury there is increasing agreement that the use of cold is the initial treatment for most conditions involving strains, sprains, and contusions. It is most commonly used immediately after injury to decrease pain and promote local vasoconstriction, thus controlling hemorrhage and **edema** (swelling).[38,43] It is also used in the acute phase of inflammatory conditions such as bursitis, tenosynovitis, and tendinitis, in which heat may cause additional pain and swelling.[38] Cold is also used to reduce pain and the reflex muscle spasm and spastic conditions that accompany it.[40] Its analgesic effect is probably one of its greatest benefits.[12,36,44-46] One explanation of the analgesic effect is that cold decreases the velocity of nerve conduction, although it does not entirely eliminate it.[11,36,37] It is also possible that cold bombards central pain receptor areas with so many cold impulses that pain impulses are lost through the gate control therapy of pain modulation. With ice treatments, the patient usually reports an uncomfortable sensation of cold followed by stinging or burning, then an aching sensation, and finally complete numbness.[26]

Cold also has been demonstrated to be effective in the treatment of **myo-**

fascial pain.[49] This type of pain is referred from active myofascial trigger points with various symptoms, including pain on active movement and decreased range of motion. Trigger points may result from muscle strain or tension, which sensitizes nerves in a localized area. A trigger point may be palpated as a small nodule or as a strip of tense muscle tissue.

Cold does depress the excitability of free nerve endings and peripheral nerve fibers, and this increases the pain threshold. This is of great value in short-term treatment. Cold applications can also enhance voluntary control in spastic conditions, and in acute traumatic conditions they may decrease painful spasms that result from local muscle irritability.[2]

Reduction in muscle spasm relative to acute athletic trauma has been observed by all active sports therapists. Literature reviewed indicates various reasons behind reduced muscle spasms with the common thought of decreased muscle spindle activity.

The initial reaction to cold is local vasoconstriction of all smooth muscle by the central nervous system in order to conserve heat.[43] Localized vasoconstriction is responsible for the decrease in the tendency toward formation and accumulation of edema,[47] probably as a result of a decrease in local hydrostatic pressure. There is also a decrease in the amount of nutrients and phagocytes (cells that eliminate debris) delivered to the area, thus reducing phagocytic activity.[47]

It has been hypothesized that when local temperature is lowered considerably for a period of about 30 minutes, intermittent periods of vasodilation occur, lasting 4 to 6 minutes. Then vasoconstriction recurs for a 15- to 30-minute cycle, followed again by vasodilation. This phenomenon is known as the *hunting response* and is necessary to prevent local tissue injury caused by cold.[9,10,34] The hunting response has been accepted for a number of years as fact; in reality, however, these investigations have talked about measured temperature changes rather than circulatory changes. Thus the hunting response is more likely a measurement artifact than an actual change in blood flow in response to cold.[27]

If a large area is cooled, the hypothalamus (the temperature-regulating center in the brain) will reflexly induce shivering, which raises the core temperature as a result of increased production of heat. Cooling of a large area might also cause arterial vasoconstriction in other remote parts of the body, resulting in an increased blood pressure.[47]

Because of the low thermal conductivity of underlying subcutaneous fat tissue, applications of cold for short periods of time will probably be ineffective in cooling deeper tissues. It has also been shown that using cold for too long may be detrimental to the healing process.[18]

The length of treatment time needed to cool tissue effectively depends on differences in subcutaneous tissue thickness. Patients with thick subcutaneous tissue should be treated with cold applications for longer than 5 minutes to produce a significant drop in intramuscular temperature. Grant[17] treated acute and chronic conditions of the musculoskeletal system and found that thin people require shorter icing periods and that response was more successful. McMaster[38] supported these findings. Recommended treatment times range from direct contact of 5 to 45 minutes to obtain adequate cooling.

It is generally believed that cold treatments are more effective in reaching deep tissue than most forms of heat. Cold applied to the skin is capable of significantly lowering the temperature of tissue at a considerable depth. The extent of this lowered tissue temperature is dependent on the type of cold applied to the skin, the duration of its application, the thickness of the subcutaneous fat, and the region of the body on which it is applied.[5]

The following physiologic effects of cold have been documented:

Decreased local temperature, in some cases to a considerable depth
Decreased metabolism
Vasoconstriction of arterioles and capillaries (at first)
Decreased blood flow (at first)
Decreased nerve conduction velocity
Decreased delivery of leukocytes and phagocytes
Decreased lymphatic and venous drainage
Decreased muscle excitability
Decreased muscle spindle depolarization
Decreased viscosity of muscle
Decreased formation and accumulation of edema
Extreme anesthetic effects

The application of cold causes decreased cell permeability, decreased cellular metabolism, and decreased accumulation of edema and should be continued in 5- to 45-minute applications for up to 72 hours following initial trauma.[24] Care should be taken to avoid aggressive treatment of this type to prevent disruption of the healing sequence.

If edema continues into the subacute phase, contrast baths (hot and cold immersion technique) may be incorporated to facilitate a capillary response for edema reduction. This consists of alternating hot and cold immersions and will be discussed in greater detail in the clinical section.

Cold has its greatest benefit in acute athletic injury.[8,18,23-28] This benefit results from vasoconstriction with a reduction of swelling that seems to lessen the hypoxia and further tissue death by decreasing cell metabolism. Cold has been used in rehabilitation programs as an important adjunct to other forms of therapeutic exercise.

EFFECTS OF TISSUE TEMPERATURE CHANGE ON CIRCULATION

Local application of heat or cold is indicated for thermal physiologic effects. The main physiologic effect is on superficial circulation because of the response of the temperature receptors in the skin and the sympathetic nervous system.

Circulation through the skin serves two major functions: (1) nutrition of the skin tissues and (2) conduction of heat from internal structures of the body to the skin, so that heat can be removed from the body.[19] The circulatory apparatus is composed of two major vessel types: (1) nutritive arteries, capillaries, and veins; and (2) vascular structures for heating the skin. Two types of vascular structures are the subcutaneous venous plexus, which holds large quantities of blood that heat the surface of the skin, and the arteriovenous anastomosis, which provides vascular communication between arteries and venous plexuses. The walls of the plexuses have strong muscular coats innervated by sympathetic vasoconstrictor nerve fibers that secrete norepinephrine. When constricted, blood flow is reduced in the venous plexus to almost nothing. When maximally dilated, there is an extremely rapid flow of warm blood into the plexuses. The arteriovenous anastomoses are found principally in the volar or palmar surfaces of the hands and feet, the lips, the nose, and the ears.

When cold is applied directly to the skin, the skin vessels progressively constrict to a temperature of about 15° C (59° F), at which point they reach their maximum constriction.[19] This constriction results primarily from increased sensitivity of the vessels to nerve stimulation, but it probably also results at least partly from a reflex that passes to the cord and then back to the vessels. At temperatures below 15° C (59° F), the vessels begin to dilate. This dilation is caused by a direct local effect of the cold on the vessels themselves, producing paralysis of the contractile mechanism of the vessel wall or block of the nerve impulses coming to the vessels. At temperatures approaching 0° C (32° F), the skin vessels frequently reach maximum vasodilation. Vasodilation associated with intense cold plays a protective role in preventing freezing of the exposed portions of the body, and it is commonly referred to as hunting response.[9]

With circulatory stress, skin plexuses are supplied with sympathetic vasoconstrictor innervation. In times of circulatory stress, such as exercise, hemorrhage, or anxiety, sympathetic stimulation of these skin plexuses forces large quantities of blood into internal vessels. Thus the subcutaneous veins of the skin act as an important blood reservoir, often providing blood to serve other circulatory functions when needed.[19]

Three types of sensory receptors are involved in the subepithelial tissue: cold, warm, and pain. The pain receptors are free nerve endings. Temperature and pain are transmitted to the brain via the lateral spinothalamic tract (Chapter 1). The nerve fibers respond differently at different temperatures. Both cold and warm receptors discharge minimally at 33° C (91.4° F). Cold receptors discharge between 10° and 41° C (50° and 105.8° F) with a maximum discharge in the 37.5° to 40° C (99.5° to 104° F) range. Above 45° C (113° F), cold receptors begin to discharge again and pain receptors are stimulated. Nerve fibers transmitting sensations of pain respond to the extremes of temperature. Both warm and cold receptors adapt rapidly to temperature change; the more rapid the temperature change, the more rapid the receptor adaptation. The number of warm and cold receptors in any given small surface area is thought to be few; therefore small temperature changes are difficult to perceive in localized areas. Larger surface areas stimulate summation of thermal signals. These larger patterns of excitation activate the vasomotor centers and the hypothalamic center.[33,35] Stimulation of the anterior hypothalamus causes cutaneous vasodilation, while stimulation of the posterior hypothalamus causes cutaneous vasoconstriction.[19,45]

The cutaneous blood flow depends on the discharge of the sympathetic nervous system. These sympathetic impulses are transmitted simultaneously to the blood vessels for cutaneous vasoconstriction and to the adrenal medulla. Both norepinephrine and epinephrine are secreted into the blood vessels and induce constriction of the vessels.[19] Most of the sympathetic constriction influences are mediated chemically through these neural transmitters. General exposure to cold elicits cutaneous vasoconstriction, shivering, piloerection, and an increase in epinephrine secretion, so vascular contraction occurs. Simultaneously, metabolism and heat production are increased to maintain the body temperature.[19]

Increased blood flow supplies additional oxygen to the area, thus explaining the analgesic and relaxation effects on muscle spasm. An increased proprioceptive reflex mechanism may explain these effects. Receptor end organs located in the muscle spindle are reflexly inhibited by heat temporarily, while sudden cooling tends to excite the receptor end organ.[33,35]

EFFECTS OF TISSUE TEMPERATURE CHANGE ON MUSCLE SPASM

Studies dealing with the effects of heat and cold in the treatment of many musculoskeletal conditions are numerous. While it is true that the use of heat as a therapeutic modality has long been accepted and documented in the literature, it is apparent that most recent research has been directed toward the use of cold. There seems to be general agreement that the physiologic mechanisms underlying the effectiveness of heat and cold treatments in reducing muscle spasm lie at the level of the muscle spindle (receptors sensitive to changes in the length of a muscle), Golgi tendon organs (receptors sensitive to changes in the tension of a muscle), and the gamma system.

Heat is believed to have a relaxing effect on skeletal muscle tone.[16] Local application of heat relaxes muscles throughout the skeletal system by simultaneously lessening the stimulus threshold of muscle spindles and by decreasing the gamma efferent firing rate. This suggests that the muscle spindles are more easily excited. Consequently, the muscles may be electromyographically silent while at rest during the application of heat, but the slightest amount of voluntary or passive movement may cause the Ia efferents to fire, thus increasing muscular resistance to stretch. If this is indeed the case, then it seems logical that increasing the afferent impulses by raising the threshold of the muscle spindles might be effective in facilitating muscle relaxation.

The rate of firing of both primary and secondary endings is directly proportional to temperature. Local applications of cold decrease neural activity locally. Annulospiral, flower-spray (small fibers located in the muscle spindle that detect changes in muscle position), and Golgi tendon organ endings all fire more slowly when cooled. Cooling actually decreases the rate of afferent activity even more, with an increase in the amount of tension on the muscle. Thus cold appears to raise the threshold stimulus of muscle spindles, and heat tends to lower it.[15]

While firing of the primary spindle afferents increases abruptly with the application of cold, a subsequent decrease in spindle afferent activity occurs and persists as the temperature is lowered.[36]

Simultaneous use of heat and cold in the treatment of muscle spasm has also been studied.[13] Local cooling with ice, while maintaining body temperature to prevent shivering, results in a significant reduction of muscle spasm, greater than that which occurs with the use of heat or cold independently. This was attributed to maintenance of body temperature, which decreases γ efferent activity while local cooling decreases afferent activity. If the core temperature of the body were not maintained, the reflex shivering would result in increased muscle tonus, thus inhibiting relaxation.

There is a substantial reduction in the frequency of action potential (stimulus intensity necessary for firing muscle fibers) firing of the motor unit when the muscle temperature is reduced. Muscle spindle activity is most significantly reduced when the muscle is cooled while normal body temperature is maintained.

Miglietta[39] presented a slightly different perspective on the effect of cold in reducing muscle spasm. He performed an electromyographic analysis of the effects of cold on the reduction of clonus (increased muscle tone) or spasticity in a group of 15 patients. After immersion of the spastic extremity in a cold whirlpool for 15 minutes, it was observed that electromyographic activity dropped significantly and in some cases disappeared altogether. The cold was thought to induce an afferent bombardment of cold impulses, which modify the cortical excitatory state and block the stream of painful impulses from the muscle. Thus relaxation of skeletal muscle is assumed to occur with the disappearance of pain.[48] It is not certain whether it is the excitability of the motor neurons or the hyperactivity of the γ system, which is changed either at the muscle-spindle level or at the cord level, that is responsible for the reduction of spasticity. However, it is certain that cold is effective in reducing spasticity by reducing or modifying the highly sensitive stretch reflex mechanism in muscle.

Another factor that may be important to the reduction of spasticity is reduction in the nerve conduction velocity as a result of the application of cold.[11] These changes may result from a slowing of motor and sensory nerve conduction velocity and a decrease of the afferent discharges from cutaneous receptors.

Several studies investigated the use of cold followed by some type of exercise in the treatment of various injuries to the musculotendinous unit.[17,29] Each of these studies indicated that the use of cold and exercise was extremely effective in the treatment of acute pathologies of the musculoskeletal system that produced restrictions of muscle action.

CLINICAL USE OF THE INFRARED MODALITIES

It must be made clear that the physiologic effects of heat and cold discussed previously are rarely the result of direct absorption of infrared energy. There is general agreement that no form of infrared energy can have a depth of penetration greater than 1 cm.[1] Thus the effects of the infrared modalities are primarily superficial and directly affect the cutaneous blood vessels and the cutaneous nerve receptors.

Absorption of infrared energy cutaneously increases and decreases circulation subcutaneously in both the muscle and fat layers. If the energy is absorbed cutaneously over a long enough period of time to raise the temperature of the circulating blood, the hypothalamus will reflexly increase blood flow to the underlying tissue. Likewise, absorption of cold cutaneously can decrease blood flow via a similar mechanism in the area of treatment.[1]

Thus if the primary treatment goal is a tissue temperature increase with a corresponding increase in blood flow to the deeper tissues, it is perhaps wiser to choose a modality, such as diathermy or ultrasound, that produces energy that can penetrate the cutaneous tissues and be directly absorbed by the deep tissues.

If the primary treatment goal is to reduce tissue temperature and decrease blood flow to an injured area, it should be clear that the superficial application of ice or cold is the only modality capable of producing such a response.

Perhaps the most effective use of the infrared modalities should be for the purpose of analgesia or reducing the sensation of pain associated with injury. The infrared modalities stimulate primarily the cutaneous nerve receptors. Through one of the mechanisms of pain modulation discussed in Chapter 1, most likely the gate control theory, hyperstimulation of these nerve receptors by heating or cooling reduces pain. Within the philosophy of an aggressive program of rehabilitation, as is standard in most sports medicine settings, the reduction of pain as a means of facilitating therapeutic exercise is a common practice. As emphasized in the preface to this text, therapeutic modalities are perhaps best used as an adjunct to therapeutic exercise. Certainly, this should be a prime consideration when selecting an infrared modality for use in any treatment program.

Continued investigation and research into the use of heat and cold is warranted to provide useful data for the athletic trainer and sports medicine professional. Heat and cold applications, when used properly and efficiently, will provide the sports therapist with the tools to enhance recovery and provide the athlete with optimal health care management. Thermotherapy and cryotherapy are only two of the tools available to assist in the well-being and reconditioning of the injured athlete.

CRYOTHERAPY TECHNIQUES

Cryotherapy is the use of cold in the treatment of acute trauma and subacute injury and for the decrease of discomfort following athletic reconditioning and rehabilitation. Tools of cryotherapy include ice packs, cold whirlpool, ice whirlpool, ice massage, commercial chemical cold spray, and contrast baths. Application of cryotherapy produces a three- to four-stage sensation. First there is an uncomfortable sensation of cold followed by a stinging, then a burning or aching feeling, and finally numbness. Each stage is related to the nerve endings as they temporarily cease to function as a result of decreased blood flow. The time required for this sequence varies, but several authors indicate that it occurs within 5 to 15 minutes.* It was noted that after 12 to 15 minutes, a reflex deep-

---

*References 3, 4, 17, 20, 26, and 40-43.

tissue vasodilation called the hunting response is sometimes demonstrable with intense cold (10° C [50° F]).[9,27,41-43] Thus a minimum of 15 minutes is necessary to achieve extreme analgesic effects.

Application of ice is safe, simple, and inexpensive. Cryotherapy is contraindicated in patients with cold allergies (hives, joint pain, nausea), Raynaud's phenomenon (arterial spasm), and some rheumatoid conditions.[3,12,17,19,22]

Depth of penetration is dependent on the amount of cold and the length of the treatment time because the body is well-equipped to maintain skin and subcutaneous tissue viability through the capillary bed by reflex vasodilation of up to 4 times normal blood flow. The body has the ability to decrease blood flow to the body segment that is supposedly losing too much body heat by shunting the blood flow. Depth of penetration is also related to intensity and duration of cold application and the circulatory response to the body segment exposed. If the person has normal circulatory responses, frostbite should not be a concern. Even so, caution should be exercised when applying intense cold directly to the skin. If deeper penetration is desired, ice therapy is most effective using ice towels, ice packs, ice massage, and ice whirlpools. Patients should be advised of the four stages of cryotherapy and the discomfort they will experience. The sports therapist should explain this sequence and advise the athlete of the expected outcome, which may include a rapid decrease in pain.[3,11,17,21]

Ice Massage

Ice massage can be applied by the sports therapist or the athlete if the athlete can reach the area of application to administer self-treatment. It is best for the first three treatments to be administered by the sports therapist to give the athlete the full benefit of the treatment. When positioning the athlete's body segment to be treated, it should be relaxed and the athlete should be made comfortable. Appropriate seating and positioning should be taken into consideration with the application of ice. Administration must be thorough to get the most out of the treatment. Ice massage is perhaps best indicated in conditions in which some type of stretching activity is to be used.

EQUIPMENT NEEDED (Figs. 5-1 and 5-2)
A. Styrofoam cups. A regular 6- to 8-ounce styrofoam hot or cold cup should be filled with water and placed in the freezer. After it is frozen, all the styrofoam on the sides should be removed down to 1 inch from the bottom. This device is preferred because it has a handle with which to hold the block of ice.
B. Popsicle ice cups. Cups are filled with water, and a wooden popsicle stick (tongue blade) is placed in each cup. The cups are then placed in the freezer. After it is frozen the paper cup is torn off. A block of ice on a stick is now ready to be used for massage purposes.
C. Paper cups. Same technique as the styrofoam cups except toweling may be needed to insulate the sports therapist's hand holding the paper cup.
D. Towels. These are used for positioning and absorbing the melting water in the area of the ice massage application.

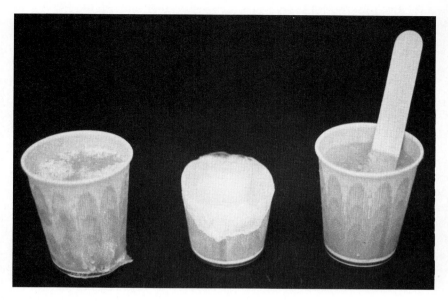

Figure 5-1. Water may be frozen in a paper cup, styrofoam cup, or on a popsicle stick for the purpose of ice massage.

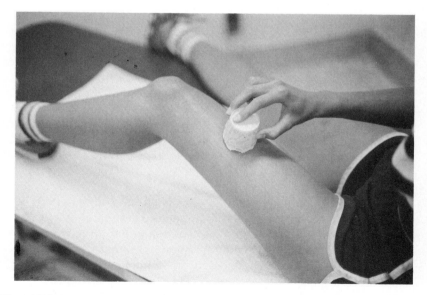

Figure 5-2. Ice massage may be applied using either circular or longitudinal strokes.

TREATMENT

A. Athlete position. Sidelying, prone, supine, hooklying, or sitting, depending on the area to be treated.

B. Self-treatment. Used when athletes can comfortably reach the area to be treated by themselves.

C. Circular motion. Application of ice massage in a circular pattern with each succeeding stroke covering half the previous stroke.

D. Longitudinal strokes. Application of ice massage in a longitudinal motion with each stroke overlapping half the previous stroke.

E. Peripheral coverage. Ice should be applied for 15 to 20 minutes; consistent patterning of circular and longitudinal strokes includes the sequence described in the clinical uses section.

PHYSIOLOGIC RESPONSES

A. Cold progression proceeds through the four stages: cold, stinging, burning, and numbness.

B. Reddening of the skin (erythema) occurs as a result of blanching or lack of blood in the capillary bed. A common example occurs when one works outside in the cold without gloves or appropriate footwear and returns inside to find the toes beet-red. The body is attempting to pool blood in the area to prevent further temperature loss.

C. Ice applications of 5 to 15 minutes and greater than 10° C (50° F) will not stimulate the hunting response and do not stimulate the reflex vasodilation that creates the body's own physically induced heat or increased blood flow.

CONSIDERATIONS

A. The time necessary for the surface area to be numbed will depend on the body area to be massaged. Approximate time will depend on how fast the ice application melts and what **thermopane** develops between the skin and ice massage.

B. Athlete comfort should be considered at all times.

C. If adequate circulation is present, frostbite should not be a concern. However, if the athlete has diabetes, the extremities, especially the toes, may require reduced temperature and adjustment of the intensity and duration of the cold.

APPLICATION. After the type of cold applicator for ice massage is selected, the athlete should be positioned comfortably and clothing should be removed from the area to be treated. The area should be set up prior to positioning the athlete. Remove the top two thirds of paper from the ice-filled paper or styrofoam cup, leaving 1 inch on the bottom of the cup as a handle for the therapist or athlete to use as a handgrip. The rough edges of the ice cup should be smoothed by gently rubbing along the edges with the therapist's hand. Ice should be applied to the exposed skin of the athlete in circular or longitudinal strokes with each stroke overlapping the previous stroke. The application should be continued until the athlete goes through the cold progression sequence of cold stinging sensation, burning, aching, and numbness. Once the skin is numb to fine touch, the ice application can be terminated. The cold pro-

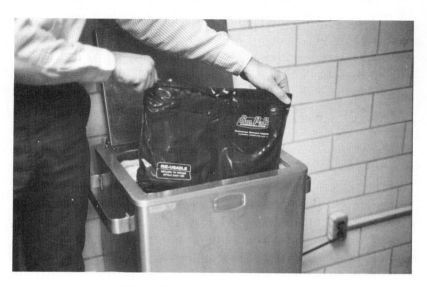

Figure 5-3. Commercial cold pack.

gression is the response of the sensory nerve fibers in the skin. The difference between cold and burning is primarily between the dropping out (sensory deficit) of the cold and warm nerve endings. Standard evening treatments allow the athlete to place cold applications every other 20 minutes, thus facilitating the hunting response. Some thermobarrier is developed during the ice massage in the layer of water directly on the skin, but this allows the ice cup to move smoothly over the skin. The time from application to numbing of the body segment depends on the size of the segment, but progression to numbing should be around 7 to 10 minutes.

Commercial (Cold) Hydrocollator Packs

Cold hydrocollator packs (Fig. 5-3) are indicated in any acute injury to a musculoskeletal structure.

EQUIPMENT NEEDED

A. Hydrocollator cold pack. This must be cooled to 8° F (−15° C); a 120-volt cycle is commercially available. It needs plastic liners or protective toweling for placement on a body segment. Petroleum distillate gel is the substance contained in the plastic pouch design.

B. Moist cold towels. Towels may be immersed in ice water and molded to the skin surface, or they can be packed in ice and allowed to remain in place. The commercial cold pack should be placed on top of a moist towel.

C. Plastic bag. The hydrocollator should be placed in the bag. Air should be removed from the bag. The plastic bag may then be molded around the body segment.

D. Dry towel. To prevent cold hydrocollator from losing heat rapidly, the towel is used as a covering to insulate the cold pack.

TREATMENT

A. Athlete position. Sidelying, prone, supine, hooklying, or sitting, depending on the area to be treated.

B. The patient must simply remain still during the treatment to maintain appropriate positioning of the cold pack.

C. Cold pack must be molded onto the skin.

D. The pack should be covered with a towel to limit loss of cold.

E. A timer should be set or time should otherwise be noted.

F. Treatment time should be 20 minutes.

PHYSIOLOGIC RESPONSE

A. Cold progression proceeds through the four stages.

B. Erythema occurs.

CONSIDERATIONS

A. Body area should be covered to prevent unnecessary exposure.

B. The physiologic response to cold treatment is immediate.

C. Athlete comfort should be considered at all times.

D. Frostbite should not be a concern unless circulation is inadequate.

APPLICATION. The athlete should be positioned with treatment area exposed and towel draped to protect clothing. The commercial cold pack should be placed against wet toweling to enhance transfer of cold to the body segment. If the injury is acute or subacute, the body segment should be elevated to reduce gravity-dependent swelling. Pack the cold pack around the joint in a manner designed to remove all air and ensure placement directly against wet toweling. Cold progression will be the same as with ice massage but not as quick, because of the toweling between the skin and cold pack. General treatment time required for numbing is about 20 minutes. The importance of a comfortable, properly positioned athlete is evident. Checking of the sensory area after application is important. Again, frostbite should not be a concern if circulation is intact. If swelling is a concern, a wet compression (elastic) wrap could be applied under the cold pack. A sequence of 20 minutes on and 20 minutes off should be repeated for 2 hours; the same sequence can be used in home treatment. Elevation is a key adjunct therapy during the sleeping hours.

Ice Packs

Like cold hydrocollator packs, ice packs (Fig. 5-4) are indicated in acute stages of injury, as well as for prevention of additional swelling after exercise of the injured part.

EQUIPMENT NEEDED

A. Small plastic bags. Vegetable or bread bags may be used.

B. Ice flaker machine. Flaked or crushed ice is easier to mold than cubed ice.

C. Moist towels. These are used to facilitate cold transmission and should be placed directly on the skin.

D. Elastic bandaging. Bandaging holds the plastic ice pack in place and applies compression. The body segment may be elevated.

E. Salt solution. This is used to increase melting temperature. Melting ice has more thermal energy than stable ice and is therefore colder.

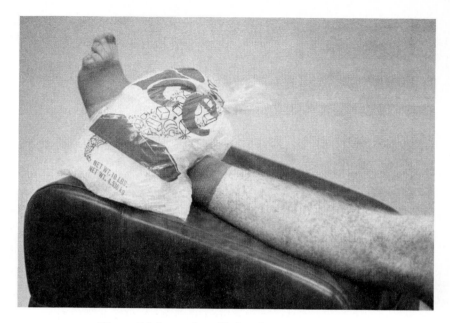

Figure 5-4. Ice pack molded to fit the injured part.

TREATMENT
A. Athlete position. Position depends on the part to be treated.
B. The patient must simply remain still during treatment.
C. Pack must be placed on skin.
D. Pack should be secured in place with toweling or elastic bandage.
E. Pack should be covered with towel to limit cold loss.
F. A timer should be set or time should otherwise be noted.
G. Treatment time should be 20 minutes.

PHYSIOLOGIC RESPONSE
A. Cold progression proceeds through the four stages.
B. Erythema occurs.

CONSIDERATIONS
A. Body area should be covered to prevent unnecessary exposure.
B. The physiologic response to cold is immediate.
C. Athlete comfort should be considered at all times.
D. Frostbite should not be a concern unless circulation is inadequate.

APPLICATION. Application of ice packs is similar to using commercial cold hydrocollator packs; the equipment to be set up in the treatment area consists of flaked or cubed ice in a plastic bag large enough for the area to be treated. The plastic bag can be applied directly to the skin and held in place by a moist or dry elastic wrap. Patient comfort is of the utmost importance during this application to facilitate relaxation on the part of the patient. The sports therapist may want to add salt to the ice to facilitate melting of the ice to create a colder slush mixture. Melting ice gives off more energy because of its less stable state, and it is therefore colder. A towel should be placed over the ice pack to de-

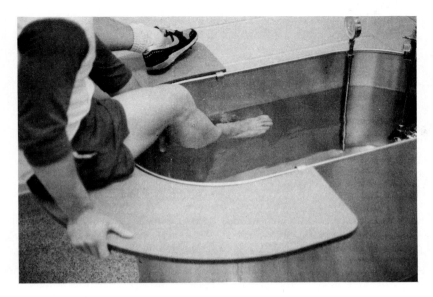

Figure 5-5. The cold whirlpool should have the ice melted before it is turned on.

crease the warming effect of the environmental air, thus facilitating the cold application. The normal physiologic response will be cold-stinging and burning-numbness, at which time the setup can be terminated. Because of the pliability of the flaked ice pack, it can be molded to the body segment treated. If cubed ice is used instead of flaked ice, it can still be molded, but it will not readily hold its position and will need to be secured via elastic wrap or toweling.

Cold Whirlpool

The cold whirlpool (Fig. 5-5) is indicated in acute and subacute conditions in which exercise of the injured part during a cold treatment is desired.

EQUIPMENT NEEDED
A. Whirlpool. The appropriate size whirlpool must be filled with cold water or ice to lower the temperature to 50° to 60° F. The therapist should use flaked ice and make sure the ice melts completely, as pieces of ice could become projectiles if a body segment is in the pool.
B. Ice machine. Flaked ice acts faster than cubed to lower the water temperature.
C. Toweling. Sufficient toweling is needed for padding the body segment on the whirlpool and for drying off after treatment.
D. Appropriate setup in area. A chair, whirlpool, and a bench in the whirlpool must be arranged before treatment.

TREATMENT
A. Temperature should be set at 50° to 60° F.
B. Body segment must be immersed.
C. For total body immersion the water temperature should be set at 65° to 80° F.
D. Treatment time should be 5 to 15 minutes.

PHYSIOLOGIC RESPONSES

A. Cold progression proceeds through the four stages.

B. Erythema occurs.

CONSIDERATIONS

A. Caution: Gravity-dependent positions should be avoided with acute and subacute injuries. Cold wet compression or elastic wrap should be put in place prior to treatment.

B. The body area treated should be completely immersed.

C. A cold whirlpool allows exercises to be done during treatment.

D. Athlete comfort should be considered at all times.

E. Frostbite should not be a concern unless circulation is inadequate.

F. A toe cap made of neoprene can be used to make the athlete more comfortable in the cold whirlpool.

APPLICATION. The unit should be turned on after it has been established that the ground fault interrupter (GFI) is functioning. The athlete should be positioned in the whirlpool area, and appropriate padding should be provided for the athlete's comfort. The timer should be set for the amount of time desired, depending on the size of the body part to be treated. Treatment time will be until the body segment becomes numb (approximately 15 minutes). Numbness is the cutaneous (skin or superficial) response. Frostbite should not be a concern unless the individual has a history of circulatory deficiencies or has diabetes. Treatment time will be between 7 and 15 minutes to allow the complete circulatory response. Caution is indicated in the gravity-dependent position because of possible additional swelling if the body segment is already swollen. This is the most intense application of cold of the cryotherapy techniques listed; therefore the first two or three treatments should be administered with the sports therapist remaining in the area. One of several reasons for the intensity of cold is that the body cannot develop a thermopane (insulating layer of water) on the skin because of the convection effect of the whirlpool. Additional benefits include the massaging and vibrating effect of the water flow. Removal of the part being treated from the whirlpool will necessitate a review of the skin surface and an assessment of edema in the extremities. If total body immersion is used, care should be taken for the intensity and duration of the whirlpool and for protection of the genitals from direct water flow. Repeated applications can be attempted following rewarming of the body segment after sensation has returned. If the cold application is administered prior to practice, it should be done before the application of preventive strapping, but enough time should also be allowed for sensation to return before taping. Studies have indicated that the reflex vasodilation lasts up to 2 hours. An athlete could practice, then return to the training room after practice and receive additional treatment without additional edema created by congestion as a result of vascular and capillary insufficiency occurring during the healing process. Increased heart rate and blood pressure are associated with cold application. Conditioned athletes should not have a problem with dizziness following cold applications, but care should be taken when transferring the athlete from the whirlpool area. To keep bacterial growth under control, whirlpool cultures of the tank and jet should be taken monthly.

Cold sprays, such as Fluori-Methane or ethyl chloride, do not provide adequate deep penetration, but they do provide adjunctive therapy for acupressure techniques to reduce muscle spasm. Physiologically this is accomplished by stimulating the A fibers involved in the gate control theory. The primary action of a cold spray is reduction of the pain spasm sequence secondary to direct trauma. It will, however, not reduce hemorrhage because it works on the superficial nerve endings to reduce the spasm via the stimulation of A fibers to reduce the so-called painful arc. Cold spray is an extremely effective technique in the treatment of myofascial trigger points. Precautions concerning the use of cold spray include protecting the face of the patient from the fumes and spraying the skin at an acute angle rather than at a perpendicular angle.[49] Cold spray is indicated when stretching of an injured part is desired along with cold treatment.

Cold Spray

EQUIPMENT NEEDED
A. Fluori-Methane.
B. Toweling.
C. Padding.

TREATMENT
A. The area to be treated should be sprayed and then stretched.
B. Spasm should be reduced.
C. Treatment should be distal to proximal.
D. A quick jetstream spray or stroking motion should be used.
E. Cooling should be superficial; no frosting should occur.
F. Cold sprays may be used in conjunction with acupressure.
G. Treatment time should be set according to body segment.

PHYSIOLOGIC RESPONSE
A. Muscle spasm is reduced.
B. Golgi tendon organ response is facilitated.
C. Muscle spindle response is inhibited.
D. Ligament and other musculoskeletal structures may be stimulated.

CONSIDERATIONS
A. Both the acute and the subacute response should be positive.
B. The room should be well ventilated to avoid the accumulation of fumes.
C. Athlete comfort should be considered at all times.

APPLICATION. The application of Fluori-Methane (Fig. 5-6) is typical of the application of other cold sprays. The following application procedures apply specifically to Fluori-Methane, but they provide an outline of the procedures, indications, and precautions applicable to all cold sprays. The sports therapist should follow the manufacturer's instructions in the use of any cold spray.

Fluori-Methane is a topical vapocoolant that produces a "touch cold sensation," acting as a counterirritant to block pain impulses of muscles in spasm. When used in conjunction with the spray and stretch technique, Fluori-Methane can break the pain cycle, allowing the muscle to be stretched to its normal length (pain-free state). The application of spray and stretch technique is a therapeutic modality that involves three stages: evaluation, spraying, and stretching. The therapeutic value of spray and stretch becomes most effective when the practitioner has mastered all stages and applies them in the proper sequence.

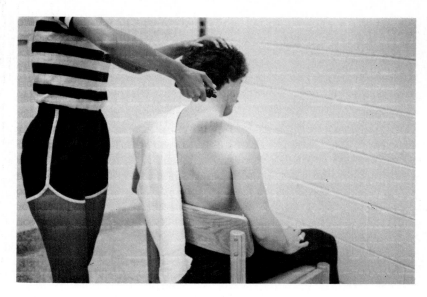

Figure 5-6. Spray and stretch technique using Fluori-Methane.

1. *Evaluation:* During the evaluation phase the cause of pain is determined as local spasm of an irritated trigger point. The method of applying spray and stretch to a muscle spasm differs slightly from application to a trigger point. The trigger point is a deep hypersensitive localized spot in a muscle that causes a referred pain pattern. With trigger points the source of pain is seldom the site of the pain. A trigger point may be detected by a snapping palpation over the muscle, causing the muscle in which the irritated trigger point is situated to "jump." In the case of muscle spasm, the source and site of pain are identical.

2. *Spraying:* To apply Fluori-Methane, (a) Patients should assume a comfortable position. (b) Take precautions to cover the patient's eyes, nose, and mouth if spraying near face. (c) Hold bottle in an upside down position (12 to 18 inches) away from the treatment surface, allowing the jetstream of vapocoolant to meet the skin at an acute angle to lessen the shock of impact. (d) Apply the spray in one direction only—not back and forth—at a rate of 4 inches (10 cm) per second. Three or four sweeps of the spray in one direction only are sufficient to extinguish the trigger point or to overcome painful muscle spasms. The skin must not be frosted due to the intense cold (15° C) of the Fluori-Methane, which can freeze the skin, causing a first degree burn similar to frostbite, and result in superficial tissue necrosis. In the case of trigger point, spray should be applied from the trigger point to the area of referred pain. If there is no trigger point, the spray should be applied from the affected muscle to its insertion. The spray should be applied in an even sweep. About two to four parallel, but not overlapping, sweeps of spray should be enough to cover this skin representation of the affected muscle.

3. *Stretching:* The stretch should begin as you start spraying from the origin to the insertion (simple muscle spasm pain) or from the trigger point to the referred pain when the trigger point is present. Spray and stretch until the muscle reaches its maximal or normal resting length. You will usually feel a gradual increase in range of motion. The spraying and stretching may re-

quire two to four spray applications to achieve the therapeutic results in any treatment session. In athletics, the athlete may have multiple treatment sessions in any one day.

The spray and stretch technique outlined above must be considered a therapeutic system. The practitioner should spend some time each day practicing until the technique is mastered.

Composition: Fluori-Methane is a combination of two chlorofluorocarbons—15% dichlorodifluoromethane, and 85% trichloromonofluoromethane. The combination is not flammable and at room temperature is only volatile enough to expel the contents from the inverted container. Fluori-Methane is supplied in amber Dispenseal bottles that emit a jetstream from a calibrated nozzle.

Indications: Fluori-Methane is a vapocoolant intended for topical application in the management of myofascial pain, restricted motion, and muscle spasm. Clinical conditions that may respond to spray and stretch include low back pain (due to muscle spasm), acute stiff neck, torticollis, acute bursitis of shoulder, muscle spasm associated with osteoarthritis, ankle sprain, tight hamstring, masseter muscle spasm, certain types of headache, and referred pain due to trigger points.

Precautions: Federal law prohibits dispensing without a prescription. Although Fluori-Methane is safe for topical application to the skin, care should be taken to minimize inhalation of vapors, especially when it is being applied to the head or neck. Fluori-Methane is not intended for production of local anesthesia and should not be applied to the point of frost formation. Freezing can occasionally alter pigmentation.*

Contrast Bath

Contrast baths are used to treat subacute swelling, gravity-dependent swelling, and vasodilation-vasoconstriction response.

EQUIPMENT NEEDED (Fig. 5-7)

A. Two containers. One container is used to hold cold water (50° to 60° F), and the other is used to hold warm water (104° to 106° F). Whirlpools may be used as one or both containers.

B. Ice machine.

C. Towels.

D. Chair.

TREATMENT

A. Hot and cold immersions are alternated.

B. Treatment time should be at least 20 minutes. Treatments should consist of five 1-minute cold immersions and five 3-minute warm immersions, although the exact ratio of cold to hot treatment is highly variable.

PHYSIOLOGIC RESPONSE

A. Vasoconstriction and vasodilation occur.

B. There is a reduction of necrotic cells at the cellular level.

C. Edema is decreased.

CONSIDERATIONS

A. The temperatures of the baths must be maintained.

B. A large area is required for treatment.

C. Athlete comfort must be considered at all times.

*Modified with permission of the Gebauer Chemical Company, Cleveland, Ohio, 44104, (800) 321-9348; Ohio, (216) 271-5252.

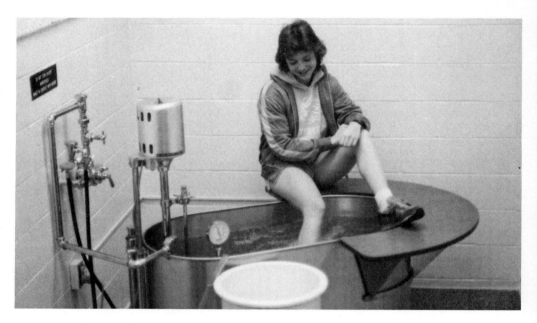

Figure 5-7. Contrast bath using a warm whirlpool and ice immersion cylinder.

APPLICATION. After the area is set up, a whirlpool can be used for either hot or cold application, with the opposite method of treatment contained in a bucket or sterile container. The temperatures of these immersion baths must be maintained (cold at 50° to 60° F, hot at 98° to 110° F) with ice additions or added warm water. It is generally easier to use a large whirlpool for the warm water application and a bucket for the cold water application. There has been considerable controversy regarding the use of contrast bath for the purpose of controlling swelling. Contrast baths are most often indicated when changing the treatment modality from cold to hot to facilitate a mild tissue temperature increase. The use of a contrast bath allows for a transitional period during which a slight rise in tissue temperature may be effective for increasing blood flow to an injured area without causing the accumulation of additional edema. The theory that contrast baths induce a type of pumping action by alternating vasoconstriction with vasodilation has little or no credibility. Contrast baths probably cause only a superficial capillary response as a result of an inability of the larger deep blood vessels to constrict and dilate in response to superficial heating.

Thus it is recommended that during the initial stages of contrast bath treatment the ratio of hot to cold treatment begins with a relatively brief period in hot, gradually increasing the length of time in the hot bath during subsequent treatments. Recommendations as to specific lengths of time are extremely variable. However, it would appear that a 3:1 ratio (3 minutes in hot, 1 minute in cold) or 4:1 for 19 to 20 minutes is fairly well accepted. Whether the treatment is ended with cold or hot depends to some extent on the degree of tissue temperature increase desired. Other sports therapists prefer to use the same ratios of 3:1 or 4:1 beginning with cold. The technique may certainly be modified to meet specific needs. Removal of the injured part following the contrast bath requires checking of skin sensation and the amount of edema accumulation to make sure that the treatment has not actually increased the amount of edema.

Ice Immersion

Ice buckets allow ease of application for the sports therapist. Again, a wet area should be selected (where spilled water is not a concern), with the patient positioned for comfort. The immersion, like the contrast bath, should be maintained until desired results are reached. If **cryokinetics** are part of the treatment, then the container should be large enough to allow for the movement of the body segment. Ice immersion is similar to cold whirlpool in that the body segment may be subject to gravity-dependent positions.

Cryokinetics

Cryokinetics is a technique that combines cryotherapy or the application of cold with exercise. The goal of cryokinetics is to numb the injured part to the point of analgesia and then work toward achieving normal range of motion through progressive active exercise.

The technique begins by numbing the body part via ice immersion, cold packs, or ice massage. Most athletes will report a feeling of numbness within 12 to 20 minutes. If numbness is not perceived within 20 minutes, the therapist should proceed with exercise regardless. The numbness usually will last for 3 to 5 minutes, at which point ice should be reapplied for an additional 3 to 5 minutes until numbness returns. This sequence should be repeated five times.

Exercises are performed during the periods of numbness. The exercises selected should be pain free and progressive in intensity, concentrating on both flexibility and strength. Changes in the intensity of the activity should be limited by both the nature of the healing process and by individual patient differences in perception of pain. However, progression always should be encouraged within the framework of those limiting factors, the ultimate goal being a return to full sport–type activities.[24]

THERMOTHERAPY TECHNIQUES

Heat is still used as a universal treatment for pain and discomfort. Much of the benefit is derived from the treatment simply feeling good. However, in the early stages following injury, heat causes increased capillary blood pressure and increased cellular permeability; this results in additional swelling or edema accumulation.[3,8,17,26,51] No athlete with edema should be treated with any heat modality until the reasons for the edema are determined. It is in the best interests of the sports therapist to use cryotherapy techniques or contrast baths to reduce the edema prior to heat applications. Superficial heat applications seem to feel more comfortable for complaints of the neck, back, low back, and pelvic areas and may be most appropriate for the athlete who exhibits some allergic response to cold applications. However, it must be remembered that the tissues in these areas are absolutely no different from those in the extremities. Thus, the same physiologic responses to the use of heat or cold will be elicited in all areas of the body.

Primary goals of thermotherapy include increased blood flow and increased muscle temperature to stimulate analgesia, increased nutrition to the cellular level, reduction of edema, and removal of metabolites and other products of the inflammatory process.

Warm Whirlpool

EQUIPMENT NEEDED

A. Whirlpool. The whirlpool must be the correct size for the body segment to be treated.

B. Towels. These are to be used for padding and drying off.

C. Chair.

D. Padding. This is to be placed on the side of the whirlpool.

TREATMENT

A. The athlete should be positioned comfortably, allowing the injured part to be immersed in the whirlpool.

B. Direct flow should be 6 to 8 inches from the body segment.

C. Temperature should be 98° to 110° F (37° to 45° C) for treatment of the arm and hand. For treatment of the leg, the temperature should be 98° to 104° F (37° to 40° C), and for full body treatment, the temperature should be 98° to 102° F (37° to 39° C).

D. Time of application should be 15 to 20 minutes.

CONSIDERATIONS

A. Athlete positioning should allow for exercise of the injured part.

B. The size of the body segment to be treated will determine whether an upper extremity, lower extremity, or full body whirlpool should be used.

C. Frequency.

APPLICATION (Fig. 5-8). The temperature range of a warm whirlpool is 100° to 110° F (39° to 45° C). It is similar in setup to a cold whirlpool. The athlete must be positioned in the whirlpool, with appropriate padding provided for the athlete's comfort. The unit should be turned on after it has been ascertained that the ground fault interrupter (GFI) is functioning. The timer should be set for the amount of time desired, depending on the size of the body part to be treated (10 to 30 minutes). Treatment time should be long enough to stimulate vasodilation and reduce muscle spasm (approximately 20 minutes). Again, caution is indicated in the gravity-dependent position in subacute athletic injuries. If some pitting edema exists (i.e., finger pressure on the skin leaves an indentation), cold or contrast baths are better indicated. In addition to increased circulation and reduction of spasm, benefits of the warm whirlpool include the massaging and vibrating effects of the water movement. On removal of the body segment from the whirlpool, it is necessary to review the skin surface and limb girth to see if the warm whirlpool increased swelling; this step is indicated even if the athlete is past the subacute stages. After allowing the body segment to cool down, the athlete can have appropriate preventive strapping or padding placed on the body segment. If the athlete receives the treatment prior to

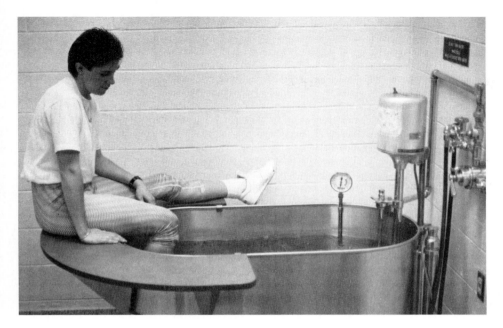

Figure 5-8. Warm whirlpool.

exercising, it is recommended that he or she gently do range of motion exercises to reduce congestion and increase proprioception (sense of position) in all joints. If the athlete is complaining of muscle soreness, it would be more appropriate to recommend swimming pool exercises. The whirlpool provides a sedative effect. It is recommended that the athlete shower or clean the body surface prior to using a whirlpool. Random access to the whirlpool is not warranted.

The warm whirlpool is an excellent postsurgical modality to increase systemic blood flow and mobilization of the affected body part. The appropriateness of whirlpool therapy needs to be addressed by the sports therapist because it is the most commonly abused physical therapy modality. An example of this abuse is the common practice of placing an individual in the whirlpool without taking the time to assess the specific physiologic responses desired (such as reflex vasodilation or reduction of inflammatory deposits). However, it is an excellent adjunctive modality when used appropriately in the sports medicine setting.

Whirlpools should be cleaned frequently to prevent the growth of bacteria. Certainly when a patient with any open or infected lesion uses the whirlpool, it should be drained and cleaned immediately. Cleaning should be done using both a disinfecting and antibacterial agent. Particular attention should be paid to cleaning the turbine by placing the intake valves in a bucket containing the disinfecting solution and turning the power on. Bacterial cultures should be monitored periodically from the tank, drain, and jets.

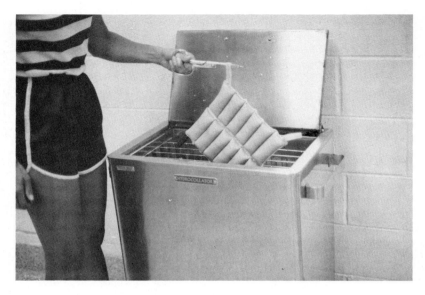

Figure 5-9. Hydrocollator packs stored in tank.

Hydrocollator Packs (Fig. 5-9)

EQUIPMENT NEEDED

A. Unit heat packs. These are canvas pouches of petroleum distillate. A thermostat maintains the high temperature (170° F) and helps prevent burns. Unit heat packs come in three sizes: (1) regular size is 12 × 12 inches for most body segments, (2) double size is 24 × 24 inches, for the back, low back, and buttocks, (3) cervical is 6 × 18 inches for the cervical spine. Packs are removed by tongs or scissor handles.

B. Towels. Regular bath towels and commercial double pad towels are required. Commercial double pad toweling has a pouch for pack placement and 1 inch thick toweling to be placed in cross fashion, tags on the edge of packs folded in, toweling overlapped on one side and four layers on the opposite side. Six layers equal 1 inch of toweling. Additional toweling may be needed depending on total body surface covered.

TREATMENT

A. Position 6 layers of toweling as described above (shown in Fig. 5-10).

B. Sufficient toweling should be provided to protect the patient from burns.

C. Athlete position should be comfortable.

D. Treatment time should be 15 to 20 minutes.

PHYSIOLOGIC RESPONSE

A. Circulation is increased.

B. Muscle temperature is increased.

C. There is an increase in tissue temperature.

D. Spasms are relaxed.

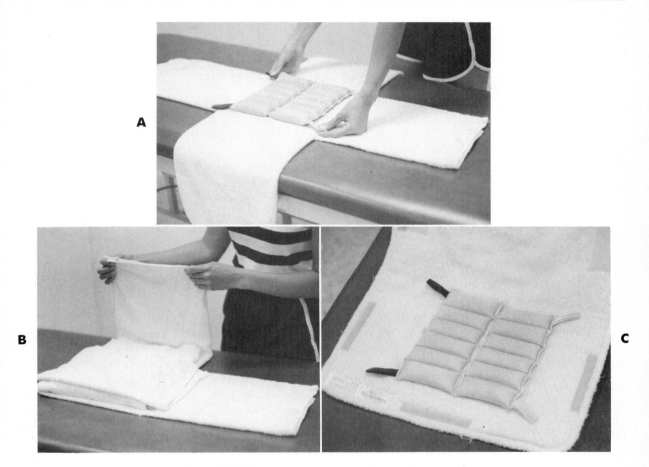

Figure 5-10. Technique for wrapping hydrocollator packs.

CONSIDERATIONS
A. The size of the body segment to be treated should determine how many packs are needed.
B. Athlete comfort is always a consideration.
C. Time of application should be 15 to 20 minutes.

APPLICATION. Appropriate toweling and positioning of the athlete is necessary for a comfortable treatment. The moist heat pack tends to stimulate the circulatory response. Dry heat, as discussed in the infrared section, has a tendency to force blood away from the cutaneous capillary bed, thus increasing the possibility of a burn with the skin's inability to dissipate heat. The patient must not be allowed to lie on the packs because this will force the silicate gel out through the seams of the fabric sleeves. If the patient cannot tolerate the weight of the moist heat pack, alternate methods, such as placing the patient sidelying with the majority of the weight of the hot pack on the side of the pack and the pack held in place by additional towels or sheets wrapped around the patient, can be used. The most common indication is for muscular spasm, back pain, or as a preliminary treatment to other modalities.

Paraffin Bath

Paraffin bath is a simple and efficient, though somewhat messy, technique for applying a fairly high degree of localized heat. Paraffin treatments provide 6 times the amount of heat available in water because the mineral oil in the paraffin lowers the melting point of the paraffin. The combination of paraffin and mineral oil has a low specific heat, which enhances the ability of the patient to tolerate heat from paraffin better than from water of the same temperature.

The risk of a burn with paraffin is substantial. The sports therapist should weigh heavily the considerations between a paraffin bath and warm whirlpool bath in the athletic setting. The majority of paraffin baths are used for chronic arthritis patients' hands and feet. If the patient-athlete has a chronic hand or foot problem, the use of paraffin instead of water usually gives longer lasting pain relief.[6,26]

EQUIPMENT NEEDED
A. Paraffin bath (Fig. 5-11, *A*).
B. Plastic bags and paper towels.
C. Towels.

TREATMENT
A. Dipping. The extremity should be dipped into the paraffin for a couple of seconds, then removed to allow the paraffin to harden slightly for a few seconds. This procedure is repeated until 10 layers have accumulated on the part to be treated.
B. Wrapping. The paraffin-coated extremity should be wrapped in a plastic bag with several layers of toweling around it to act as insulation (Fig. 5-11, *B*).
C. Treatment time should be 20 to 30 minutes.

PHYSIOLOGIC RESPONSES
A. There is an increase in tissue temperature.
B. Pain relief occurs.
C. Thermal hyperthermia occurs.

CONSIDERATIONS
A. Some units are equipped with thermostats that may elevate the temperature to 212° F, thus killing any bacteria that may grow in the paraffin. Otherwise the temperature should be set at 126° F.
B. If the paraffin becomes soiled, it should be dumped and replaced at no longer than 6-month intervals.

APPLICATION. The purchase of a paraffin bath for the training room requires that the bath have a built-in thermostat. Prior to treatment, the athlete's body segment should be cleaned thoroughly with soap, water, and finally alcohol to remove any soap residue. This will prevent bacterial build-up in the bottom of the paraffin bath, which is an excellent medium for culture growth.

The mixture ratio of paraffin to mineral oil is 1 gallon of mineral oil to 2 pounds of paraffin. The mineral oil reduces the ambient temperature of the paraffin, which is 126° F (at which temperature a burn could occur). This is impor-

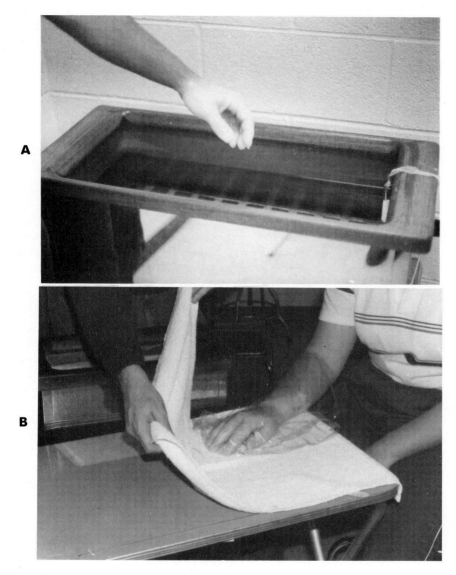

Figure 5-11. A, Hand being dipped in paraffin bath. **B,** After being dipped in paraffin, the hand should be wrapped in plastic bags and toweling.

tant because when dipping the extremity in the paraffin, if the second layer of paraffin is allowed to get between the skin and the first layer of paraffin, the heat will not dissipate and the athlete could be burned. Therefore, it is important to build 6 layers of paraffin, with the first layer highest on the body segment and each successive layer lower than the previous one. Because heat is retained in the body and heat is also radiated from the paraffin, there is an increase in capillary dilation and blood supply in the treated segment. Care is indicated to place the athlete in a comfortable position and to enclose the paraffin in paper towels, plastic bags, and toweling to maintain the heat. Treatment is applied for approximately 20 to 30 minutes. Removal of the paraffin calls for extra care not to contaminate the used portion so that it does not contaminate the entire bath when it is returned.

Removal of paraffin involves removing towels, plastic bag, and paper towels, then using a tongue depressor to split the paraffin to allow easy removal. If the paraffin has not touched the floor, remove the paraffin cast over the open paraffin bath. It will dissolve on returning to the remaining liquid paraffin. Clean the body segment with soap and water or, if a postsurgical patient is being treated, give a massage, as the mineral oil will make the skin moist and supple. When cleaning the skin, the therapist must examine the surface for burns or mottling. The thermostat will raise the temperature of the paraffin to 212° F, destroy any bacteria, and maintain a sterile contact medium. Paraffin baths require a large amount of supervision to prevent contamination, but they do provide a special type of treatment well-adapted to the athletic patient with injuries of the hands and feet.

Infrared Lamps

When talking about infrared modalities, the sports therapist most typically thinks of the infrared lamp. The biggest advantage of an infrared lamp is the superficial tissue temperature rise and the fact that the unit does not touch the patient. However, radiant heat is seldom used because it is limited in depth of skin penetration to less than 1 mm. Dry heat from an infrared lamp tends to elevate superficial skin temperatures more than moist heat; however, moist heat probably has a greater depth of penetration.

Superficial skin burns occasionally occur because of intense infrared radiation and the reflector becoming extremely hot (4000° F). It is recommended that a warm moist towel be placed over the body segment to be treated to enhance the heating effects. Dry towels should cover the remainder of the body not being treated. This will allow a greater blood/tissue exchange by trapping the heat build-up in the moist towel and reducing the stagnant air over the body segment. Caution should be used, and the skin should be checked every few minutes for mottling.

Infrared generators may be divided into two categories: luminous and nonluminous. Nonluminous generators consist of a spiral coil of resistant metal wire wound around a cone-shaped piece of nonconducting material. The resistance of the wire to the electric flow produces heat and a dull red glow. A properly shaped reflector then radiates the heat to the body. All incandescent bodies and tungsten and carbon filament lamps are in the category of luminous generators. No nonluminous lamps are being manufactured these days since it was shown that because of a certain unique characteristic of human skin, infrared at a wavelength of 12,000 A will penetrate slightly more deeply than either longer or shorter waves. Tungsten filament and special quartz red sources produce significant amounts of infrared heat at 12,000 A. Flare as a result of reflection off the skin can be a real problem.

EQUIPMENT NEEDED

A. Infrared lamp.

B. Dry toweling. This is to be used for draping the parts of the body not being treated.

C. Moist toweling. Moist towels are used to cover the area to be treated.

D. A ground fault interrupter should be used with an infrared lamp.

TREATMENT

A. The athlete should be positioned 20 inches from the source.

B. Protective toweling should be put in place.

C. Treatment time should be 15 to 20 minutes.

D. Skin should be checked every few minutes for mottling.

E. Areas that are not to be treated must be protected.

PHYSIOLOGIC RESPONSE

A. A superficial rise in tissue temperature occurs.

B. There is some decrease in pain.

C. Moisture and sweat appear on the skin surface.

CONSIDERATIONS

A. To avoid a generalized temperature rise, only that portion that is injured should be treated.

B. The infrared lamp should be used primarily when a patient cannot tolerate pressure from another type of modality (e.g., hydrocollator packs).

C. Caution must be exercised to avoid burns.

APPLICATION (Fig. 5-12). The athlete should be placed in a comfortable position. Moist heat should be used to stimulate blood flow, and it is recommended to prevent blood from being forced away from the area as with dry heat; a moist, warm towel should be applied to the area to be treated. A squirt bottle is needed to keep the towel moist. All areas not to be treated should be draped. The distance from the area to be treated to the lamp should be adjusted according to treatment time: the standard formula is 20 inches distance = 20 minutes treatment time. However, the inverse square law dictates that if a 10-inch distance is used, a 5-minute treatment time is required. Because of superficial heating, care and continual observation is mandatory to prevent superficial skin burns. After treatment, the skin surface should be assessed. This type of treatment has a tendency to force the blood away from the capillary bed and should be used only in superficial skin complaints related to dry heat requirements.

Fluidotherapy

Fluidotherapy is a unique, multifunctional physical medicine modality. The fluidotherapy unit is a dry heat modality that uses a suspended air stream, which has the properties of a liquid. Its therapeutic effectiveness in rehabilitation and healing is based on its ability to simultaneously apply heat, massage, sensory stimulation for desensitization, levitation, and pressure oscillations. Unlike water, the dry, natural medium does not irritate the skin or produce thermal shocks. This allows for much higher treatment temperatures than with aqueous or paraffin heat transfer. The pressure oscillations may actually minimize

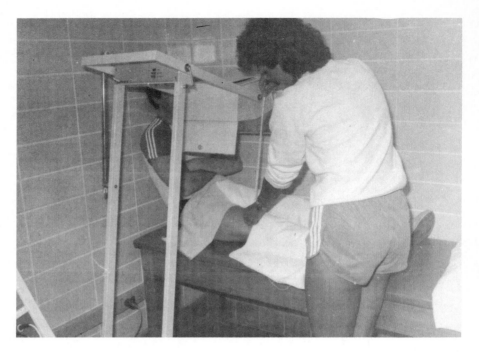

Figure 5-12. Measuring the treatment distance with far positioning of the infrared baker.

edema, even at very high treatment temperatures. Outstanding clinical success has been reported in treatment of pain, range of motion, wounds, acute injuries, swelling, and blood flow insufficiency. Fluidotherapy treatment of the hand at 115° F (46.2° C) results in a sixfold increase in blood flow and a fourfold increase in metabolic rates in a normal adult.[6] These properties will increase blood flow, sedate, decrease blood pressure, and promote healing by accelerating biochemical reactions.[6]

Counterirritation, through **mechanoreceptor** and **thermoreceptor** stimulation, reduces pain sensitivity, thus permitting high temperatures without painful heat sensations. Pronounced **hyperthermia** accelerates the chemical metabolic processes and stimulates the normal healing process. The high temperatures enhance tissue elasticity and reduce tissue viscosity, which improves musculoskeletal mobility. Vascular responses are stimulated as a result of the long-lasting hyperthermia and pressure fluctuations, resulting in increased blood flow to the injured area.

EQUIPMENT NEEDED

A. Fluidotherapy model 104 (Fig. 5-13).

B. Toweling.

TREATMENT

A. The patient must be positioned for comfort.

B. The patient should place the body segment to be treated (hand or foot) in the fluidotherapy unit.

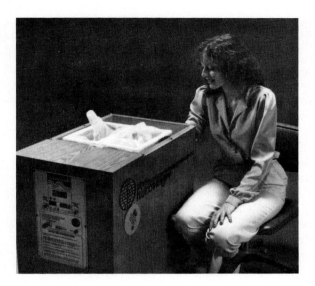

Figure 5-13. Fluidotherapy treatment.
(Photo courtesy of Fluidotherapy Corporation, 6113 Aletha Lane, Houston, TX 77081.)

C. Protective toweling must be placed at the unit interface and body segment.
D. Treatment time should be 15 to 20 minutes.

PHYSIOLOGIC RESPONSES

A. Tissue temperature increases.
B. Pain relief occurs.
C. Thermal hyperthermia occurs.

CONSIDERATIONS

A. Fluidotherapy unit must be kept clean.
B. All knobs must be returned to zero following treatment.

APPLICATION. The patient should be positioned comfortably. The treated body segment should be submerged in the medium before the unit is turned on. There is no thermal shock when heat is applied. Treatments are approximately 20 minutes. Recommended temperature varies by body part and patient tolerance, with a range of 110° to 125° F (43° to 53° C). Maximum temperature rise in the treated part occurs after 15 minutes of treatment. Unless contraindicated, active and passive exercise is encouraged during treatment.

In case of open lesions or infections, a protective dressing is recommended to prevent soiling or contaminating the cloth entry ports. Patients with splints, bandages, tape, orthopedic pins, plastic joint replacement, and artificial tendons may be treated with fluidotherapy. The medium is clean and will not soil clothing. It is not necessary to disrobe to get the full benefit of heat and massage; however, direct contact between skin and the medium is desirable to maximize heat transfer.

In treating the hands, muscles, ankles, and conditions that manifest themselves relatively near the surface of the skin, appreciably higher body temperatures can be achieved using superficial heating modalities.[6] Further, the superficial modalities treat a larger area of the body than ultrasound or microwave diathermies, thus the total amount of heat absorbed will be much higher. Fluidotherapy, hydrotherapy, and paraffin cause about the same amount of temperature increase.[12]

CONCLUSIONS

Infrared sources transmit thermal energy to or from the athlete. In most cases they are simple, efficient, and inexpensive. Sports therapists who choose to compare modalities and use the most appropriate technique for their athletes will be providing quality care for that athlete. A haphazard approach to the use of infrared modalities will only reflect a haphazard regard for the health care of the student athlete.

Questioning, thinking sports therapists will determine which procedure is best and most appropriate clinically. They will take responsibility for seeing that the most appropriate therapeutic modality is applied to enhance the athlete's reconditioning and rehabilitation. This chapter has provided various methods and modalities, their physiologic responses, and special considerations for the sports medicine practitioner.

Regardless of what infrared modality sports therapists choose, they should be aware of (1) the physiologic implications relative to circulation, (2) the ease of application, and (3) the short- and long-term benefits of treatment.

Additional areas of concern relate to the (1) benefits of the infrared modality application, whether cryotherapy or thermotherapy, (2) economy of modality application, and (3) repeatability of applications. Common sense in the application of these modalities will provide optimum injury management and optimum modality usage for tissue healing of athletic trauma.

SUMMARY

1. Any modality that radiates energy with wavelengths and frequencies that fall into the classification of the infrared region of the electromagnetic spectrum are referred to as infrared modalities.
2. When infrared modalities are applied to connective tissue or muscle and soft tissue, they will cause either a tissue temperature lowering or tissue temperature rise.
3. The primary physiologic effect of heat is vasodilation of capillaries with increased blood flow, increased metabolic activity, and relaxation of muscle spasm.
4. The primary physiologic effect of cold is vasoconstriction of capillaries with decreased blood flow, decreased metabolic activity, and analgesia with reduction of muscle spasm.
5. The infrared energies have a depth of penetration of less than 1 cm, thus the

physiologic effects are primarily superficial and directly affect the cutaneous blood vessels and nerve receptors.

6. Examples of thermotherapy are whirlpools, moist heat packs, infrared lamps, heating pads, and fluidotherapy.
7. Examples of cryotherapy are ice packs, ice massage, commercial ice packs, ice whirlpools, and cold sprays.

GLOSSARY

ablution Washing or bathing.

analgesia Loss of sensibility to pain.

anesthesia Loss of sensation.

atonic Without tone.

cold-induced vasodilation Vasodilation following cold application.

conduction Heat loss or gain through direct contact.

congestion Presence of an abnormal amount of blood in the vessels as a result of an increase in blood flow or obstructed venous return.

contraindication Special symptom or circumstance that renders the use of a remedy or procedure inadvisable.

contrast bath Hot (106° F) and cold (50° F) treatments in a combined sequence to stimulate superficial capillary vasodilation or vasoconstriction.

convection Heat loss or gain through the movement of air or water molecules across the skin.

conversion Changing of one energy into another.

cryokinetics The use of cold and exercise in the treatment of pathology or disease.

cryotherapy The use of cold in the treatment of pathology or diseases.

douche A current of water directed against the skin surface (e.g., scotch douche alternating hot and cold water).

edema Excessive fluid in cells.

erythema Redness of the skin; inflammation. A redness of the skin caused by capillary dilation.

evaporation Loss of volume of liquid by changing into vapor; loss of heat by this process; heat transfer.

fluidotherapy A modality of dry heat using a finely divided solid suspended in an air stream with the properties of liquid.

Hubbard tank An immersion tank for the whole body, may have vertical depth for walking or supine treatment.

hunting response A reflex vasodilation that occurs in response to cold approximately 15 minutes into the treatment. This has been demonstrated to be only an increase in temperature and not necessarily a change in blood flow.

hydrocollator A synthetic hot (170° F) or cold (0° F) gel used as an adjunctive modality to stimulate tissue temperature rise or tissue temperature lowering.

hydrogymnastics Exercises using the buoyant properties of immersion in water.

hydrotherapy Cryotherapy and thermotherapy techniques that use water as the medium for heat transfer.

hyperemia Presence of an increased amount of blood in part of the body.

indication The reason to prescribe a remedy or procedure.

infrared That portion of the electromagnetic spectrum associated with thermal changes; located adjacent to the red portion of the visible light spectrum. That part of the electromagnetic spectrum dealing with infrared wavelengths.

metabolites Waste products of metabolism or catabolism.

myofascial pain A type of referred pain associated with trigger points.

nutrients Essential or nonessential food substance.

paraffin bath A combined paraffin and mineral oil immersion technique in which the paraffin substance is heated to 126° F for conductive heat gains; commonly used on the hands and feet for distal temperature gains in blood flow and temperature.

radiation The process of emitting energy from some source in the form of waves. A method of heat transfer through which heat can either be gained or lost.

secondary vasodilation Dilation following exposure to cold to sustain viable tissues.

sterile technique Maintenance of a sterile environment; aseptic; free from all living microorganisms; preventing contamination.

thermal Pertaining to heat.

thermopane An insulating layer of water next to the skin.

thermotherapy The use of heat in the treatment of pathology or disease.

vasoconstriction Narrowing of the blood vessels.

vasodilation Dilation of the blood vessels.

REFERENCES

1 Abramson, D.I., Tuck, S., Lee, S.W., Richardson, G., and Chu, L.S.W.: Vascular basis for pain due to cold, Arch. Phys. Med. Rehabil. 47:300-305, 1966.

2 Basset, S.W., and Lake, B.M.: Use of cold applications in management of spasticity, Phys. Ther. Rev. 38(5):333-334, 1958.

3 Behnke, R.: Cold therapy, Athl. Train. 9(4):178-179, 1974.

4 Behnke, R.: Cryotherapy and vasodilation, Athl. Train. 8(3):106, 1973.

5 Bierman, W., and Friendlander, M.: The penetrative effect of cold, Arch. Phys. Med. Rehabil. 21:585-592, 1940.

6 Chambers, R.: Clinical uses of cryotherapy, J. Am. Phys. Ther. Assoc. 49(3):145-149, 1969.

7 Clarke, D.H.: Effect of immersion in hot and cold water upon recovery of muscular strength following fatiguing isometric exercise, Arch. Phys. Med. Rehabil. 44:565-568, 1963.

8 Clarke, D.H., and Stelmach, G.E.: Muscle fatigue and recovery curve parameters at various temperatures, Res. Q. 37(4):468-479, 1966.

9 Clarke, R.S.J., Hellon, R.E., and Lind, A.R.: Vascular reactions of the human forearm to cold, Clin. Sci. 17:165-179, 1958.

10 Clarke, R.S.J., and Hellon, R.F.: Hyperaemia following sustained and rhythmic exercise in the human forearm at various temperatures, J. Physiol. 145:447-458, 1959.

11 DeJong, R.H., Hershey, W.M., and Wagman, I.H.: Nerve conduction velocity during hypothermia in man, Anes. 27:805-810, 1966.

12 Downer, A.H.: Physical therapy procedures, ed. 3, Springfield, 1978, Charles C Thomas Publishers.

13 Domtigny, R., and Sheldon, K.: Simultaneous use of heat and cold in treatment of muscle spasm, Arch. Phys. Med. 43:235-237, 1962.

14 Downey, J.A.: Physiological effects of heat and cold, J. Am. Phys. Ther. Assoc. 44(8):713-717, 1964.

15 Eldred E., Lindsley D.F., and Buchwald, J.S.: The effect of cooling on mammalian muscle spindles, Exp. Neurol. 2:144-157, 1960.

16 Fischer, E., and Soloman, S.: Physiologic responses to heat and cold. In Licht, S., editor. Therapeutic heat, New Haven, 1965, Elizabeth Licht.

17 Grant, A.E.: Massage with ice (cryokinetics) in the treatment of painful conditions of the musculoskeletal system, Arch. Phys. Med. Rehabil. 45:233-238, 1964.

18 Griffin, J.E., Karselis, T.C.: Physical agents for physical therapists, ed. 2, Springfield, 1982, Charles C Thomas Publishers.

19 Guyton, A.C.: Medical physiology, ed. 6, Philadelphia, W.B. Saunders Co., Chapters 29 and 72.

20 Hayden, C.: Cryokinetics in an early treatment program, J. Am. Phys. Ther. Assoc. 44:11, 1964.

21 Hedenberg, L.: Functional improvement of the spastic hemiplegic arm after cooling, Scand. J. Rehabil. Med. 2:154-158, 1970.

22 Hocutt, J.E., Jr., Jaffe, R., Rylander, C.R., and Beebe, J.K.: Cryotherapy in ankle sprains, Am. J. Sports Med. 10(5): 1982.

23 Knight, K.L.: Effects of hypothermia on inflammation and swelling, Athl. Train. 11:7-10, 1976.

24 Knight, K.L.: Cryotherapy in sports medicine. In Scribner, K., and Burke, E.J., editors: Relevant topics in athletic training, New York, 1978, Movement Publications, pp. 52-59.

25 Knight, K.L.: Ankle rehabilitation with cryotherapy, Phys. Sportsmed. 7(11):133, 1979.

26 Knight, K.L., Aquino, J., Johannes, S.M., and Urban, C.D.: A reexamination of Lewis' cold induced vasodilation in the finger and the ankle, Athl. Train. 15:248-250, 1980.

27 Knight, K.L., and Londeree, B.R.: Comparison of blood flow in the ankle of uninjured subjects during therapeutic applications of heat, cold, and exercise, Med. Sci. Sport Exer. 12(1):76-80, 1980.

28 Knight, K.L.: Ice for immediate care of injuries, Phys. Sportsmed. 10(2):137, 1982.

29 Knott, M., and Barufaldi, D.: Treatment of whiplash injuries, Phys. Ther. Rev. 41:8, 1961.

30 Knutsson, E., and Mattson, E.: Effects of local cooling on monosynaptic reflexes in man, Scand. J. Rehabil. Med. 1:126-132, 1969.

31 Knutsson, E.: Topical cryotherapy in spasticity, Scand. J. Rehab. Med. 2:159-163, 1970.

32 Knutsson, E., Lindblom, U., and Martensson, A.: Differences in gamma and alpha spasticity induced by the GABA derivative Baclofen (Lioresal), Brain 96:29-46, 1973.

33 Lehman, J.F.: Therapeutic heat and cold, ed. 3, Baltimore, 1982, Williams & Wilkins.

34 Lewis, T.: Observations upon the reactions of the vessels of the human skin to cold, Heart 15:177-208, 1930.

35 Licht, S.: Therapeutic heat and cold, New Haven, 1965, Elizabeth Licht, Chapters 4 and 21.

36 Lippold, O.C.J., Nicholls, J.G., and Redfearn, J.W.T.: A study of the afferent discharge produced by cooling a mammalian muscle spindle, J. Physiol. 153:218-231, 1960.

37 Lowdon, B.J., and Moore, R.J.: Determinants and nature of intramuscular temperature changes during cold therapy, Am. J. Phys. Med. 54(5):223-233, 1975.

38 McMaster, W.C.: A literary review on ice therapy in injuries, Am. J. Sports Med. 5(3):124-126, 1977.

39 Miglietta, O.: Electromyographic characteristics of clonus and influence of cold, Arch. Phys. Med. Rehabil. 45:508, 1964.

40 Moore, R., Nicolette, R., and Behnke, R.: The therapeutic use of cold (cryotherapy) in the care of athletic injuries, Athl. Training 2:6-13, 1967.

41 Moore, R.: Uses of cold therapy in the rehabilitation of athletes, recent advances, Proceedings 19th American Medical Association National Conference on the medical aspects of sports, San Francisco, June 1977.

42 Murphy, A.J.: The physiological effects of cold application, Phys. Ther. Rev. 40(2):112-115, 1960.

43 Olson, J.E., and Stravino, V.: A review of cryotherapy, Phys. Ther. 52(8):840-853, 1972.

44 Prentice, W.E.: An electromyographic analysis of the effectiveness of heat or cold and stretching for inducing relaxation in injured muscle, J. Orthoped. Sports Phys. Ther. 3(3):133-146, 1982.

45 Rocks, J.A.: Intrinsic shoulder pain syndrome, Phys. Ther. 59(2):153-159, 1979.

46 Roy, S., and Irvin, R.: Sports medicine prevention, evaluation, management, and rehabilitation, Englewood Cliffs, N.J., 1983, Prentice-Hall, Inc., pp. 104-107.

47 Stillwell, K.: Therapeutic heat and cold. In Krusen, F., Kootke, F., and Ellwood, P.: Handbook of physical medicine and rehabilitation, Philadelphia, 1971, W.B. Saunders Co.

48 Travell, J.: Rapid relief of acute "stiff neck" by ethyl chloride spray, J. Am. Med. Wom. Assoc. 4(3):89-95, 1949.

49 Travell, J.: Ethyl chloride spray for painful muscle spasm, Arch. Phys. Med. Rehabil. 32:291-298, 1952.

50 Travell, J., and Simons, D.: Myofascial pain and dysfunction. The trigger point manual, Baltimore, 1983, Williams & Wilkins.

51 Zankel, H.: Effect of physical agents on motor conduction velocity of the ulnar nerve, Arch. Phys. Med. Rehabil. 47(12):787-792, 1966.

SUGGESTED READINGS

Abraham, E.: Whirlpool therapy for treatment of soft tissue wounds complicated by extremity fractures, J. Trauma 4:222, 1974.

Abraham, W.M.: Heat vs cold therapy for the treatment of muscle injuries, Athl. Train. 9(4):177, 1974.

Abramson, D.I., et al.: Changes in blood flow, O_2 uptake and tissue temperatures produced by therapeutic physical agents, III. Effect of indirect or reflex vasodilation, Am. J. Phys. Med. 405:5, 1961.

Abramson, D.I., et al.: Changes in blood flow, oxygen uptake and tissue temperatures produced by a topical application of wet heat, Arch. Phys. Med. Rehabil. 42:305, 1961.

Abramson, D.I., et al.: The effect of altering limb position on blood flow, O_2 uptake and skin temperature, J. Appl. Physiol. 17:191, 1962.

Abramson, D.I., et al.: Effect of paraffin bath and hot fomentation on local tissue temperature, Arch. Phys. Med. Rehabil. 45:87, 1965.

Abramson, D.I., et al.: Indirect vasodilation in thermotherapy, Arch. Phys. Med. Rehabil. 46:412, 1965.

Abramson, D.I.: Physiologic basis for the use of physical agents in peripheral vascular disorders, Arch. Phys. Med. Rehabil. 46:216, 1965.

Abramson D.I., et al.: Effect of tissue temperatures and blood flow on motor nerve conduction velocity, J.A.M.A. 198:1082, 1966.

Abramson, D.I., et al.: Comparison of wet and dry heat in raising temperature of tissues, Arch. Phys. Med. Rehabil. 48:654, 1967.

Arnheim, D.: Modern principles of athletic training, ed. 6, St. Louis, 1985, C.V. Mosby Co.

Ascenzi, J.: The need for decontamination and disinfection of hydrotherapy equipment, vol. 1, Surgikos, Inc, 1980, Asepsis Monograph.

Austin, K.F.: Diseases of immediate type hypersensitivity. In Isselbacher, K.J., et al., editors: Harrison's principles of internal medicine, ed. 9, New York, 1980, McGraw-Hill.

Barnes, L.: Cryotherapy: putting injury on ice, Phys. Sportsmed. 7(6):130-136, 1979.

Basur, R., Shephard, E., and Mouzos, G.: A cooling method in the treatment of ankle sprains, Practitioner 216:708, 1976.

Beasley, R., and Kester, N.: Principles of medical-surgical rehabilitation of the hand, Med. Clin. North Am. 53:645, 1969.

Benson, T.B., and Copp, E.P.: The effects of therapeutic forms of heat and ice on the pain threshold of the normal shoulder, Rheumatol. Rehabil. 13:101, 1974.

Berne, R., and Levy, M.N.: Cardiovascular physiology, ed 4, St. Louis, 1981, C.V. Mosby Co.

Bickle, R.J.: Swimming pool management, Physiotherapy 57:475, 1971.

Bierman, W.: Therapeutic use of cold, J.A.M.A. 157:1189-1192, 1955.

Boes, M.C.: Reduction of spasticity by cold, J. Am. Phys. Ther. Assoc. 42(1):29-32, 1962.

Boland, A.L.: Rehabilitation of the injured athlete. In Strauss, R.A., editor: Physiology, Philadelphia, 1979, W.B. Saunders Co., pp. 228-229.

Borrell, R.M., Parker, R., Henley, E.J., Masley, D., and Repinecz, M.: Comparison of in vivo temperatures produced by hydrotherapy, paraffin wax treatment, and fluidotherapy, Phys. Ther. 60(10):1273-1276, 1980.

Borrell, R.M., et al.: Fluidotherapy: evaluation of a new heat and modality, Arch. Phys. Med. Rehabil. 58:69, 1977.

Boyer, J.T., Fraser, J.R.E., and Doyle, A.E.: The haemodynamic effects of cold immersion, Clin. Sci. 19:539, 1980.

Boyle, R.W., Balisteri, F., and Osborne, F.: The value of the Hubbard tank as a diuretic agent, Arch. Phys. Med. Rehabil. 45:505, 1964.

Chastain, P.B.: The effect of deep heat on isometric strength, Phys. Ther. 58:543, 1978.

Claus-Walker, J., et al.: Physiological responses to cold stress in healthy subjects and in subjects with cervical cord injuries, Arch. Phys. Med. Rehabil. 55:485, 1974.

Clendenin, M.A., and Szumski, A.J.: Influence of cutaneous ice application on single motor units in humans, Phys. Ther. 51(2):166-175, 1971.

Clarke, K., editor: Fundamentals of athletic training: physical therapy procedures, Chicago, 1971, AMA Press, pp. 228-229.

Cobb, C.R., et al.: Electrical activity in muscle pain, Am. J. Phys. Med. 54:80, 1975.

Cobbold, A.F., and Lewis, O.J.: Blood flow to the knee joint of the dog: effect of heating, cooling and adrenaline, J. Physiol. **132:**379, 1956.

Cohen, A., Martin, G., and Wakim, K.: The effect of whirlpool bath with and without agitation on the circulation in normal and diseased extremities, Arch. Phys. Med. Rehabil. **30:**212, 1949.

Conolly, W.B., Paltos, N., and Tooth, R.M.: Cold Therapy—an improved method, Med. J. Aust. **2:**424, 1972.

Cordray, Y.M., and Krusen, E.M.: Use of hydrocollator packs in the treatment of neck and shoulder pains, Arch. Phys. Med. Rehabil. **39:**105, 1959.

Crockford, G.W., and Hellon, R.F.: Vascular responses of human skin to infra-red radiation, J. Physiol. **149:**424, 1959.

Crockford, G.W., Hellon, R.F., and Parkhouse, J.: Thermal vasomotor response in human skin mediated by local mechanism, J Physiol. **161:**10, 1962.

Currier, D.P., and Kramer, J.F.: Sensory nerve conduction: heating effects of ultrasound and infrared, Physiother. Can. **34:**241, 1982.

Dawson, W.J., et al.: Evaluation of cardiac output, cardiac work, and metabolic rate during hydrotherapy exercise in normal subjects, Arch. Phys. Med. Rehabil. **46:**605, 1965.

Day, M.J.: Hypersensitive response to ice massage: report of a case, Phys. Ther. **54:**592, 1974.

DeLateur, B.J., and Lehmann, J.F.: Cryotherapy. In Lehmann, J.F., editor: Therapeutic heat and cold, ed 3, Baltimore, 1982, Williams & Wilkins.

DeVries, H.: Quantitative electromyographic investigation of the spasms theory of muscle pain, Am. J. Phys. Med. **45:**119, 1966.

Drez, D., Faust, D.C., and Evans, J.P.: Cryotherapy and nerve palsy, Am. J. Sports Med. **9:**256, 1981.

Edwards, H.T., et al.: Effect of temperature on muscle energy metabolism and endurance during successive isometric contractions, sustained to fatigue, of the quadriceps muscle in man, J. Physiol. **220:**335, 1972.

Epstein, M.: Water immersion: modern researchers discover the secrets of an old folk remedy, Sciences, **205:**12, 1979.

Eyring, E.J., and Murray, W.R.: The effect of joint position on the pressure of intra-articular effusion, J. Bone Joint Surg. **46A**(6):1235, 1964.

Farry, P.J., and Prentice, N.G.: Ice treatment of injured ligaments: an experimental model, N.Z. Med. J. **9:**12, 1980.

Folkow, B., et al.: Studies on the reactions of the cutaneous vessels to cold exposure, Acta Physiol. Scand. **58:**342, 1963.

Fountain, F.P., Gersten, J.W., and Senger, O.: Decrease in muscle spasm produced by ultrasound, hot packs and IR, Arch. Phys. Med. Rehabil. **41:**293, 1960.

Fox, R.H.: Local cooling in man, Br. Med. Bull. **17**(1):14-18, 1961.

Fox, R.H., and Wyatt, H.T.: Cold-induced vasodilation in various areas of the body surface in man, J. Physiol. **162:**289, 1962.

Gammon, G.D., and Starr, I.: Studies on the relief of pain by counterirritation, J. Clin. Invest. **20:**13, 1941.

Gieck, J.: Precautions for hydrotherapeutic devices, Clinical Management **3:**44, 1983.

Golland, A.: Basic hydrotherapy, Physiotherapy **67:**258, 1981.

Greenberg, R.S.: The effects of hot packs and exercise on local blood flow, Phys. Ther. **52:**273, 1972.

Halkovich, I.R., et al.: Effect of Fluori-Methane® spray on passive hip flexion, Phys. Ther. **61:**185, 1981.

Harrison, R.A.: Tolerance of pool therapy by ankylosing spondylitis patients with low vital capacity, Physiotherapy **67:**296, 1981.

Harrison, A.S., et al.: The effect of heat and stretching on the range of hip motion, J. Ortho. Sports Phys. Ther. **6:**110, 1984.

Head, M.D., and Helms, P.A.: Paraffin and sustained stretching in the treatment of burn contractures, Burns **4:**136, 1977.

Hellerbrand, T., Holutz, S., and Eubank, I.: Measurement of whirlpool temperature, pressure and turbulence, Arch. Phys. Med. Rehabil. **32:**17, 1950.

Hendler, E., Crosbie, R., and Hardy, J.D.: Measurement of heating of the skin during exposure to infrared radiation, J. Appl. Physiol. **12:**177, 1958.

Hocutt, J.E., et al.: Cryotherapy in ankle sprains, Am. J. Sports Med. **10:**316, 1982.

Holmes, G.: Hydrotherapy as a means of rehabilitation, Br. J. Phys. Med. **5:**93, 1942.

Horton, B.T., Brown, G.E., and Roth, G.M.: Hypersensitiveness to cold with local and systemic manifestations of a histamine-like character: its amenability to treatment, J.A.M.A. **107:**1263, 1936.

Horvath, S.M., and Hollander, J.L.: Intra-articular temperature as a measure of joint reaction, J. Clin. Invest. **28:**469, 1949.

Hunter, J., and Mackin, E.: Edema and bandaging. In Hunter, J., et al, editors: Rehabilitation of the hand, ed. 1, St. Louis, 1978, C.V. Mosby.

Jessup, G.T.: Muscle soreness: temporary distress of injury? Athl. Train. **15**(4):260, 1980.

Jezdinsky, J., Marek, J., and Ochonsky, P.: Effects of local cold and heat therapy on traumatic oedema of the rat hind paw. I. Effects of cooling on the course of traumatic oedema, Acta Universitatis Palackianae Olomucensis Facultatis Medicae **66:**185, 1973.

Johnson, D.J., et al.: Effect of cold submersion on intramuscular temperature of the gastrocnemius muscle, Phys. Ther. **59:**1238, 1979.

Johnson, J., and Leider, F.E.: Influence of cold bath on maximum handgrip strength, Percept. Mot. Skills **44:**323, 1977.

Kessler, R.M., and Hertling, D.: Management of common musculoskeletal disorders, Philadelphia, 1983, Harper & Row.

Kowal M.A.: Review of physiological effects of cryotherapy, J. Orth. Sports Phys. Ther. **5**(2):66-73, 1983.

Kramer, J.F., and Mendryk, S.W.: Cold in the initial treatment of injuries sustained in physical activity programs, Can. Assoc. Health Phys. Ed. Rec. J. **45**(4):27-29, 38-40, 1979.

Krusen, E.M. et al.: Effects of hot packs on peripheral circulation, Arch. Phys. Med. **31:**145, 1950.

Landen, B.R.: Heat or cold for the relief of low back pain? Phys. Ther. **47:**1126, 1967.

Lane, L.E.: Localized hypothermia for the relief of pain in musculoskeletal injuries, Phys. Ther. **51:**182, 1971.

Lee, J.M., Warren, M.P., and Mason, S.M.: Effects of ice on nerve conduction velocity, Physiotherapy **64**:2, 1978.

Lehmann, J.F.: Effect of therapeutic temperatures on tendon extensibility, Arch. Phys. Med. Rehabil. **51**:481, 1970.

Lehmann, J.D., Brunner, G.D., and Stow, R.W.: Pain threshold measurements after therapeutic application of ultrasound, microwaves and infrared, Arch. Phys. Med. Rehabil. **39**:560, 1958.

Lehmann, J.F., et al.: Temperature distributions in the human thigh produced by infrared, hot pack and microwave applications, Arch. Phys. Med. Rehabil. **47**:291, 1966.

Levine, M.G., et al.: Relaxation of spasticity by physiological techniques, Arch. Phys. Med. Rehabil. **35**:214, 454.

Lundgren, C., Muren, A., and Zederfeldt, B.: Effect of cold vasoconstriction on wound healing in the rabbit, Acta. Chir. Scand. **118**:1, 1959.

Magness, J., Garrett, T., and Erickson, D.: Swelling of the upper extremity during whirlpool baths, Arch. Phys. Med. Rehabil. **51**:297, 1970.

Major, T.C., Schwinghamer, J.M., and Winston, S.: Cutaneous and skeletal muscle vascular responses to hypothermia, Am. J. Physiol. **240** (Heart Circ. Physiol. **9**):H868, 1981.

Marek, J., Jezdinsky, J., and Ochonsky, P.: Effects of local cold and heat therapy on traumatic oedema of the rat hind paw. II. Effects of various kinds of compresses on the course of traumatic oedema. Acta Universitatis Palackianae Olomucensis Facultatis Medicae **66**:203, 1973.

Matsen, F.A., Questad, K., and Matsen A.L.: The effect of local cooling on post fracture swelling, Clin. Orthop. **109**:201, 1975.

McGown, H.L.: Effects of cold application on maximal isometric contraction, Phys. Ther. **47**:185, 1967.

McGray, R.E., and Patton, N.J.: Pain relief at trigger points: a comparison of moist heat and shortwave diathermy, J. Ortho. Sports Phys. Ther. **5**:175, 1984.

McMaster, W.C.: Cryotherapy, Physician Sports Med. **10**(11):112-119, 1982.

McMaster, W.C., and Liddle, S.: Cryotherapy influence on posttraumatic limb edema, Clin. Orthop. **150**:283-287.

McMaster, W.C., Liddle, S., and Waugh, T.R.: Laboratory evaluation of various cold therapy modalities, Am. J. Sports Med. **6**(5):291-294, 1978.

Mennel, J.M.: The therapeutic use of cold, J. Am. Osteopathic Assoc. **74**:1146-1157, 1975.

Mense, S.: Effects of temperature on the discharges of muscle spindles and tendon organs, Pflugers Arch. **374**:159, 1978.

Miglietta, O.: Action of cold on spasticity, Am. J. Phys. Med. **52**(4):198-205, 1973.

Michalski, W.J., and Sequin, J.J.: The effects of muscle cooling and stretch on muscle spindle secondary endings in the cat, J. Physiol. **253**:341-356, 1975.

Newton, M.J., and Lehmkuhl, D.: Muscle spindle response to body heating and localized muscle cooling: implications for relief of spasticity, J. Am. Phys. Ther. Assoc. **45**(2):91-105, 1965.

Nylin, J.: The use of water in therapeutics, Arch. Phys. Med. Rehabil. **13**:261, 1932.

Oliver, R.A.: Johnson, D.J., Wheelhouse, W.W., and Griffin,

P.P.: Isometric muscle contraction response during recovery from reduced intramuscular temperature, Arch. Phys. Med. Rehabil. **60**:126-129, 1979.

Perkins, J., et al.: Cooling and contraction of smooth muscle, Am. J. Physiol. **163**:14, 1950.

Petajan, J.H., and Watts, N.: Effects of cooling on the triceps surae reflex, Am. J. Phys. Med. **42**:240-251, 1962.

Pope, C.: Physiologic action and therapeutic value of general and local whirlpool baths, Arch. Phys. Med. Rehabil. **10**:498, 1929.

Randall, B.F., Imig, C.J., and Hines, H.M.: Effects of some physical therapies on blood flow, Arch. Phys. Med. **33**:73, 1952.

Randt, G.A.: Hot tub folliculitis, Physician Sports Med. **11**:75, 1983.

Ritzmann, S.E., and Levin, W.C.: Cryopathies: a review, Arch. Intern. Med. **107**:186, 1961.

Roberts, P.: Hydrotherapy: its history, theory and practice, Occupational Health **235**:5, 1981.

Schaubel, H.H.: Local use of ice after orthopedic procedures, Am. J. Surg. **72**:711, 1946.

Schultz, K.: The effect of active exercise during whirlpool on the hand, unpublished thesis. San Jose, CA, 1982, San Jose State University.

Shelley, W.B., and Caro, W.A.: Cold erythema: a new hypersensitivity syndrome, J.A.M.A. **180**:639, 1962.

Simonetti, A., Miller, R., and Gristina, J.: Efficacy of povidone-iodine in the disinfection of whirlpool baths and hubbard tanks, Phys. Ther. **52**:450, 1972.

Steve, L., Goodhart, P., and Alexander, J.: Hydrotherapy burn treatment: use of chloramine-T against resistant microorganisms, Arch. Phys. Med. Rehabil. **60**:301, 1979.

Stewart, J.B., and Basmajian, J.V.: Exercises in water. In Basmajian, J.V., editor: Therapeutic exercise, ed 3, Baltimore, 1978, Williams & Wilkins.

Strandness, D.E.: Vascular diseases of the extremities. In Isselbacher, K.J., et al., editors: Harrison's principles of internal medicine, ed. 9, New York, 1980, McGraw-Hill.

Travell, J.G., and Simons, D.G.: Myofascial pain and dysfunction. The trigger point manual, Baltimore, 1983, Williams & Wilkins.

Urbscheit, N., Johnston, R., and Bishop, B.: Effects of cooling on the ankle jerk and H-response in hemiplegic patients, Phys. Ther. **51**:983, 1971.

Wakim, K.G. Porter, A.N., and Krusen, K.H.: Influence of physical agents and of certain drugs on intra-articular temperature, Arch. Phys. Med. **32**:714, 1951.

Walsh, M.: Relationship of hand edema to upper extremity position and water temperature during whirlpool treatments in normals, Unpublished thesis. Philadelphia, 1983, Temple University.

Warren, C.G.: The use of heat and cold in the treatment of common musculoskeletal disorders. In Kessler, R.M., and Hertling, D.: Management of common musculoskeletal disorders, Philadelphia, 1983, Harper & Row.

Warren, G.C., Lehmann, J.F., and Koblanski, J.N.: Heat and stretch procedures: an evaluation using rat tail tendon, Arch. Phys. Med. Rehabil. **57**:122, 1976.

Watkins, A.L.: A manual of electrotherapy, ed. 3, Philadelphia, 1972, Lea & Febiger, pp. 7-32.

Waylonis, G.W.: The physiological effect of ice massage, Arch. Phys. Med. Rehabil. **48:**37-42, 1967.

Wessman, M.S., and Kottke, F.J.: The effect of indirect heating on peripheral blood flow, pulse rate, blood pressure and temperature, Arch. Phys. Med. Rehabil. **48:**567, 1967.

Whyte, H.M., and Reader, S.R.: Effectiveness of different forms of heating, Ann. Rheum. Dis. **10:**449, 1951.

Wickstrom, R. and Polk, C.: Effect of whirlpool on the strength endurance of the quadriceps muscle in trained male adolescents, Am. J. Phys. Med. **40:**91, 1961.

Wolf, S.L., and Basmajian, J.V.: Intramuscular temperature changes deep to localized cutaneous cold stimulation, Phys. Ther. **53**(12):1284-1288, 1973.

Wolf, S.L., and Letbetter, W.D.: Effect of skin cooling on spontaneous EMG activity in triceps surae of the decerebrate cat, Brain Res. **91:**151-155, 1975.

Wright, V., and Johns, R.J.: Physical factors concerned with the stiffness of normal and diseased joints, Bull. Johns Hopkins Hosp. **106:**215, 1960.

Wyper, D.J., and McNiven, D.R.: Effects of some physiotherapeutic agents on skeletal muscle blood flow, Physiotherapy **62:**83, 1976.

Yackzan, L., Adams, C., and Francis, K.T.: The effects of ice massage in delayed muscle soreness, Am. J. Sports Med. **12**(2):159-165, 1984.

Zankel, H.T.: Effect of physical agents on motor conduction velocity of the ulnar nerve, Arch. Phys. Med. Rehabil. **47:**787, 1966.

Zeiter, W.J.: Clinical application of the paraffin bath, Arch. Phys. Ther. **20:**469, 1939.

Zislis, J.: Hydrotherapy. In Krusen, F., editor: Handbook of physical medicine and rehabilitation, ed 2, Philadelphia, 1971, W.B. Saunders Co.

Ultrasound

6

John C. Spiker

OBJECTIVES

Following completion of this chapter, the student will be able to:

- Explain the mechanics of the ultrasound machine.

- List tissues and conditions that are most affected by ultrasound and indications for its use.

- Administer proper treatment.

- List all contraindications to the use of ultrasound.

- Explain phonophoresis and list the indications for its use.

Ultrasound has become an accepted modality in the treatment of athletic injuries during the last three to four decades. Its use continues to become more judicious as we learn more about the healing process and the effect of ultrasound on that process.

Ultrasound is truly a therapeutic modality that aids sports therapists in their attempts to return athletes to preinjury status. Before being administered, however, it must be preceded by an orthopedic evaluation to determine the tissues involved, the degree of injury, and the status of the healing process.

Ultrasound must be respected for the significant effects it produces on a variety of tissues and for its depth of penetration. It is generally classified as a deep heating modality. In the hands of individuals who do not understand its effects and those who would administer it before an appropriate musculoskeletal examination, it is a modality that could be more of a liability than a benefit.

Ultrasound falls under the classification of the acoustic spectrum rather than the electromagnetic spectrum. Sound waves that are at a higher frequency than are detectable by the human ear are termed *ultrasound*. Therefore frequencies above 16,000 to 20,000 **hertz** (Hz) are defined as ultrasound. Standard therapeutic units used on the musculoskeletal system operate at a frequency between 800,000 and 1,000,000 cycles per second (Hz).[3] Many applications of ultrasound with quite varied frequencies are used in industry and medicine today. Uses range from fish finding and burglar alarms to diagnosing tumors and examining a fetus. For the sports therapist, the major purpose for using ultrasound is the treatment of soft tissue injury. The propagation of ultrasonic energy in biologic tissue depends on the absorption characteristics of the tissue, as well as on the density of the tissue.[6] A major advantage of ultrasound is its capability of heating deeper tissues without producing significant heating of the more superficial tissues.

ANATOMY OF EQUIPMENT

Ultrasound machines are not as mechanically and electrically complex as many other therapeutic modalities. A high-frequency generator provides electricity via a **coaxial cable** to the "hot" electrode in the **transducer.** The transducer contains a **crystal** made of quartz or a synthetic ceramic. The sound head also includes an insulator and a metal front plate that serves as the surface of the applicator (Fig. 6-1).

The unit also contains a timer directly linked to the on-off switch and either a digital display or meter that shows the output of the total number of watts and the watts per square centimeter of the surface of the sound head (Fig. 6-2).

Physics

The transducer is the key part of the ultrasound machine. It is the device that converts one form of energy to another. The transducer in the ultrasound machine converts electrical energy to acoustic energy, resulting in mechanical deformation of the crystal. Crystals (2 to 3 mm thick) of certain materials are such that when voltage is applied to them, they change shape. The opposite is also true, in that when the crystal material is compressed, a voltage is developed across it. This phenomenon of crystal vibration when an electrical field is applied to it is known as the **piezoelectric effect.** The most common piezoelectric material used in the crystal is quartz. Other materials that may be used as the crystal are lead zirconate titanate, barium titanate, nickel, and nickel-cobalt ferrite. When quartz is used, a high amount of voltage is necessary because it is a high-impedance substance. Thick, well-insulated cables (coaxial) are used to deliver the electricity.[10]

As the electrical energy is received by the electrode in the transducer, re-

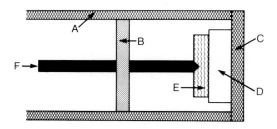

Figure 6-1. Anatomy of an ultrasound applicator: *(A)* metal housing, *(B)* insulator, *(C)* front plate, *(D)* quartz crystal, *(E)* active electrode and reflecting chamber, and *(F)* coaxial cable.

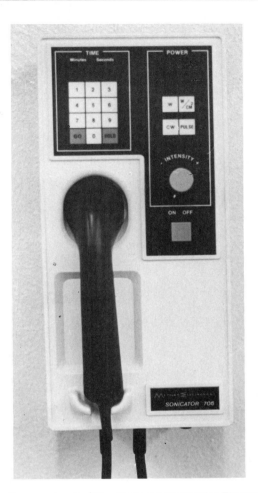

Figure 6-2. Portable ultrasound unit. (Manufactured by Mettler Electronics, Anaheim, Calif.)

peated changes occur in the thickness of the crystal proportional to the frequency of the unit. This frequency ranges from 800,000 to 1,000,000 times per second and is specified on the unit. The result of this alternation of size of the crystal is a mechanical vibratory motion that is passed on through the transducer head to the various tissues in the local area being treated.[14]

Sound waves, unlike electromagnetic radiations, are most effectively transmitted through dense materials. They travel through biologic tissues at an average of about 1540 meters per second, with a wavelength of 1.5 mm. At a frequency of 1 MHz there is little divergence of the sound wave, and consequently energy is concentrated in a limited area. As the sound wave travels through the various tissues, there is **attenuation** or a decrease in energy owing to both absorption and dispersion of the sound wave. Absorption increases as the frequency increases, thus less energy is transmitted to the deeper tissues.[22]

The amount of energy absorbed or reflected is dependent on the different acoustic impedances of the tissues. Interfaces such as bone-muscle produce high impedance values. Significant variations in tissue density are reported to exist in homogeneous tissues, resulting in varied amounts of absorption and reflection of ultrasonic energy within and between tissue types.

Ultrasound is an extremely effective clinical modality in a sports medicine setting. Its effectiveness may be attributed to a combination of both thermal and mechanical factors.

EFFECTS

Physiologic effects that occur because of heating of tissues are referred to as *thermal*. Ultrasound is used primarily by the sports therapist for the purpose of elevating temperature in deep tissues to a depth of 5 cm or greater. Many of the effects of ultrasound are attributed to heat, as was reviewed in Chapter 5. It is generally accepted that heat produces the following results:

1. Increases the extensibility of collagen tissue
2. Decreases joint stiffness
3. Increases the pain threshold
4. Reduces muscle spasm
5. Assists in mobilizing inflammatory infiltrates, edema, and exudates
6. Increases blood flow
7. Increases local metabolism
8. Increases nerve conduction velocities[11]

The effects listed are obviously beneficial and necessary in the rehabilitation process. If ultrasound produced only these thermal effects, it would still be a worthwhile modality.

When energy is added to the body in the form of sound waves, it is absorbed, transmitted, reflected, or refracted.[8] Penetration and absorption are inversely related (Table 6-1). Tissues of high water content have a low rate of absorption (thereby a high rate of penetration) while tissues of high protein content have a high rate of absorption. Fat has a relatively low absorption rate, and muscle absorbs considerably more. Bone that is rather superficial absorbs more ultrasonic energy than any of the other tissues. This is thought to be because of

TABLE 6-1

Relationship between Absorption and Penetration (Ultrasonic Frequency = 1 Megacycle)

Media	Absorption	Penetration
Water	1	1200
Blood plasma	23	52
Whole blood	60	20
Fat	390	4
Skeletal muscle	663	2
Peripheral nerve	1193	1

From Griffin, J.E.: J. Am. Phys. Ther. **46**(1):18-26, 1966. Reprinted with permission of the American Physical Therapy Association.

the high protein content and density of bone compared with other tissue. Pohlman[19] has shown a reflection rate of 35% when the energy was directed perpendicular to the bone. Peripheral nerve absorbs at a rate approximately twice that of muscle. It has been concluded that soft tissue in close proximity to bone receives more of the effects of ultrasound because of a rebound phenomenon. Therefore, joint structures such as the **periosteum,** capsule, tendon, and **extracapsular ligament** are significantly affected by ultrasound treatment. Gersten[4] has shown more thermal effects on or near bone than in fat. It has also been demonstrated that ultrasound raises the temperature in the collagen tissues of tendon.[4] Increases in the extensibility of tight capsular tissue and in the mobility of mature scar tissue have been proven with ultrasound and exercise.[1]

The effects of the high absorption rate on peripheral nerve have been a source of controversy. Research is available that demonstrates increases in the nerve conduction velocity of peripheral nerves, while other studies demonstrate a decrease in the conduction velocity. It is not yet clearly understood whether the thermal or mechanical effects of ultrasound cause the changes in the conduction velocity of peripheral nerve.[11]

Ultrasound produces the desirable therapeutic effects of any deep-heat modality. The effect of ultrasound that may be the most distinguishable is its ability to selectively increase temperature in local, well-circumscribed areas.

Effects at the cellular level that are the result of the vibratory motion are referred to as **mechanical effects. Cavitation** is the mechanical vibration of small gas bubbles located in blood or fluids. The expansion and contraction of these bubbles alters the permeability of cell membranes and thus cell function.[17] It should also be added that if the intensity of this vibration is great enough, the bubbles may collapse and tissue damage may result. Cavitation results within the intensity ranges used with therapeutic ultrasound.

Few studies provide evidence of isolated mechanical effects. Acceleration in the rate of **diffusion** across membranes has, however, been shown to be a result of mechanical vibration.[16] This results in increased blood flow and consequently absorption of the by-products of the healing process, thus facilitating that process. This in itself is significant to consider when an injury is in an acute or subacute phase.

TECHNIQUES

The machine should be turned on with the intensity at the lowest allowable setting. Only after the **coupling agent** has been spread over the area with the head should the intensity be adjusted to the desired level. Having the intensity turned up when the head is not in contact with the coupling agent can result in damage to the crystal.

The theory behind the development and use of pulsed ultrasound is that the mechanical effects can be produced without thermal effects. The pulsed beams, as compared with continuous beams, allow for a rest period for cooling purposes. As more research becomes available to support the isolated benefits of the mechanical effects, this method should gain more popularity. The primary indication for such a treatment would be when the thermal effects are undesirable. If a duty cycle of 20% is selected there will be only a slight temperature increase. As the duty cycle increases, tissue temperatures will also increase.

Stationary versus Moving Transducer

Ultrasound may be administered by either moving the transducer or holding it stationary (Fig. 6-3). The moving technique is recommended with continuous ultrasound so that energy will be distributed as evenly as possible in the treatment area. The applicator is moved very slowly (4 centimeters per second) in either a circular or longitudinal pattern. With the moving technique, the total energy delivered to the treatment area will be decreased. However, there is less danger of creating **hot spots** or areas where tissue is heated excessively, thus causing damage. The area being treated should be considerably larger than the size of the particular head so that one area is not receiving continuous administration. For this reason, it is advisable to have a unit with a small sound head (2 to 5 square centimeters) and a large one (approximately 10 square centimeters) (Fig. 6-4). The head should be held so that it is all in contact with the body area being treated. This is difficult over irregular surfaces. The administrator of the treatment need not deliver pressure by pressing the head tightly to the body part.

The stationary technique is sometimes used when treating a small area or when the surface contour is uneven. This technique is thought to produce an uneven distribution of energy in the tissues, which may result in hot spots.

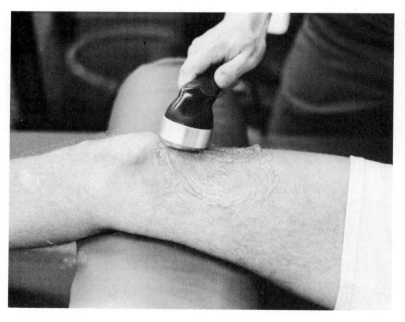

Figure 6-3. Technique of ultrasound administration to the anterior thigh.

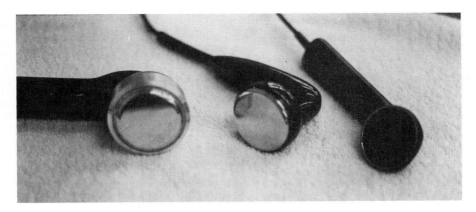

Figure 6-4. Various sizes of ultrasound applicator heads.

Pulsed ultrasound is most often used with the stationary technique. The use of continuous ultrasound is contraindicated with this technique except at extremely low intensities.

Since sound waves rely on molecular collision for transmission, a coupling agent must be used to reduce the attenuation at the tissue/air interface. The coupling medium must have good lubricating qualities so that the applicator can glide against the skin on even very hairy individuals without significant friction. There are many commercial gels on the market to serve as this medium. Studies have been done that showed no significant difference between the common commercial gels, mineral oil, and degassed water.[21] Conflicting evidence was made available by Griffin's study,[9] which compared the transmissiveness of ultrasonic energy through large volumes of tap water, glycerin, and mineral oil and showed a significantly better transmissiveness through water than through the other two substances. Griffin also found that the glycerin and mineral oil produced a significantly greater increase in tissue temperature than was produced when using water.

Lehmann et al.[15] found in their studies that the temperature of the coupling medium has a significant effect on the response to ultrasound. The study demonstrated that coupling mediums at 18° C (64.4° F) or less were most effective at increasing the temperatures of the deeper tissues. Cooling the sound head prior to treatment may result in more effective results because of this phenomenon. One might surmise from this that ultrasound would be less effective when used following a superficial hot pack application. Those who do use hot packs prior to ultrasound argue that the increased blood flow from the superficial heat cools the tissues enough that the subsequent ultrasound treatment is still effective in heating deep tissues.

One may conclude then, from this evidence, that because of the greater temperature gradient, the application of ice prior to ultrasound would provide

Coupling Agents

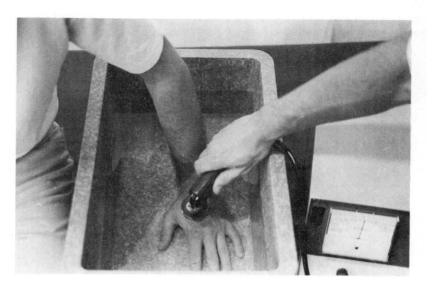

Figure 6-5. Application of ultrasound under water. The sound transducer should not be in contact with the skin.

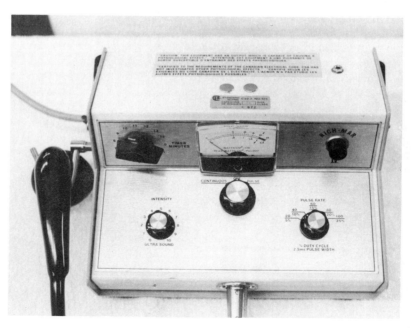

Figure 6-6. Ultrasound unit capable of either pulsed or continuous ultrasound. (Manufactured by Rich-Mar, Tulsa, OK.)

the most deep-heating effects. One must be aware, however, that such application may produce an **anesthesia** (loss of sensation) that is undesirable, eliminating the normal feedback that is necessary to determine correct intensity settings.

Underwater Application

Ultrasound can be used effectively under water to treat irregular surfaces such as a hand (Fig. 6-5). The sound head need not be in contact with the body part and is moved in a circular fashion. The applicator should be approximately ½ inch from the body part, and the intensity setting is the same as for regular application. Bubble formation sometimes occurs over the head as a result of gaseous separation and needs to be wiped off by the person administering the treatment. This degassing process is done by simply rubbing the bubbles off with the fingers and proceeding with the treatment.

Safety precautions such as those indicated in Chapter 3 should be taken to be certain that there is no electrical short anywhere within the system. Such a condition could obviously result in either the patient or administrator being shocked or even electrocuted.

Continuous versus Pulsed

Most ultrasound units are capable of producing either continuous or pulsed ultrasound (Fig. 6-6). With continuous ultrasound the intensity of the sound remains constant throughout the treatment, whereas pulsed ultrasound is periodically interrupted. The term *duty cycle* refers to the percentage of time that ultrasound is on during a pulse period. The mathematical calculation of the duty cycle is as follows:[22]

$$\text{Duty cycle} = \frac{\text{time on (duration of pulse)}}{\text{time on + time off (pulse period)}}$$

Most ultrasound machines have duty cycles preset at either 20% or 50%.

Dosage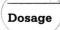

Care must be taken to determine the proper dosage when administering ultrasound. The meter on the machine shows the watts per square centimeter and the total watts being administered. Specific settings, however, do not predict the effectiveness of the treatment. Intensities may range between 0.5 and 3.0 watts per square centimeter. Higher settings (above 1.5 watts per square centimeter) often need to be used for heating deep tissues. Much lower settings (as low as 0.5 watts per square centimeter) may be used for superficial problems. Structures with little soft tissue or bone near the surface need to be treated with lower intensities. Settings that are too high for the area being treated produce periosteal pain.

Most advocates of ultrasound state that the patient should feel nothing more than movement of the sound head over the area. Some clinicians, however, feel that the intensity should be set so that mild warmth is felt locally by the patient. The treatment should not produce reports of pain from the patient. If the patient reports that the transducer feels hot at the skin surface, either the coupling agent is inadequate or the crystal has been damaged and the sound head is overheating.

Tissue treatments are recommended to be from 5 to 10 minutes, depending on the size of the area being treated. A very local area such as the common extensor tendon of the elbow would be treated for 5 minutes, while a significantly larger area could be treated for up to 10 minutes.

COMMON INDICATIONS

Ultrasound has been scientifically proven to be effective in some situations. In many other situations, pure scientific evidence may be lacking but experienced practitioners are confident in their results using this modality. Studies done by a variety of people have proven the increase in tissue temperature. Research by Gersten demonstrated that ultrasound had a significant effect on the extensibility of connective tissue, which is located in adhesions, tendon, fibrotic muscle, and joint capsule.[4] Most practitioners follow ultrasound treatment with appropriate stretching exercises to increase joint motion.

Ultrasound is the treatment of choice when it is desirable to provide deep heat. It is particularly effective in obese individuals since fatty tissue does not absorb a great amount of ultrasound. The effective power can, therefore, reach the structures desired.

There are many injuries that occur in athletics that respond quite well to ultrasound. The most common of these are **overuse syndromes** that occur to tendons. This is because of the high affinity of ultrasound for protein, which is abundant in tendons. Ultrasound is an appropriate modality to use on Achilles, patellar, and other tendinous structures that frequently suffer from overuse trauma.

Muscle spasms, such as those commonly seen in the rhomboids, erector spinae, and trapezius in athletes, are treated effectively with ultrasound, heat or ice, and appropriate exercise. Muscle spasm is the pathologic condition in athletes to which ultrasound has traditionally been applied the most.

Undesirable joint tightness that is not the result of a fracture is treated effectively with ultrasound. When such stiffness occurs in a joint that has a fracture that is not yet calcified, it should not be treated because ultrasound may cause breakdown of the new **calcification** of the fracture site. Tight joint capsule structures, such as occur with adhesive capsulitis in the shoulder, are helped to return to normal with the use of ultrasound.

Areas of mature, undesired calcification are often effectively treated with ultrasound. **Calcific bursitis** in the subdeltoid bursae of the shoulder is one such condition. **Myositis ossificans** that is usually caused by repeated contusions to the midhumerus and the anterior femur can be treated effectively if these areas are no longer being continually irritated and appear as mature bone radiographically.

One of the most dramatic and conclusive cases in which I have used ultrasound was with an athlete who had an **exostosis** (calcific growth) on his tibia that became intermittently symptomatic. Approximately eight ultrasound treatments relieved the symptoms and allowed full participation in two separate episodes approximately 2 years apart. Although a number of case reports support this observation, there are no scientific investigations that verify this use.

Ultrasound is effective at breaking down adhesions. It also is effective in reducing the symptoms from an inflamed synovial **plica** (fold in synovial membrane medial to patella) in the knee.

Pain reduction is a goal of ultrasound treatment in some instances. The reduction of pain following treatment is seldom dramatic and is difficult to document. Pain reduction from ultrasound treatments is usually secondary to the reduction of muscle spasm.

Ultrasound has been reported to be effective in the treatment of plantar warts. Treatment regimens have recommended 0.6 watts/per square centimeter for 15 minutes with from 2 to 15 treatment sessions.[2]

DANGERS AND CONTRA-INDICATIONS

The use of ultrasound is contraindicated in acute and postacute injuries. Care must be taken to avoid using any deep heating modality until the possibility of bleeding and swelling no longer exists. There are a number of other conditions in which ultrasound is contraindicated. No part of the central nervous system (brain or spinal cord) or reproductive organs should be treated with ultrasound. Patients with **thrombophlebitis** (blood clot within an inflamed vein) should not be treated with ultrasound because of the possible dislodging of a clot that could result in an obstruction in a vital organ.[18] Vascular problems are uncommon in athletes, but it is dangerous to administer ultrasound to a person with such a condition because of the possibility of an emboli. Any acute **sepsis** of tissue should not be treated with ultrasound. Infectious conditions and tumors or cysts should also not be treated with ultrasound. No part of the abdomen should be treated on any woman who may be pregnant because of the possibility of fetal damage. No one with cardiac disease should be treated over the **cervical ganglia, stellate ganglion,** the thorax in the region of the heart, or the **vagus nerve** because a reflex action could occur with a resultant change in the cardiac rate. People with diabetes who receive ultrasound treatments should be encouraged to rest after treatment because a slight reduction in blood sugar has been reported during the treatment.[18]

A common mistake made by practitioners is the use of ultrasound too soon. There is no place for continuous ultrasound in acute injury treatment, although pulsed ultrasound may be used immediately after injury for pain. Use of continuous ultrasound in this phase may lead to an exacerbation of symptoms in the form of pain or swelling. A situation in which this principle is often violated and results in complications is an acute thigh contusion. Treatment with ultrasound prior to the complete calcification process of bone results in increased inflammation and often contributes to the development or irritation of an already existing **hematoma** in the involved muscle. This also contributes to the likelihood of undesirable bone formation in the hematoma. Orthopedic surgeons generally agree that it requires many months for new calcification to become mature. If myositis ossificans is still in the developmental stages as documented radiographically, ultrasound is contraindicated.

Ultrasound should also not be administered immediately after exercise of an injured area. Any inflammation that the exercise may have produced would only be increased by the ultrasound.

Healing fractures should never be treated with ultrasound. Such a treatment could retard the calcification process of the healing bone.

Inappropriate administration of ultrasound is sometimes a problem. No pain should be felt during the time that ultrasound is administered. Pain felt when the intensity is set too high or the sound head is being moved too slowly comes from the periosteum and indicates incorrect technique. Patients without normal sensation in the area should not be treated with ultrasound because this feedback is essential. Oakley reports that "pins and needles" may be felt by the patient if the bone in the area being treated is overheated.[18] A burning sensation is reported by the patient if the administration is not appropriate and the area is overheated.

Caution should be exercised when using ultrasound at high intensities over epiphyseal areas in children. Normal therapeutic intensities appear to cause no harm; however, intensities above 3 watts per square centimeter have been shown to produce retardation of growth and bone demineralization.[20]

Metal Implants

It has been assumed by many clinicians that metal implants provide a contraindication to the use of ultrasound in a local area. Studies by Gersten[5] and Lehmann[15] indicate that metal carries the heat away so quickly that it causes no danger to the surrounding tissue. This is because of the low specific heat of metals. Ultrasound is, therefore, not contraindicated for people with **metal implants.** However, research has yet to be done to prove how much heat is absorbed by modern joint replacement synthetics.

PHONOPHORESIS

Phonophoresis is a technique in which a topical application of a selected medication is driven to deep tissue. The first reporting of this technique of driving in whole molecules of medication appeared in the 1960s and 1970s, but it is still considered to be a rather new treatment approach. In athletics, it is probably safe to say that it has been used commonly only in the past decade.

Phonophoresis has proved to be an effective treatment approach to get medication to an area without having to undergo painful and sometimes poorly placed injections. The risks of injection and the anxiety accompanying them are, therefore, avoided.

The technique involves using a **hydrocortisone** cream or ointment in the coupling agent for the application of ultrasound (Fig. 6-7). The technique of administering this treatment is no different from that of conventional ultrasound with the exception of the medium.

Griffin et al.[7] conducted a double-blind study comparing the effects of hydrocortisone phonophoresis and the use of ultrasound with conventional technique. In this series of 102 patients with chronic inflammatory conditions of peripheral joints, 68% became pain free and gained full active range of motion when it had been limited before; 18% were partially improved with the hydrocortisone treatment.

Caution must be exercised when using hydrocortisone cream over joint structures. A recent study by Hereford showed that repeated ultrasound treatments with hydrocortisone appeared to result in degeneration of the articular

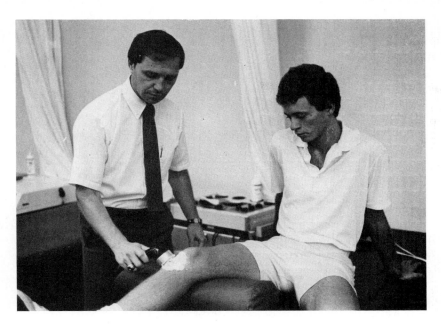

Figure 6-7. Phonophoresis uses ultrasound to drive ions into an injured area.

cartilage and that the effects may be more severe than those occurring with in-tra-articular injection.[12]

Studies have been done comparing 1% and 10% hydrocortisone cream when using phonophoresis. In a study of 285 patients treated for a variety of common inflammatory conditions, the 10% preparation was definitely superior to the 1% preparation at producing desired results.[13]

Questions have been raised concerning the possible weakening of tendons with the use of phonophoresis, as has been reported following repeated **percutaneous injections.** No clinical evidence is presently available to indicate that the levels of cortisone in the treated tendons place the structures in jeopardy.

Various protocols are used in the administration of phonophoresis. It is generally agreed by clinicians that this treatment should not go on indefinitely. Most clinicians use the treatment for 3 or 4 consecutive days (one time per day) to determine if positive effects are occurring. For those individuals who are obtaining a desirable response, treatment is continued on a daily basis over the next week or so. Stopping at a total of 10 treatments is reasonable and usually produces a desired result. It should be pointed out that ice massage and stretching exercises are often used concurrently.

Common extensor tendon inflammation (tennis elbow) has been shown to respond quite well to this treatment. Achilles, patellar, and bicipital tendonitis also respond favorably to this treatment.

Chronic suprahumural impingement in the shoulder responds quite well to the administration of 9 minutes of phonophoresis; 3 minutes each to the anterior, lateral, and posterior aspects is recommended. The arm is held in internal rotation and adduction to help expose the supraspinatus tendon when administering the treatment to the lateral aspect of the shoulder.

The use of 10% hydrocortisone cream added to a neutral cream (e.g., Unibase) seems to provide the best medium for the treatment. Other substances such as white petroleum, Eucerin, and Aquaphor are sometimes used.

Various other medications have been driven into tissue with ultrasound. Local anesthetics and salicylates are recommended by some practitioners.

ULTRASOUND IN COMBINATION WITH OTHER MODALITIES

In a sports medicine environment, it is not uncommon to combine modalities to accomplish a specific treatment goal. Ultrasound is frequently used with other modalities including hot packs, cold packs, and electrical stimulating currents.

Hot packs and ultrasound are a useful combination because of the relaxing effects of hot packs in muscle spasm or muscle guarding. However, increasing circulation cutaneously may reduce the depth of penetration of the ultrasound, because the medium for transmission is not as dense.

Cold packs may facilitate the penetration of the sound energy to the deeper tissues, because blood will be shunted away from the cutaneous layers. Cold also has a strong analgesic effect; thus caution must be exercised to prevent burning or damage to the tissues owing to decreased sensation.

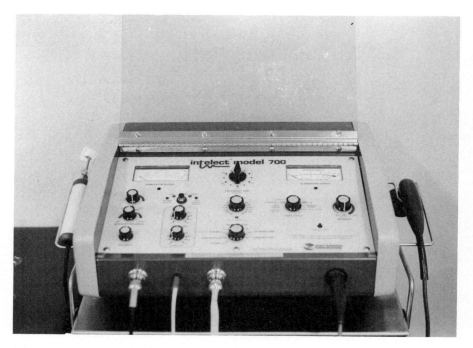

Figure 6-8. Combination ultrasound and electrical stimulator unit. (Manufactured by Chattanooga Corporation, Chattanooga, TN.)

Ultrasound is frequently used with electrical stimulating currents and is thought to be particularly effective in treating trigger points and acupuncture points. Ultrasound increases the blood flow to the deep tissues while the electrical currents can produce a muscle contraction or modulate pain associated with an injury (Fig. 6-8).

SUMMARY

1. Ultrasound is a therapeutic modality that aids sports therapists in their attempts to return the athlete to preinjury status. Before being administered, it must be preceded by an appropriate orthopedic evaluation.
2. Ultrasound must be respected for the significant effects it produces on a variety of tissues and its depth of penetration. In the hands of individuals who do not understand its effects, it is a modality that is quite dangerous.
3. Ultrasound therapy involves a series of electrical and mechanical phenomena that cause thermal and mechanical effects on cells at both superficial and deep levels.
4. There are several indications for ultrasound in the postacute stage of injury. Overuse syndromes and pathologies that involve undesirably tight articular structures are some of the most common indications.
5. Knowing the contraindications is critically important for anyone administering ultrasound. Acute injuries, healing fractures, infection, and treatment over vital organs are all contraindications.
6. The actual administration of ultrasound is not difficult. Dosage is based on the specific situation.
7. Phonophoresis is an effective treatment for a variety of overuse syndromes; 10% hydrocortisone is generally agreed to be appropriate.

GLOSSARY

adhesions Fibrous bands that hold together tissues that are normally separated.

anesthesia Loss of sensation.

articular Dealing with two or more bones joining together to form a joint.

attenuation A decrease in energy due to either absorption or scattering of the sound wave.

calcific bursitis Hardening of the bursa sack.

calcification Hardening of tissue that results from deposits of lime salts.

cavitation The mechanical vibration of small gas bubbles in blood or body fluids.

cervical ganglia A mass of nerve cells located at the cervical portion of the sympathetic trunk.

coaxial cable Heavy, well-insulated electrical wire.

coupling agent A substance used as a medium for the transfer of sound waves.

crystal The part of the ultrasound head that vibrates and changes shape.

diffusion Transfer of a substance from an area of greater to lesser concentration.

exostosis Bony growth that arises from the surface of a bone.

extracapsular ligament Ligament found outside of the joint capsule.

hematoma An area of swelling containing blood, usually clotted.

hertz A unit of frequency equal to one cycle per second.

hot spots Areas of tissue that may be overheated during an ultrasound treatment.

hydrocortisone An antiinflammatory steroid.

mechanical effects Ultrasonic effects that involve movement as a result of vibratory motion.

metal implant Any metal device placed within tissue.

myositis ossificans Inflammation of muscle tissue with bony formation of the muscle.

overuse syndromes Injury to a tissue by working it

harder than it is prepared to work over a period of time.

percutaneous injection Injection in which fluid is forced beneath the skin.

periosteum Fibrous covering of bone.

phonophoresis Driving of medication into tissue by ultrasound.

piezoelectric effect Vibration of a crystal as a result of receiving electrical current.

plica Thickened synovial fold.

pulsed ultrasound Method of administering ultrasound in which the conduction of sound waves is intermittent.

sepsis A pathologic state that involves toxic substance in the blood steam.

stellate ganglion Ganglion (group of nerve cell bodies) formed by the first thoracic ganglion and the inferior cervical ganglion.

thrombophlebitis Inflammation of a vein with a blood clot formed within a blood vessel.

transducer A device that changes energy from one type to another.

ultrasound A portion of the acoustic spectrum located above audible sound. Sound waves higher than the 16,000 to 20,000 Hz detectable by the human ear.

vagus nerve Tenth cranial nerve; this nerve innervates cardiac muscle and some smooth and striated muscle.

REFERENCES

1 Bierman, W.: Ultrasound in the treatment of scars, Arch. Phys. Med. Rehab. **35**:209-214, 1954.

2 Delacerda, F.: Ultrasonic techniques for the treatment of plantar warts in athletes, J. Ortho. Sports Phys. Ther. **1**:100, 1979.

3 Downer, A.: Ultrasound, Athletic Training **10**(3):138-139, 1975.

4 Gersten, J.: Effect of ultrasound on tendon extensibility, Am. J. Phys. Med. **34**:362-369, 1955.

5 Gersten, J.: Effect of metallic objects on temperature rises produced in tissue by ultrasound, Am. J. Phys. Med. **37**:75-82, 1958.

6 Gieck, J., Bamford, M., Stewart, H., and Ferguson, B.: Therapeutic ultrasound: technology, performance standards, biological effect, and clinical application, HHS Publication FOA 84-XXXX, August, 1984.

7 Griffin, J.E.: Phonophoresis, as presented at the International Symposium on Therapeutic Ultrasound, Winnipeg, Manitoba, Canada, September, 1981.

8 Griffin, J.E.: Physiological effects of ultrasonic energy as it is used clinically, J. Am. Phys. Ther. Assoc. **46**(1):18–26, 1966.

9 Griffin, J.E.: Transmissiveness of ultrasound through tap water, glycerin, and mineral oil, Phys. Ther. **60**(8):1010-1016, 1980.

10 Haar, G.: Basic physics of therapeutic ultrasound, Physiotherapy **64**(4):100-102, 1978.

11 Halle, J., Scoville, C., and Greathouse, D.: Ultrasound's effect on the conduction latency of the superficial radial nerve in man, Phys. Ther. **61**(3):345-350, 1981.

12 Hereford, J.: The effects of phonophoretically driven hydrocortisone acetate on the morphology of the rabbit knee joint, Abstr. Phys. Ther. **68**(5):812, 1988.

13 Kleinkort, J.A., and Wood, F.: Phonophoresis with one percent versus ten percent hydrocortisone, Phys. Ther. **55**(12):1320-1324, 1975.

14 Lehmann, J.F.: Ultrasound therapy. In Therapeutic heat and cold, ed. 2, Baltimore, 1965, Williams & Wilkins.

15 Lehmann, J.F., Delateur, B., and Silverman, D.R.: Selective heating effects of ultrasound in human beings, Arch. Phys. Med. Rehabil. **47**:331-338, 1966.

16 Lehmann, J.F., and Delateur, B.J.: Therapeutic heat. In Therapeutic heat and cold, ed. 3, Baltimore, 1982, Williams & Wilkins.

17 Lehmann, J., and Guy, A.: Ultrasound therapy. In Reid, J., and Sikov, M., editors: Interaction of ultrasound and biological tissues, Washington, D.C., 1971, DHEW Pub. (FDA) 73-8008, Session 3:8, pp. 141-152.

18 Oakley, E.M.: Application of continuous beam ultrasound at therapeutic levels, Physiotherapy **64**(6):169-172, 1978.

19 Pohlman, R.: Uber dic absorption des ultra shalls im meneschlichen Schadelknochen und ihre Abhandigkut von der frequenz, Physik. Z. **40**:159, 1939.

20 Vaughen, J., and Bender, L.: Effects of ultrasound on growing bone, Arch. Phys. Med. Rehabil. **35**:555, 1954.

21 Vaughn, D.: Direct method versus underwater method in the treatment of plantar warts with ultrasound, Phys. Ther. **53**(4):396-397, 1973.

22 Ziskin, M., and Michlovich, S.: Therapeutic ultrasound. In Michlovich, S., editor: Thermal agents in rehabilitation, Philadelphia, 1986, F.A. Davis Co.

SUGGESTED READINGS

Abramson, D.I., et al.: Changes in blood flow, oxygen uptake and tissue temperatures produced by therapeutic physical agents. I. Effect of ultrasound, Am. J. Phys. Med. **39**:51, 1960.

Aldes, J., and Grabine, S.: Ultrasound in the treatment of intervertebral disc syndrome, Am. J. Phys. Med. **37**:199-201, 1958.

Allen, K.G., and Battye, C.K.: Performance of ultrasonic therapy instruments, Physiotherapy **64**(6):174-179, 1978.

Baldes, E., Herrick, J.F., and Stroebell, C. III: Biological effects of ultrasound, Arch. Phys. Med. **39**:111-112, 1958.

Bearzy, H.J.: Clinical applications of ultrasonic energy in the treatment of acute and chronic subacromial bursitis, Arch. Phys. Med. Rehabil. **34**:228, 1953.

Bender, L.F., Janes, J.M., and Herrick, J.F.: Histologic studies following exposure of bone to ultrasound, Arch. Phys. Med. Rehabil. **35**:555, 1954.

Bickford, R.H., and Duff, R.S.: Influence of ultrasonic irradiation on temperature and blood flow in human skeletal muscle, Circ. Res. **1**:534, 1953.

Bierman, W.: Ultrasound in the treatment of scars, Arch. Phys. Med. Rehabil. **35**:209, 1954.

Braatz, J.H., McAlistar, B.F., and Broaddus, M.D.: Ultrasound and plantar warts: a double blind study, Milit. Med. **139**:199, 1974.

Buchtala, V.: The present state of ultrasonic therapy, Br. J. Phys. Med. **15**:3, 1952.

Bundt, F.B.: Ultrasound therapy in supraspinatus bursitis, Phys. Ther. Rev. **38**:826, 1958.

Cherup, N., Urben, J., and Bender, L.F.: The treatment of plantar warts with ultrasound, Arch. Phys. Med. Rehabil. **44**:602, 1963.

Cline, P.D.: Radiographic follow-up of ultrasound therapy in calcific bursitis, Phys. Ther. **43**:16, 1963.

Coakley, W.T.: Biophysical effects of ultrasound at therapeutic intensities, Physiotherapy **64**(6):166-168, 1975.

Currier, D., Greathouse, D., and Swift, T.: Sensory nerve conduction: effect of ultrasound, Arch. Phys. Med. Rehab. **59**:181-185, 1978.

Currier, D., and Kramer, J.F.: Sensory nerve conduction: heating effects of ultrasound and infrared, Physiother. Can. **34**:241, 1982.

DeForest, R.E., Herrick, J.F., and Janes, J.M.: Effects of ultrasound on growing bone: an experimental study, Arch. Phys. Med. Rehabil. **34**:21, 1953.

Downer, A.: Physical therapy procedures, Springfield, Ill, 1978, Charles C Thomas Publishers, pp. 75-91.

Downing, D., and Weinstein, A.: Ultrasound therapy of subacromial bursitis (abstr). Arthritis Rheum. **26** (Suppl):587, 1983.

Dunn, F.: Physical mechanisms of the action of intense ultrasound on tissue, Arch. Phys. Med. Rehabil. **39**:148-151, 1958.

Dyson, M., et al.: The stimulation of tissue regeneration by means of ultrasound, Clin. Sci. **35**:273, 1968.

Dyson, M., et al.: The production of blood cell stasis and endothelial damage in the blood vessels of chick embryos treated with ultrasound in a stationary wave field, Ultrasound Med. Biol. **11**:133, 1974.

Dyson, M., and Brookes, M.: Stimulation of bone repair by ultrasound (abstr), Ultrasound Med. Biol. **8** (Suppl 50):50, 1982.

Dyson, M., and Suckling, J.: Stimulation of tissue repair of ultrasound: a survey of the mechanism involved, Physiotherapy **64**(4):105-108, 1978.

Dyson, M., and ter Haar, G.R.: The response of smooth muscle to ultrasound (abstr). In Proceedings from an International Symposium on Therapeutic Ultrasound, Winnipeg, Manitoba (Canada), September 10-12, 1981.

Echternach, J.L.: Ultrasound: an adjunct treatment for shoulder disability, Phys. Ther. **45**:865, 1965.

Feibel, A., and Fast, A.: Commentary: deep heating of joints, a reconsideration, Arch. Phys. Med. Rehabil. **57**:513-514, 1976.

Fountain, F.P., Gersten, J.W., and Sengu, O.: Decrease in muscle spasm produced by ultrasound, hot packs and IR, Arch. Phys. Med. Rehabil. **41**:293, 1960.

Fyfe, M.C., and Chahl, L.A.: The effect of ultrasound on experimental oedema in rats, Ultrasound Med. Biol. **6**:107, 1980.

Grieder, A., et al.: An evaluation of ultrasonic therapy for temperomandibular joint dysfunction, Oral Surg. **31**:25, 1971.

Griffin, J.E., et al.: Patients treated with ultrasonic driven cortisone and with ultrasound alone, Phys. Ther. **47**:594, 1967.

Griffin, J.E., Echternach, J., and Bowmaker, K.: Results of frequency differences in ultrasonic therapy, Phys. Ther. **50**(4):481-485, 1970.

Griffin, J.E., Echternach, J.L., Price, R.E., and Touchstone, J.C.: Patients treated with ultrasonic driven hydrocortisone and with ultrasound alone, Phys. Ther. **47**(7):594-601, 1967.

Hamer, J., and Kirk, J.A.: Physiotherapy and the frozen shoulder: a comparative trial of ice and ultrasonic therapy, N.Z. Med. J. **83**:191, 1972.

Harvey, W., et al.: The stimulation of protein synthesis in human fibroblasts by therapeutic ultrasound, Rheumatol. Rehabil. **14**:237, 1975.

Hogan, R.D., et al.: The effect of ultrasound on microvascular hemodynamics in skeletal muscle: effect on arterioles, Ultrasound Med. Biol. **8**:45, 1982.

Hogan, R.D., Burke, K.M., and Franklin, T.D.: The effect of ultrasound on microvascular hemodynamics in skeletal muscle: effects during ischemia, Microvasc. Res. **23**:370, 1982.

Inaba, M., and Piorkowski, M.: Ultrasound in treatment of painful shoulders with hemiplegia, Phys. Ther. **52**(7):737-741, 1972.

Isselbacher, K.J.: Harrison's principles of internal medicine, ed. 9, New York, 1980, McGraw-Hill.

Kent, H.: Plantar wart treatment with ultrasound, Arch. Phys. Med. Rehabil. **40**:15, 1959.

Kramer, J.F.: Ultrasound: evaluation of its mechanical and thermal effects, Arch. Phys. Med. Rehabil. **65**:223, 1984.

Kuitert, J.H., and Harr, E.T.: Introduction to clinical application of ultrasound, Phys. Ther. Rev. **35**:19, 1955.

Kuiwert, J.H.: Ultrasonic energy as an adjunct in the management of radiculitis and similar referred pain, Am. J. Phys. Med. **33**:61, 1954.

LaBan, M.M.: Collagen tissue: implications of its response to stress in vitro, Arch. Phys. Med. Rehabil. **43**:461, 1962.

Lehmann, J.F., et al: Comparative study of the efficiency of shortwave, microwave and ultrasonic diathermy in heating the hip joint, Arch. Phys. Med. Rehabil. **40**:510, 1959.

Lehmann, J.F., et al: Ultrasonic effects as demonstrated in live pigs with surgical metallic implants, Arch. Phys. Med. Rehabil. **40**:483, 1959.

Lehmann, J.F., et al.: Clinical evaluation of a new approach in the treatment of contracture associated with hip fracture after internal fixation, Arch. Phys. Med. Rehabil. **42**:95, 1961.

Lehmann, J.F., et al.: Heating produced by ultrasound in bone and soft tissue, Arch. Phys. Med. Rehabil. **48**:397, 1967.

Lehmann, J.F., et al.: Therapeutic temperature distribution produced by ultrasound as modified by dosage and volume of tissue exposed, Arch. Phys. Med. Rehabil. **48**:662, 1967.

Lehmann, J.F., et al.: Heating of joint structures by ultrasound, Arch. Phys. Med. Rehabil. **49**:28, 1968.

Lehmann, J.F., and Biegler, R.: Changes of potentials and temperature gradients in membranes caused by ultrasound, Arch. Phys. Med. Rehabil. **35**:287, 1954.

Lehmann, J.F., Brunner, G.D., and Stow, R.W.: Pain threshold measurements after therapeutic application of ultrasound, microwaves and infrared, Arch. Phys. Med. Rehabil. **39**:560, 1958.

Lehmann, J.F., and Guy, A.W.: Ultrasound therapy, In Proc. Workshop on Interaction of Ultrasound and Biological Tissues. Washington, HEW (FDA 73:8008), Sept. 1972.

Lehmann, J.F., and Herrick, J.F.: Biologic reactions to cavitation, a consideration for ultrasonic therapy, Arch. Phys. Med. Rehabil. **34**:86, 1953.

Lehmann, J.F., and Johnson, E.W.: Some factors influence the temperature distribution in thighs exposed to ultrasound, Arch. Phys. Med. Rehabil. **39**:347-355, 1958.

Lehmann, J.F., and Krusen, F.: Therapeutic application of ultrasound in physical medicine, Arch. Phys. Med. Rehabil. **39**:173-180, 1958.

Lota, M.J., and Darling, R.C.: Change in permeability of the red blood cell membrane in a homogeneous ultrasonic field, Arch. Phys. Med. Rehabil. **36**:282, 1955.

Lundborg, G., and Rank, F.: Experimental intrinsic healing of flexor tendons based upon synovial fluid nutrition, J. Hand Surg. **3**:21, 1978.

Markham, D.E., and Wood, M.R.: Ultrasound for Dupuytren's contracture, Physiotherapy, **66**(2):55-58, 1980.

Michlovich, S.: Thermal agents in rehabilitation, Philadelphia, 1986, F.A. Davis Co.

Reid, J.M., and Silov, M.R., editors: Interaction of ultrasound and biologic tissues, DHEW Publication (FDA) 73-8008, BRH/DBE 73-1, 1972.

Michlovitz, S.L., Lynch, P.R., and Tuma, R.F.: Therapeutic ultrasound: its effects on vascular permeability (abstr), Fed. Proc. **41**:1761, 1982.

Middlemast, S., and Chatterjee, D.J.: Comparison of ultrasound and thermotherapy for soft tissue injuries, Physiotherapy **64**(11):331-332, 1978.

Mueller, E.E., Mead, S., Schultz, B.F., and Vadin, M.R.: A placebo-controlled study of ultrasound treatment for perioarthritis, Am. J. Phys. Med. **33**:31-35, 1954.

Munting, E.: Ultrasonic therapy for painful shoulders, Physiotherapy **64**(6):180-181, 1978.

NCRP Report No 74: Effects of ultrasound: mechanisms and clinical implications, Bethesda, MD, 1983, National Council on Radiation Protection and Measurements, p 197.

Newman, M.D., Kill, M., and Frampton, G.: Effects of ultrasound alone and combined with hydrocortisone injections by needle or hypospray, Arch. Phys. Med. Rehabil. **38**:206-209, 1957.

Nwuga, V.C.B.: Ultrasound in treatment of back pain resulting from prolapsed intervertebral disc, Arch. Phys. Med. Rehabil. **64**:88, 1983.

Oakley, E.M.: Dangers and contraindications of therapeutic ultrasound, Physiotherapy **64**(6):173-174, 1978.

Paaske, W.P., Hanne, H., and Sejrsen, P.: Influence of therapeutic ultrasonic irradiation of blood flow in human cutaneous, subcutaneous, and muscular tissues, Scand. J. Clin. Lab. Invest. pp. 389-394, 1973.

Paul, E.D., and Imig, C.J.: Temperature and blood flow studies after ultrasonic irradiation, Am. J. Phys. Med. **34**:370, 1955.

Quade, A.G., and Radzyminski, S.F.: Ultrasound in verruca plantaris, J. Am. Podiatry Assoc. **56**:503, 1966.

Quillen, W.S.: Phonophoresis: a review of the literature and technique, Athletic Training **15**(2):109-110, 1980.

Reid, D.C., and Cummings, G.E.: Factors in selecting the dosage of ultrasound with particular reference to the use of various coupling agents, Physiother. Can. **63**:255, 1973.

Roberts, M., Rutherford, J.H., and Harris, D.: The effect of ultrasound on flexor tendon repairs in the rabbit, Hand **14**:17, 1982.

Rowe, R.J., and Gray, J.M.: Ultrasound treatment of plantar warts, Arch. Phys. Med. Rehabil. **46**:273, 1965.

Siegel, E., et al.: Cellular attachment as a sensitive indicator of the effects of diagnostic ultrasound exposure on cultured human cells, Radiology **133**:175, 1979.

Soren, A.: Nature and biophysical effects of ultrasound, J. Occup. Med. **7**:375, 1965.

Stewart, H., Herman, G., Robinson, R., Haran, M., McCall, G., Carless, G., and Rees, D.: Survey of use and performance of ultrasonic therapy equipment in Pennellas County, FL, Phys. Ther. **54**(7):707-714, 1974.

Summer, W., and Patrick, M.K.: Ultrasonic therapy, New York, 1964, American Elsevier.

Tabers Cyclopedia Medical Dictionary, ed. 14, Philadelphia, 1985, F.A. Davis Co.

Vaughen, J.L., and Bender, L.F.: Effects of ultrasound on growing bone, Arch. Phys. Med. Rehabil. **40**:158, 1959.

Vaughn, D.T.: Direct method versus underwater method in treatment of plantar warts with ultrasound, Phys. Ther. **53**:396, 1973.

Warren, C.G., Koblanski, J.N., and Sigelmann, R.A.: Ultrasound coupling media: their relative transmissivity, Arch. Phys. Med. Rehabil. **57:**218-222, 1976.

Warren, C.G., Lehmann, J.F., and Koblanski, J.N.: Heat and stretch procedures: an evaluation using rat tail tendon, Arch. Phys. Med. Rehabil. **57:**122, 1976.

Wells, P.N.T.: Biomedical ultrasonics, London, 1977, Academic Press.

Wyper, D.J., McNiven, D.R., and Donnelly, T.J.: Therapeutic ultrasound and muscle blood flow, Physiotherapy **64:**321, 1978.

Zarod, A.P., and Williams, A.R.: Platelet aggregation in vivo by therapeutic ultrasound, Lancet **1:**1266, 1977.

Shortwave and Microwave Diathermy

7

Phillip B. Donley

OBJECTIVES

Following completion of this chapter, the student will be able to:

- Define diathermy, shortwave diathermy, and microwave diathermy.

- Explain the physiologic effects of diathermy.

- Explain the types of diathermy electrodes and characteristics of each.

- Describe the methods of application and precautions.

- Explain the indications and contraindications.

- Identify body areas and conditions for student practice.

Diathermy is the application of high-frequency electrical energy that is used to generate heat in body tissues; this heat is caused by resistance of the tissue to the passage of the energy. The tissue temperature must be elevated to between 40° and 45° C (104° and 113° F) if the diathermy is to be effective.[7] Diathermy treatment doses are not precisely controlled, and the amount of heating the patient receives cannot be accurately prescribed or directly measured.

Diathermy as a therapeutic agent may be classified as two distinct modalities: shortwave diathermy and microwave diathermy. The effectiveness of a shortwave or microwave diathermy treatment depends on the sports therapist's ability to tailor the treatment to the athlete's needs. This requires that the sports therapist have an accurate evaluation or diagnosis of the athlete's condition and knowledge of the heating patterns produced by various **applicators.** Many sports therapists feel that neither shortwave nor microwave diathermy produces heating at the depths desired for the treatment of athletic injuries, although the depth of penetration is greater than with the infrared modalities. Sports therapists who are knowledgeable in the physics and biophysics of diathermy, as well as its applications to a variety of cases, tend to achieve good results. Sports therapists who work with shortwave diathermy must spend considerable time experimenting with a variety of machines with both condenser and induction type techniques on a variety of uninjured parts of the body if they are to develop the skills necessary to use diathermy effectively on injured tissue.

PHYSIOLOGIC RESPONSES TO DIATHERMY

The physiologic effects of diathermy are primarily thermal and nonthermal, resulting from high-frequency vibration of molecules. The diathermies are not capable of producing depolarization and contraction of skeletal muscle since the wavelength is much too short in duration. The primary benefits of diathermy are those of heat in general, such as tissue temperature rise, increased blood flow, dilation of the blood vessels, increased filtration and diffusion through the different membranes, increased tissue metabolic rate, changes in some enzyme reactions, alterations in the physical properties of fibrous tissues (such as those found in tendons, joints, and scars), a certain degree of muscle relaxation, and a heightened pain threshold.[3,7,8] Why certain pathologic conditions respond better to diathermy than other forms of deep heat is not well understood or documented. It probably is more directly related either to the skill of the operator applying the modality or to some placebo effects associated with tissue temperature increase than it is to the specific effects of diathermy itself.

SHORTWAVE DIATHERMY

A shortwave diathermy unit is basically a radio transmitter. The Federal Communications Commission (FCC) assigned three frequencies to shortwave diathermy units: the first is 27.12 MHz with a wavelength of 11 meters; the second is 13.56 MHz with a wavelength of 22 meters; and the third is 40.68 MHz with a wavelength of 7.5 meters (see Fig. 2-2).

Any device that generates an electrical current will generate both an **electrical field** and a **magnetic field**.[4] The ratio of electrical field to magnetic field depends on the characteristics of the different units and some of the characteristics of electrodes or applicators.

Shortwave diathermy may be set up using two different methods of energy transfer: an electrostatic or condenser field method or the electromagnetic or induction field method.

In **electrostatic or condenser field** heating the patient is placed between two electrodes and becomes part of the circuit. The tissue between the two electrodes is in series (see Chapter 3). The tissue that offers the greatest resistance to current flow (i.e., skin and fat) tends to overheat.

In **electromagnetic or induction field** heating the patient is in a magnetic field and is not part of the circuit. Tissues that are high in electrolytic content (i.e., blood and muscle) respond best to the magnetic field by producing heat. The tissues are in a parallel circuit (see Chapter 3), thus the greatest current flow is through the tissues with least resistance.

Tissues that have a high fat content tend to insulate and resist the passage of an electric field. These tissues, particularly subcutaneous fat, tend to overheat when an electrical field is used, which is characteristic with a condenser type of electrode application. When a magnetic field is used with an induction type setup, the fat does not provide nearly as much resistance to the flow of the energy. The frequency of 13.56 MHz tends to give a stronger magnetic field than does the frequency of 27.12 MHz. The latter is the more commonly found frequency on shortwave diathermy units. It is important to remember that if the energy is primarily electromagnetic, heating may not be as obvious to the patient because the magnetic field will not provide nearly as much sensation of warmth in the skin as an electric field. There are few commercial units that have a frequency of 13.56 MHz.[3]

The **capacitor setup,** a type of electrostatic heating, is characteristic of a space plate or pad application. It provides a strong electrical field and is an example of a high-frequency oscillating current that is passed through each plate millions of times per second. When one plate is overloaded, it discharges to the other plate of the lower potential, and this is reversed millions of times per second.[3]

Equipment

The shortwave diathermy unit consists of a power supply that provides power to a radio frequency oscillator (Fig. 7-1). This radio frequency oscillator provides stable, drift-free oscillations at the required frequency. The power amplifier generates the power required to drive the different types of electrodes (Fig. 7-2). The output resonant tank tunes in the patient as part of the circuit and allows maximum power to be transferred to the patient.

Figure 7-3 diagrammatically shows the control panel of a shortwave diathermy unit. The output intensity knob controls the percentage of maximum power transferred to the patient circuit. This is similar to the volume control on a radio. The tuning control adjusts the output circuit for maximum energy transfer from the radio frequency oscillator, which is similar to tuning in a station on a radio. The output power meter monitors only the current that is drawn from the power supply and *not* the energy in the patient circuit. Thus it is only an indirect measure of the energy reaching the patient.

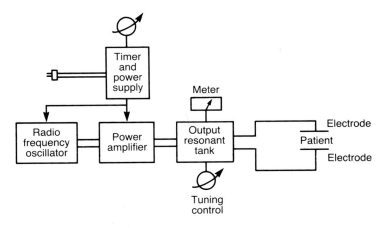

Figure 7-1. The component parts of a shortwave diathermy unit.

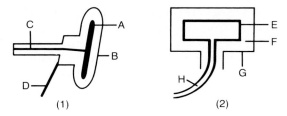

Figure 7-2. Commonly used shortwave diathermy electrodes. (1) Air space plate: *(A)* electrode plate, *(B)* plastic guard, *(C)* adjusting handle, *(D)* lead cord, (2) drum electrode: *(E)* coil, *(F)* dead air space, *(G)* housing, *(H)* lead cord.

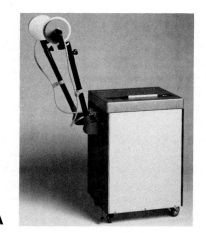
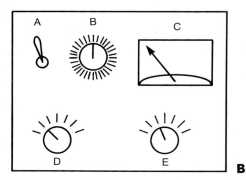

Figure 7-3. A, Shortwave diathermy unit. (Courtesy of Elmed Inc., 60 West Fay Avenue, Addison, Illinois) **B,** Control panel of a shortwave diathermy unit. *(A)* Power switch, *(B)* timer, *(C)* output power meter (monitors current drawn from power supply only and not in patient circuit), *(D)* output intensity (controls the percentage of maximum power transferred to the patient), *(E)* tuning control (tunes output circuit for maximum energy transfer from radio frequency oscillator).

If the machine is not an automatically tuning type, with the electrodes in place the output intensity should be set at 30% to 40%. The tuning control should be adjusted until the output power meter moves to the maximum and then it should be adjusted down to patient tolerance, which is usually about 50% to 60% of maximum output.

The power output of a shortwave diathermy unit should produce sufficient energy to raise the tissue temperature into a therapeutic range, 40° to 45° C. This is referred to as the *specific absorption rate* (SAR) and represents the rate of energy absorbed per unit of tissue mass. This has been roughly determined to be 170 watts per kilogram. Many units are not capable of this. They are safe, but they are ineffective.[6] The shortwave diathermy unit should have several types of applicators or electrodes. In other words, it should have the capability of providing energy through a coil or cable, an induction drum, and condenser plate or pads. It is important to remember that the tissue temperature rise with diathermy units can be offset dramatically by an increase in blood flow, which has a cooling effect in the tissue being energized. Therefore, units should be able to generate enough power to provide for an excess of this power absorption to about 130 watts per kilogram.[6] Patient sensation is probably the most common criterion for regulation of heat generation. It varies considerably with different patients. A very good evaluation of several shortwave diathermy units was published in June 1979.[6]

The lower frequencies in diathermy currents provide for deeper penetration because the wavelength is longer.[1] The contention is that as the frequency is increased, the magnetic field will increase to somewhere between 10 to 15 MHz. Beyond that, the magnetic field will decrease.[3]

PAD ELECTRODES. Pad electrodes are not commonly used in athletics; however, they may be available for some units. They are true capacitor-type electrodes, and they must have uniform contact pressure on the body part if they are to be effective in producing deep heat, as well as avoiding skin burns (Fig. 7-4). The patient is part of the external circuit. Several layers of toweling are necessary to make sure that there is sufficient spacing between the skin and the pads. The pads should be separated in such a way that they are at least as far apart as the cross-sectional diameter of the pads. In other words, if the pads are 15 cm across, then there should be at least 15 cm between the pads. There will be more heat buildup directly under the pads than there will

Electrodes

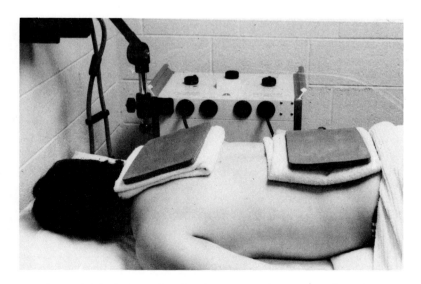

Figure 7-4. Pad electrodes showing correct placement and spacing.

be in the deeper tissues. The part of the body to be treated should be centered between the pads.[3,4,6,7]

AIR SPACE PLATES. Air space plates are another example of a capacitor (strong electric field) setup or a capacitor electrode (Fig. 7-5). The patient is a part of the external circuit. The depth of penetration is inversely proportional to the distance from the plate to the skin, particularly as long as the plate guard is in contact with the towel, which is in contact with the skin. The sensation of heat tends to be in direct proportion to the distance of the plate from the skin. The closer the plate is to the skin, the better the energy penetration because there will be less reflection of the energy. However, it should be remembered that the closer plate will also generate more surface heat in the skin and the subcutaneous fat in that area. Just as the pads should be further apart than the cross-sectional diameter, so too should the plates be placed in such a manner that they are at least as far apart as the cross-sectional diameter of the plate (Fig. 7-6). In fact, more distance between the plates is much better. The area to be treated should be centered between the two plates. The greatest surface heat will be under the electrodes. The deeper heat is between the electrodes. Parts of the body that are low in subcutaneous fat content (e.g., hands, feet, wrists, and ankles) are best treated by this method. Athletes who have a very low subcutaneous fat content can be effectively treated on other body areas.[2] In my experience, the hamstrings, quadriceps, calf muscles, and the muscles about the shoulders and upper extremities can be treated effectively with the condenser technique when the individual has a very low subcutaneous fat content. This technique is also very effective for treating the spine and the ribs.

DRUM ELECTRODES. The drum electrode is made up of one or more mono-planer coils that are rigidly fixed inside some kind of housing (Fig. 7-7). If a

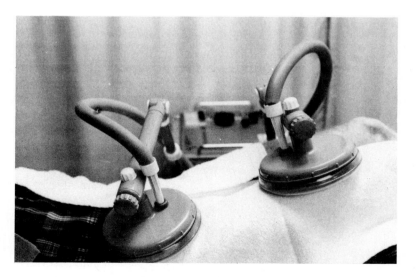

Figure 7-5. Air space plates.

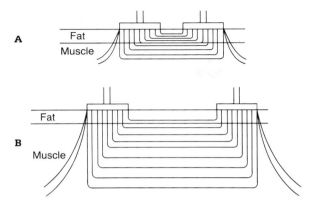

Figure 7-6. Correct spacing of shortwave electrodes. They must be separated by a distance of at least the diameter of the electrode: **A,** too close together; **B,** proper spacing.

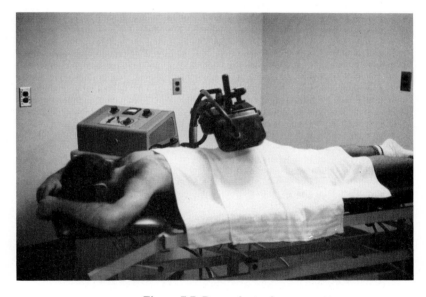

Figure 7-7. Drum electrodes.

small area is to be treated, particularly a small flat area, then a one-drum setup is fine. However, if the area is contoured, then two or more drums, which may be on a hinged apparatus or hinged arm, may be more suitable. In this type of application, there is more electromagnetic energy than electrical energy being used. The patient is not part of the electrical circuit. The electromagnetic energy is being induced into the tissue. The electromagnetic energy creates a circular electrical field of eddy currents, and the intramolecular oscillation (vibration of tissue molecules) of tissue contents causes heat generation. Tissues that are high in water content such as muscle, blood, and bone are more easily heated. Electromagnetic penetration tends to be on the order of 2 to 3 cm if the skin is no more than 1 to 2 cm away from the drum.[1] The electromagnetic field may be significant up to 5 cm away from the drum. A light towel must be kept in contact with the skin and between the drum and the skin. The towel is used to absorb moisture because an accumulation of water droplets would tend to overheat and cause hot spots on the surface. If there is more than 2 cm of fat, there probably will be no great tissue temperature rise under the fat with a drum setup. The maximum penetration of shortwave diathermy with a drum electrode is 3 cm provided there is no more than 2 cm of fat beneath the skin. For best absorption of energy, the housing of the drum should be in contact with the towel that is covering the skin.[2]

CABLE ELECTRODES. The **cable electrode** is an inductance type electrode or an electromagnetic energy application (Fig. 7-8). There are two basic types of arrangements: the pancake and the wraparound coil. If a pancake arrangement is used, the size of the smaller circle should be greater than 6 inches in diameter. In either arrangement, there should be at least 1 cm of toweling between the cable and the skin. Stiff spacers should be used to keep the coils or the turns of the pancake or the wraparound coil between 5 and 10 cm between turns of the cable, thus providing spacing consistency. The pancake and the wraparound coils often provide more even heating because they both are more able to follow the contours of the skin than are the drum or the space plates. It is important that the cables not touch each other because they will short out and cause excessive heat buildup. Diathermy units that operate on a frequency of 13.56 MHz are probably best suited to cable electrode type applications. This

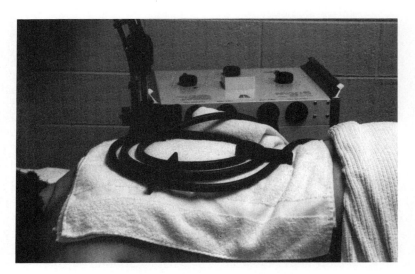

Figure 7-8. Pancake cable electrodes.

is primarily because the lower frequency provides better production of electromagnetic energy.[2]

Heating occurs in proportion to the square of the current and in direct proportion to the resistance. If tissues are arranged parallel with electrodes, the greatest current flow will occur through the tissue with the least resistance (such as muscle). When applied to an extremity such as with a capacitor application or in a parallel circuit, with the face plates facing the same direction (as though treating the anterior thigh with both face plates on the anterior thigh), then the greatest current flow will occur through those tissues with the least resistance (Fig. 7-9). If the tissues are arranged in series (capacitor setup with the face plates facing each other as on the medial and lateral side of the knee), then the tissue with the greatest resistance, such as subcutaneous fat, will be heated the most (Fig. 7-10). When the subcutaneous fat is minimal, such setups are very effective. This is particularly true with the knee, ankle, foot, hand, and wrist. Induction drums should be located so that they are in contact with the towel between the skin and the drum.[2]

It is very important to use shortwave and microwave diathermy units at a safe distance from other therapy equipment that is transistorized. Transcutaneous electrical nerve stimulation units and other low-frequency current units often have transistor type circuits, and these can be very easily damaged by the reflected or stray radiation that is produced by shortwave and microwave diathermy units.[4]

A single layer of toweling should be used with both the drum and with space plates. However, with other types of applicators, such as pads and cables, the toweling should be more dense and thicker: up to about 1 cm or more.[3]

Techniques

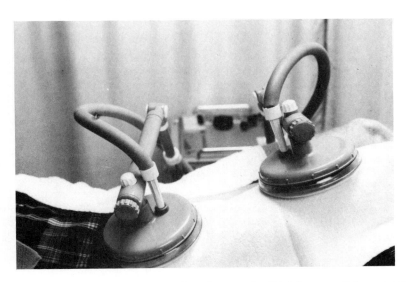

Figure 7-9. Air space plates being used on the anterior thigh in a parallel arrangement.

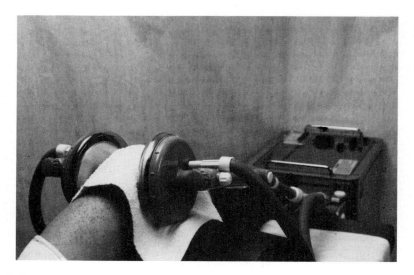

Figure 7-10. Air space plates being used on the medial and lateral knee in a series arrangement.

There should be no overlapping of skin surfaces. If the buttock area is to be treated, then a towel should be placed in the cleavage between the buttocks. If the shoulder area is to be treated, a towel should be placed between the skin folds in the axilla.

The patient should not come in contact with any of the cables with the drum, face plate, or cable setups. There should be no crossover of the lead cables with any electrode setup.

There should be no metal touching the surface of the athlete, and there should be no metal chairs or metal tables used to support the athlete during treatment. The area being treated should also be free of metal implants. Women wearing intrauterine devices should not be treated in the low back or lower abdomen. There should be no watch or jewelry in the area because the electromagnetic energy will tend to magnetize the watch and both electrical and electromagnetic energy may heat up the jewelry.

The athlete must remain in a reasonably comfortable position for the duration of the treatment so that the field does not change because of movement during treatment. It is also important that no clothing be permitted in the exposed area. Many of the synthetic fabrics worn today allow for no evaporation of moisture. These fabrics serve as a vapor barrier and allow moisture to accumulate. This moisture can create extremely hot spots with diathermy treatments.

As skin temperature goes up, impedance goes down; therefore the unit should be retuned after 5 to 10 minutes of treatment.

Tuning

Because the patient's electrical impedance becomes a part of the patient's circuit impedance, it is necessary to tune the patient's circuit to resonance with the oscillating circuit of the unit. This is done by adjusting a variable capacitor in the machine's circuit. The meter on the machine is used to determine the peak tuning readings, and it should not be confused as a reading of the power received by the patient. If more than 50% of the available power on the meter is used, then the patient's setup is out of tune or out of resonance.[1] Some shortwave diathermy units have manual tuning; others have an automatic tuning device. Those with automatic tuning turn off the power when the patient circuit is out of tune.

Treatment Time

A 20-to-30-minute treatment for one body area is probably all that is necessary to reach maximum physiologic effects. Treatments in excess of 30 minutes or those that are in excess of 45 to 60 minutes may create a circulatory rebound phenomenon in which the digital temperature may drop after the treatment because of reflex vasoconstriction.[8] If a sports therapist finds that a diathermy unit has been left on in excess of 30 minutes, it would be wise to check the temperature of the toes or the fingers, depending on which extremity has been treated.

A mild treatment is categorized as a general feeling of warmth by the athlete, and it is used in a subacute type of condition. A vigorous treatment is one in which the pain threshold of the athlete has been found, and then the energy has been backed off to just below the pain level. Because diathermy selectively heats tissues that are high in water content, it would be wise not to use diathermy over a joint effusion. The increase in temperature may cause an increase in synovitis. The skin should be inspected before and after a diathermy treatment. It is recommended that the part being treated either be horizontal or elevated during the treatment.

Indications

For the most part, shortwave diathermy is best used for long-term pain, local relaxation, increases in circulation, and subacute pain. The effects seem to last for about 30 minutes. This is particularly true of the circulatory effects. The unit must be used for at least 20 minutes to get maximum benefits, and a 30-minute treatment is considered to be the maximum.[2] Anytime that heat, particularly deep heat, is desirable—such as when skin conditions may be exacerbated by moisture—then diathermy is desirable. If the skin is very tender and will not tolerate the loading of a moist heat pack, then again shortwave diathermy may be desirable. Whenever heat is required at a depth greater than that which can be acquired by surface heating, shortwave diathermy is desirable. The sports therapist should never underestimate the psychologic effects that a treatment with a large machine may be capable of producing.

Pulsed diathermy is a relatively new form of diathermy. Nonthermal effects of diathermy have been documented, but they do not appear to be therapeutically important.[5] Pulsed diathermy is claimed to have therapeutic value and to produce both thermal and nonthermal effects, depending on the intensity of the application. When pulsed diathermy is used in acute conditions, a mild elevation in temperature may occur that will produce less swelling than other forms of heat. Studies that use pulsed diathermy do not normally compare it with continuous diathermy but rather with a control group that has received no heat treatment.[7] When pulsed diathermy is used in intensities that create an increase in tissue temperature, its effects are no different from those of continuous diathermy.[2,7]

Contraindications

Shortwave diathermy is known to produce a tissue temperature rise and may be contraindicated in conditions where this increased temperature may produce negative or undesired effects. The following is a list of contraindications for shortwave diathermy: metal implants, IUDs, pacemakers, malignancy, wet dressings, gonads, anesthetized areas, adhesive taped areas, acute muscle and ligament injuries, and pregnancy. There should be no vigorous heating of the epiphysis in children. Shortwave diathermy should not be applied to the pelvic area of the female who is menstruating. It should not be used around the eyes for any prolonged periods of time or for repeated treatments. It should not be used over contact lenses.

Caution should be exercised when treating an athlete who has a high percentage of body fat, particularly when using electrostatic or condenser field heating. As indicated earlier, tissues such as fat that offer resistance to current flow tend to overheat in an electrical field.

Common Uses of Shortwave Diathermy

Sports therapists should take the opportunity to examine several different types of diathermy units, as well as the different applicators available with each unit. They should not only practice using the different applicators on healthy tissue, but they should also experience the sensation themselves. In particular, they should recognize or experience the difference between the energy flow with an induction type application as opposed to the capacitor type application. The following is a list of conditions and commonly injured body parts that may be best treated using shortwave diathermy:

1. Blocker's exostosis (induction)
2. Rectus femoris strains (condenser or induction)
3. Sartorius strains (condenser or induction)
4. Gracilis strains (condenser or induction)
5. Hamstring strains (condenser or induction)
6. Tensor fascia lata strains (condenser or induction)
7. Strains of the gluteus maximus (condenser proximal and distal)
8. Contusions to the crest of the ilium such as a hip pointer (induction)
9. Contusions or strains to the quadratus lumborum, to the thoracic spine, to costal cartilages or the intercostal muscles, and to the mid forearm (induction)
10. Subacute conditions in which there is no swelling, such as those related to sprains of the knee, ankle, elbow, glenohumeral joint, wrist, costochondral joints (induction)
11. Subacute or chronic bronchitis and subacute pleurisy (induction)

In each of these conditions, I have found diathermy at one time or another to be effective and the treatment of choice.

Microwave diathermy has two FCC-assigned frequencies in this country: 2456 MHz and 915 MHz. Microwave has a much higher frequency and a shorter wavelength than shortwave diathermy. It has an advantage in that there is less than 10% of the energy lost from the machine as it is applied to the athlete. The microwave antenna or director beams energy toward the patient, and its wavelength is short enough to have the properties of light, which means that it is easily reflected (see Fig. 7-14). Bone tends to absorb more shortwave and microwave energy than any type of soft tissue. Heating is caused by the intramolecular vibration of molecules that are high in polarity. If the subcutaneous fat is greater than 1 cm, the fat temperature will rise to a level that is too uncomfortable before there is a tissue temperature rise in the deeper tissues.[3] This is less of a problem if the microwave diathermy is of the frequency of 915 MHz.[7] However, there are very few commercial units operating on that frequency. Almost all of the older units have the higher frequency of 2456 MHz. If the subcutaneous fat is 0.5 cm or less, microwave diathermy can penetrate and cause a tissue temperature rise up to 5 cm deep in the tissue.

MICROWAVE DIATHERMY

Equipment

The microwave diathermy unit consists of a power supply that energizes the magnetron and timing circuitry. The magnetron control regulates output power by varying the magnetron operating voltage. The magnetron oscillator uses an electromagnetic field to produce high-frequency currents (Fig. 7-11).

Figure 7-12 represents the control panel of a microwave unit. The power output can be adjusted to patient tolerance. The output meter indicates the relative output in watts or transmitted and unabsorbed energy. There are two indicator lamps: the amber lamp indicates that the machine is still warming up, and the red lamp indicates that the machine is ready to output energy.

Applicators

Electrodes for microwave diathermy are called **applicators.** The microwave energy can only be beamed to one surface at a time. The contour of that surface must be very flat; otherwise there will be considerable reflection of the energy. Bath toweling on the area is not necessary. Those microwave diathermy units operating on the frequency 2456 MHz will have a specified air space required between the applicator and the skin. The manufacturer-suggested distances and power output should be followed closely. In units that have a frequency of

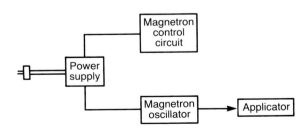

Figure 7-11. Component parts of a microwave diathermy unit.

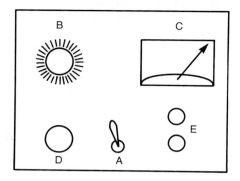

Figure 7-12. Control panel of a microwave diathermy unit: *(A)* power switch, *(B)* timer, *(C)* output meter (indicates relative output in watts of transmitted energy), *(D)* power output level, *(E)* indicator lamps (amber—standby, magnetron accelerating, red—output, microwaves available).

915 MHz, the applicators are placed on the skin and the air space between the antenna and the skin is built into the applicator. Newer units with this type of director have an advantage in that stray radiation is reduced.[7] Units that operate on the higher frequency may have one or more directors of various shapes and configurations.

There are two types of applicators that may be used with microwave diathermy: circular shaped and rectangular shaped. The circular-shaped applicators are either 4 or 6 inches in diameter. With circular-shaped electrodes, the maximum temperature is produced at the periphery of each radiation field (Fig. 7-13, *A*).

Rectangular-shaped applicators are either 4½ × 5 inches or 5 × 21 inches and produce the maximum temperature at the center of the radiation field (Fig. 7-13, *B*).

Technique

Microwave diathermy units require a period of time to warm up. This is normally built into the circuitry so that the unit power cannot be turned on until the unit is sufficiently warmed. This warm-up time is a good time for the sports therapist to position the director and the athlete (Fig. 7-14). The director should be located so that the maximum amount of energy will be penetrating at a right

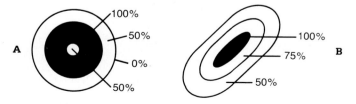

Figure 7-13. A, Circular-shaped microwave electrode. **B,** Rectangular-shaped microwave electrodes.

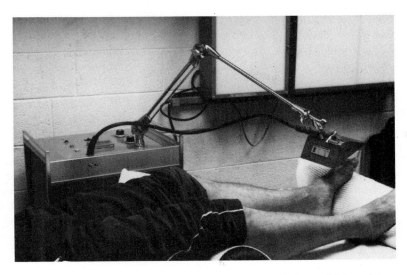

Figure 7-14. Microwave diathermy applied to the metatarsophalangeal joint of the great toe.

angle or perpendicular to the skin. Any angle greater or less than perpendicular will create reflection of the energy and significant loss of absorption (cosine law). Microwave diathermy is best used to treat conditions that exist in those areas of the body that are covered with low subcutaneous fat content. The tendons of the foot, hand, and wrist are well treated, as are the acromioclavicular and sternoclavicular joints, the patellar tendon, the distal tendons of the hamstrings, the Achilles tendon, and the costochondral joints and sacroiliac joints in lean individuals.

Indications and Contraindications

The same precautions and contraindications that were listed for shortwave diathermy apply to microwave diathermy. It is important to keep in mind that the power meter on the unit does not indicate the energy entering the tissues; therefore the sports therapist must rely on the sensation of pain for a warning that the athlete's tolerance levels have been exceeded. As with shortwave diathermy, if vigorous heating is desirable, the sports therapist should keep the output just below the pain threshold. For mild heating, the sports therapist should encourage a mild feeling of warmth.[7]

At no time should the antenna within the applicator ever come in contact with the skin. This would cause a buildup of energy sufficient to cause a severe burn.

Microwave diathermy has been very effective in the treatment of fibrous muscular contractures, as well as tendinitis and chronic tenosynovitis. If microwave diathermy is to be used to its maximum potential with its effect on the extensibility of collagen tissue, the tissue should be placed on a stretch while the treatment is in progress.[2]

Microwave diathermy may also be used to treat tender myofibrocytic nodules and myofascial trigger points. As with shortwave diathermy, there have been nonthermal effects documented with microwave diathermy; however, there does not appear to be any evidence that these nonthermal effects have any significant role in the medical application of microwave diathermy.[5]

Common Uses of Microwave Diathermy

As with shortwave diathermy, microwave diathermy must be practiced in its applications on healthy tissue, and it must be experienced by the sports therapist to appreciate its many applications. The conditions listed in this summary could be used as a guide for practice areas. There is significant risk of causing a burn when using either microwave or shortwave diathermy. For this reason, there are probably more contraindications for the use of either shortwave or microwave diathermy than for any of the other physical agents in the training room. It is also important to keep in mind that any employees in the institution who have a cardiac pacemaker should not be permitted to circulate around the area where microwave or shortwave diathermy units are being used. It is also important to keep transistorized units, such as transcutaneous electrical nerve stimulation units and other low-frequency and high-voltage units for muscle stimulation that have transistorized circuits, away from the diathermy units. Stereo receivers, digital watches, and calculators should be kept 5 to 10 feet away from the units.

SUMMARY

1. The principal effects of diathermy are those of heat in general. Even when maximum depth of penetration is achieved, it is still the effectiveness of tissue temperature that stimulates the large diameter nerve afferents to affect pain and promote the other effects of heat. When properly applied, there is less surface heating than with conductive heating agents. There is less skin pressure than with conductive heating agents. Diathermy provides heating at greater depths than conductive agents. These are all positive effects.

2. Diathermy is more expensive, harder to apply, has more contraindications, and has more precautions than any other form of heating agents. Some units have excessive stray radiation.

3. The most common shortwave diathermy setup is induction. It has been very useful in treating hip pointers, costochondral sprains, bronchitis, pleurisy, shoulder strains, quadriceps strains, and hamstring strains. The condenser setup has worked well with low back and other spinal sprains and strains. In each of these conditions heat was indicated, but when conductive agents were not effective, shortwave diathermy produced better results.

4. Microwave diathermy is used for chronic joint dysfunction in the sternoclavicular, acromioclavicular, wrist, distal radial ulnar joints, and for chronic tendinitis where the tendons are located superficially (i.e., patellar tendon, Achilles, and flexor and extensor tendons of the fingers and toes). It has been most successful when used in combination with ultrasound or phonophoresis, or both.

5. The body can become accustomed to the application of the diathermies, and

a lessened response will occur if overexposure is provided.

6. Effective treatments require practice in application and adjustment of techniques to the individual patient.

GLOSSARY

air space plate   A capacitor type electrode in which the plates are separated from the skin by the space in a glass case. Used with shortwave diathermy.

applicator   The electrode used to transfer energy in microwave diathermy.

cable electrodes   An inductance type electrode in which the electrodes are coiled around a body part, creating an electromagnetic field.

capacitor setup   A type of magnetic field heating that uses air space plates or pads.

condenser electrodes   An electrical current is conducted back and forth between the two electrodes. Highest concentration is under the electrodes, which may be pads or space plates. Highest concentration is also in fat tissue. Deeper absorption of current (deep heating effect) occurs between the electrodes.

diathermy   The application of high-frequency electrical energy that is used to generate heat in body tissues as a result of the resistance of the tissue to the passage of energy.

electrical field   A technique of heating the tissues in shortwave diathermy in which the patient is part of the electrical circuit.

electromagnetic or induction field   The patient is heated in a magnetic field and is not part of the circuit. Current flows through the tissues of least resistance.

electrostatic or condenser field   The patient is placed between electrodes and becomes a part of a series circuit.

Federal Communications Commission (FCC)   Federal agency charged with assigning frequencies for all radio transmitters including diathermies.

induction electrodes   Electrical current is passed through a coil that in turn gives off eddy currents of electromagnetic energy. This energy is absorbed by the tissues and heating occurs as a result of the resistance of the tissues.

intermolecular vibration   Movement between molecules that produces friction and thus heat.

magnetic field   A technique of heating the tissues in shortwave diathermy in which the patient is not part of the electrical circuit.

pad electrodes   Capacitor type electrode used with shortwave diathermy.

REFERENCES

1 DeLateur, B.J., Lehmann, J.F., Stonebridge, J.B., Warren, C.G., and Guy, A.W.: Muscle heating in human subjects with 915 MHz microwave contact applicator, Arch. Phys. Med. **51:**147-151, 1970.

2 Griffin, J.: Update on selected physical modalities, Paper presented in Chicago, Dec., 1981.

3 Griffin, J.E., and Karselis, T.C.: The diathermies. In Physical agents for physical therapist, ed. 2, pp. 177-216. Charles C Thomas Publishers, 1982.

4 Griffin, J., Santiesleban, A.J., and Kloth, L.: Electrotherapy for instructors, Paper presented in Lacrosse, WI, Aug., 1982.

5 Guy, A.W., and Lehmann, J.F.: On the determination of an optimum microwave diathermy frequency for a direct contact applicator, Inst. Electrical Electronics Engineers Transactions, Biomedical Engineering **13:**76-87, 1966.

6 Health devices shortwave diathermy units. Proceedings of the Emergency Care Research Institute, Meeting in Plymouth, PA, June, 1979, pp. 175-193.

7 Lehman, J.F.: Therapeutic heat and cold, ed. 3, Baltimore, 1982, Williams & Wilkins, Chapters 6, 7, 10.

8 Lehmann, J.F., and deLateur, B.J.: Diathermy and superficial heat and cold. In Krusen, F.H., editor: Krusen's handbook of physical medicine & rehabilitation, ed. 3, Philadelphia, 1982, W.B. Saunders Co., pp. 275-351.

SUGGESTED READINGS

Abramson, D.I.: Physiologic basis for the use of physical agents in peripheral vascular disorders, Arch. Phys. Med. Rehabil. **46:**216, 1965.

Allberry, J.: Shortwave diathermy for herpes zoster, Physiotherapy **60:**386, 1974.

Barnett, M.: SWD for herpes zoster, Physiotherapy **61:**217, 1975.

Daels, J.: Microwave heating of the uterine wall during parturition, J. Microwave Power **11:**166, 1976.

Doyle, J.R., and Smart, B.W.: Stimulation of bone growth by shortwave diathermy, J. Bone Joint Surg. **45A:**15, 1963.

Engel, J.P., et al.: The effects of microwaves on bone and bone marrow and adjacent tissues, Arch. Phys. Med. Rehabil. **31:**453, 1950.

Feibel, H., and Fast, H.: Deepheating of joints: a reconsideration, Arch. Phys. Med. Rehabil. **57**:513, 1976.

Fischer, C., and Solomon, S.: Physiological responses to heat and cold. In Licht, S., editor: Therapeutic heat and cold, New Haven, 1958, Elizabeth Licht.

Guy, A.W.: Analyses of electromagnetic fields induced in biological tissues by thermographic studies on equivalent phantom models, IEEE Trans. Microwave Theory Tech. Vol MTT **19**:205, 1971.

Guy, A.W., and Lehmann, J.F.: On the determination of an optimum microwave diathermy frequency for a direct contact applicator, Institute of Electrical and Electronic Engineers Trans. Biomed. Eng. **13**:76, 1966.

Guy, A.W., Lehmann, J.F., and Stonebridge, J.B.: Therapeutic applications of electromagnetic power, Proc. Institute of Electrical and Electronic Engineers **62**:55, 1974.

Guy, A.W., Lehmann, J.F., Stonebridge, J.B., and Sorensen, C.C.: Development of a 915 MHz direct contact applicator for therapeutic heating of tissues, Inst. Electrical Electronics Engineers on Microwave Theory and Techniques **26**:550-556, 1978.

Hall, E.L.: Diathermy generators, Arch. Phys. Med. Rehabil. **33**:28, 1952.

Harris, R.: Effect of shortwave diathermy on radio-sodium clearance from the knee joint in the normal and in rheumatoid arthritis, Phys. Med. Rehabil. **42**:241, 1961.

Herrick, J.F., Jelatis, D.G., and Lee, G.M.: Dielectric properties of tissues important in microwave diathermy, Fed. Proc. **9**:60, 1950.

Herrick, J.F., and Krusen, F.H.: Certain physiologic and pathologic effects of microwaves, Electrical Engineers **72**:239, 1953.

Hollander, J.L., et al.: Joint temperature measurement in evaluation of antiarthritic agents, J. Clin. Invest. **30**:701, 1951.

Hutchinson, W.J., and Burdeaux, B.D.: The effects of shortwave diathermy on bone repair, J. Bone Joint Surg. **33A**:155, 1951.

Johnson, C.C., and Guy, A.W.: Nonionizing electromagnetic wave effects in biological materials and systems, Proc. Institute of Electrical and Electronic Engineers **66**:692, 1972.

Jones, S.L.: Electromagnetic field interference and cardiac pacemakers, Phys. Ther. **56**:1013, 1976.

Kantor, G.: Evaluation and survey of microwave and radio frequency applicators, J. Microwave Power (2) **16**:135, 1981.

Kantor, G., and Witters, D.M.: The performance of a new 915 MHz direct contact applicator with reduced leakage—a detailed analysis, HHS Publication (FDA) S3-8199, April, 1983.

Kloth, L.: Shortwave and microwave diathermy. In Michlovich, S., editor: Thermal agents in rehabilitation, Philadelphia, 1986, F.A. Davis Co.

Kloth, L.C., Morrison, M., and Ferguson, B.: Therapeutic microwave and shortwave diathermy—a review of thermal effectiveness, safe use, and state-of-the-art—1984, Center for Devices and Radiological Health, DHHS, FDA 85-8237, December, 1984.

Lehmann, J.F.: Diathermy. In Krusen, F.H., editor: Handbook of physical medicine and rehabilitation, Philadelphia, 1966, W.B. Saunders Co.

Lehmann, J.F.: Therapeutic heat and cold, ed 3, Baltimore, 1982, Williams & Wilkins.

Lehmann, J.F., et al.: Comparison of relative heating patterns produced in tissues by exposure to microwave energy at frequencies of 2450 and 900 megacycles, Arch. Phys. Med. Rehabil. **46**:307, 1965.

Lehmann, J.F., et al.: Modification of heating patterns produced by microwaves at the frequencies of 2456 and 900 mc by physiologic factors in the human, Arch. Phys. Med. Rehabil. **46**:307, 1965.

Lehmann, J.F., et al.: Review of evidence for indications, techniques of application, contraindications, hazards and clinical effectiveness for shortwave diathermy, DHEW/FDA HFA-510, 5600 Fischers Lane, Rockville, MD 20852, 1974.

Lehmann, J.F., et al.: Microwave therapy: stray radiation, safety and effectiveness, Arch. Phys. Med. Rehabil. **60**:578, 1979.

Lehmann, J.F., DeLateur, B.J., and Stonebridge, J.B.: Selective muscle heating by shortwave diathermy with a helical coil, Arch. Phys. Med. Rehabil. **50**:117, 1969.

Lehman, J.F., Guy, A.W., deLateur, B.J., Stonebridge, J.B., and Warren, C.G.: Heating patterns produced by shortwave diathermy using helical induction coil applicators, Arch. Phys. Med. **49**:193-198, 1968.

Lehmann, J.F., Warren, C.G., and Scham, S.M.: Therapeutic heat and cold, Clin. Orthop. **99**:207, 1974.

Licht, S., editor: Therapeutic heat & cold, ed. 2, New Haven, Connecticut, 1972; Elizabeth Licht, Chapters 3, 11, and 12.

McNiven, D.R., and Wyper, D.J.: Microwave therapy and muscle blood flow in man, J. Microwave Power **11**:168-170, 1976.

Millard, J.B.: Effect of high frequency currents and infra-red rays on the circulation of the lower limb in man, Ann. Phys. Med. **6**:45, 1961.

Mosely, H., and Davison, M.: Exposure of physiotherapists to microwave radiation during microwave diathermy treatment, Clin. Phys. Physiol. Meas. No. 3. **2**:217, 1981.

Nelson, A.J.M., and Holt, J.A.G.: Combined microwave therapy, Med. J. Aust. **2**:88-90, 1978.

Osborne, S.L., and Coulter, J.S.: Thermal effects of shortwave diathermy on bone and muscle, Arch. Phys. Ther. **38**:281-284, 1938.

Paliwal, B.R., et al.: Heating patterns produced by 434 MHz erbotherm UHF69, Radiology **135**:511, 1980.

Pasila, M., Visuri, T., and Sundholm, A.: Pulsating shortwave diathermy: value in treatment of recent ankle and foot sprains, Arch. Phys. Med. Rehabil. **59**:383, 1978.

Pätzold, J.: Physical laws regarding distribution of energy for various high frequency methods applied in heat therapy, Ultrasonics Bio. Med. **2**:58, 1956.

Rae, J.W., Herrick, J.F., Wakim, K.G., and Krusen, F.H.: A comparative study of the temperature produced by MWD and SWD, Arch. Phys. Med. Rehabil. **30**:199, 1949.

Richardson, A.W., et al.: The relationship between deep tissue temperature and blood flow during electromagnetic irradiation, Arch. Phys. Med. Rehabil. **31**:19, 1950.

Rubin, A., and Erdman, W.I.: Microwave exposure of the human female pelvis during early pregnancy and prior to conception, Am. J. Phys. Med. **38**:219, 1959.

Schliephake, E.: Carrying out treatment. In Thom, H: Introduction to shortwave and microwave therapy, ed 3. Springfield, IL, 1966, Charles C Thomas Publishers.

Schwan, H.P., and Piersol, G.M.: The absorption of electromagnetic energy in body tissues. Part I, Am. J. Phys. Med. **33**:371, 1954.

Schwan, H.P., and Piersol, G.M.: The absorption of electromagnetic energy in body tissues. Part II, Am. J. Phys. Med. **34**:425, 1955.

Silverman, D.R., and Pendleton, L.: A comparison of the effects of continuous and pulsed shortwave diathermy on peripheral circulation, Arch. Phys. Med. **49**:429, 1968.

Smyth, H.: The pacemaker patient and the electromagnetic environment, J.A.M.A. **227**:1412, 1974.

Stuchly, M.A., et al.: Exposure to the operator and patient during shortwave diathermy treatments, Health Phys. **42**:341, 1982.

Thom, H.: Introduction to shortwave and microwave therapy, ed 3, Springfield, IL, 1966, Charles C Thomas Publishers.

Van Ummersen, C.A.: The effect of 2450 mc radiation on the development of the chick embryo. In Peyton, M.F., editor: Biological effects of microwave radiation, Vol 1, New York, 1961, Plenum Press.

Ward, A.R.: Electricity fields and waves in therapy, Science Press, Australia, 1980, NSW.

Wilson, D.H.: Comparison of shortwave diathermy and pulsed electromagnetic energy in treatment of soft-tissue injuries, Physiotherapy **60**:309, 1974.

Wilson, D.H., et al.: The effects of pulsed electromagnetic energy on peripheral nerve regeneration, Ann. N.Y. Acad. Sci. **238**:575, 1975.

Wise, C.S.: The effect of diathermy on blood flow, Arch. Phys. Med. Rehabil. **29**:17, 1948.

Witters, D.M., and Kantor, G.: An evaluation of microwave diathermy applicators using free space electric field mapping, Phys. Med. Biol. **26**:1099, 1981.

Worden, R.E., et al.: The heating effects of microwaves with and without ischemia, Arch. Phys. Med. Rehabil. **29**:751, 1948.

Ultraviolet Therapy

8

J. Marc Davis

OBJECTIVES

Following completion of this chapter, the student will be able to:

- Describe the position of ultraviolet radiation (UVR) in the electromagnetic spectrum and the relationship of UVR to other forms of electromagnetic energy.

- Understand how UVR raises energy levels within irradiated objects.

- Understand the effect of UVR on individual cells and human tissue and explain the tanning process.

- Describe the effect of long-term exposure to UVR and the effect of UVR on the eyes.

- Explain the physical setup and procedures for operating a UVR device, including safety precautions, the skin test, the inverse square law, and the cosine law.

- Understand various clinical uses of UVR.

Ultraviolet radiation (UVR) is one of the oldest medical modalities. The physicians of ancient Egypt and Greece attributed many healing powers to sunlight, and in fact life itself would not be possible without the interaction of solar UVR and plant photosynthesis. Prior to this century the sun was the only satisfactory source of UVR, but now a wide selection of UVR generators is available.

The purpose of this chapter is to familiarize the student with the properties of UVR, to explain how UVR affects human tissue, and to explore different UVR treatment apparatus and treatment techniques. Subsequently, the sports therapist should be able to understand why UVR therapy can be effective in treating certain maladies, and therefore be able to correctly choose UVR therapy when it is the appropriate treatment for a given problem.

UVR is the portion of the electromagnetic spectrum that ranges from 2000 to 4000 A and is bordered below 2000 A by x-ray and above 4000 A by visible light (see Fig. 2-2). The UVR portion of the electromagnetic spectrum is further divided into three sections: UV-A, UV-B, and UV-C. UV-C (also called shortwave UV, extreme UV, and far UV) ranges from 2000 to 2900 A and is bactericidal.[14,20] UV-B (called middle UV and the sunburn spectrum) ranges from 2900 to 3200 A and is associated with sunburn and age-related skin changes.[13-19] UV-A (near UV) ranges from 3200 to 4000 A and until recently little or no physiologic effect was attributed to UV-A, but recent research and clinical use of UV-A are showing possible benefits and hazards for UV-A exposure. The UVR apparatus most likely to be encountered in an athletic training or sports medicine setting would generate UVR in the UV-B or UV-C range, or in both ranges.

The beneficial effects of UVR as a treatment modality are mediated by its limited absorption; UVR is absorbed within the first 1 to 2 mm of human skin and most of the physiologic effects are superficial.[5] Therefore the most effective use of UVR therapy is in the treatment of various skin disorders such as acne and psoriasis.[8]

EFFECT ON CELLS

UVR is a form of energy and as such when it contacts any surface, skin included, it must be either reflected or absorbed and transmitted. If UVR strikes the skin at a 90-degree angle, 90% to 95% of the energy will be absorbed. Most will be absorbed within the epidermis of the skin (80% to 90%) while the rest will reach the dermis.[5] As the UVR is absorbed within the tissue it causes the energy level of exposed atoms to increase. These atoms will quickly return to their normal energy state; however, the presence of excess energy causes chemical excitation within the cells of the exposed tissue. This chemical excitation is the cause of the various effects of UVR on living cells and tissue. Even a single exposure to UVR will cause chemical excitation within exposed cells, which leads to physiologic changes within these cells.

These physiologic changes are the result of a photochemical event that is the end product of the UVR-induced chemical excitation. This photochemical event results in an alteration of cell biochemistry and cellular metabolism. The synthesis of **DNA** and **RNA** is affected, leading to alterations in protein and enzyme production. As a consequence, cell protein structure can be altered, and this alteration of cellular protein and DNA may leave the cell inactive or dead.[14-19]

Fortunately, defenses have evolved that protect microorganisms and cells that are exposed to a constant barrage of UVR from the sun. The damaged cells may be restored by enzymatic action or by simple deterioration of the damaged portion, the damaged segment may be replaced by normal material, or it may be bypassed when the cell reproduces.[14] DNA synthesis within cells of the human epidermis is suppressed for 24 to 48 hours following exposure to UVR in the range of 2500 to 2700 A and is then followed by a period of increased DNA synthesis.[14-19]

Normal human skin consists of two layers, the superficial epidermis and the underlying dermis (Fig. 8-1). The epidermis is avascular and composed mostly of well-organized layers of **keratinocytes.** These produce **keratin,** the fibrous protective protein of the skin. The keratinocytes are produced from cells of the basal layer of the epidermis and then move upward through the epidermis. The dermis is divided into two layers, the papillary layer that contains a rich blood supply, and the reticular layer that is composed of heavy connective tissue and contains fibroblasts, histiocytes, and most cells.

When human skin is exposed to UVR, the individual cells react as previously described. However, the skin is a protective organ, covering the entire human exterior, and it will respond in a generalized manner over the entire area that is irradiated. This generalized response culminates in the development of an acute inflammatory reaction. The end results of an active inflammation within the skin are **erythema** (the reddening of the skin associated with sunburn), pigmentation (tanning), and increased epidermal thickness.[5,9,14,19]

Inflammation is the response of any human tissue, skin included, to an irritating or injurious substance or event. In the case of UVR exposure the irritating substances are the end products of the previously described photochemical event and may include damaged DNA, RNA, and cell proteins. The purpose of the inflammatory process is to remove these injurious and irritating substances from the skin. Since the appearance of these irritating substances does not occur immediately following UVR exposure, the inflammatory response is delayed. Normally it begins several hours after irradiation and peaks 8 to 24 hours following exposure.[14]

This inflammatory response is characterized by local vasodilation and increased capillary permeability. Theoretically this is caused by (1) the absorption of UVR by keratinocytes, leading to the release of substances that diffuse to the

EFFECT ON
NORMAL
HUMAN TISSUE
Short-Term Effect
On Human Skin

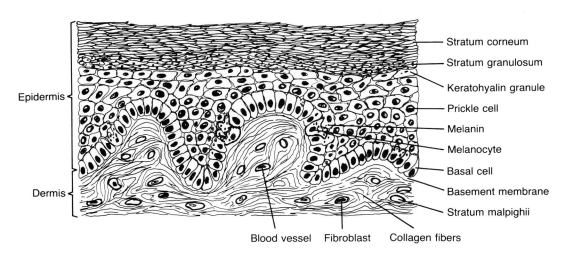

Figure 8-1. A cross section of the skin showing the layers of epidermis and dermis.

papillary dermis and cause vasodilation, or (2) the absorption of UVR by mast cells in the dermis that in turn release histamine, resulting in vasodilation.[5,9,14] Erythema is caused by this vasodilation and the subsequent increase of blood within the dermis. The increased capillary permeability permits certain proteins to move from the capillaries and into the dermis. This results in a change in osmotic pressure; consequently water is drawn into the area and edema occurs. Leukocytes, lymphocytes, and monocytes pass into the dermis and to a small degree into the epidermis. These cells phagocytize (consume or engulf) dead cells and other debris. At 24 hours the inflammatory process is completed, and at 30 hours the rebuilding begins. The reparative process is characterized by increased activity of the keratinocytes and results in a thickening of the epidermis **(hyperplasia)**.[14] This is protective; areas covered with a thick epidermis, such as the soles of the feet, do not sunburn.

The acute effects of UVR exposure can be exacerbated if certain chemicals or medications are present on the skin or in the body. Photosensitization is a process in which a person becomes overly sensitive to UVR as a result of the excitation of a chemical by UVR exposure.[5] Any person taking a photosensitizing medication is very susceptible to the effects of UVR and should be treated accordingly. It should be noted that such an adverse reaction can occur even after limited exposure to natural sunlight. A list of common photosensitizing agents follows:

ANTIBACTERIAL AND MICROBIAL AGENTS
Tetracyclines—a group of broad spectrum antibiotics
Sulfonamides—a group of synthetic antimicrobial drugs
Griseofulvin (Fulvicin, Grifulvin, Grisactin)—an antibiotic with an additional antifungal action
THIAZIDE DIURETICS. A group of drugs that act on the kidney to increase sodium and water in the urine
Chlorothiazide (Diuril)
Hydrochlorothiazide (Hydrodiuril, Oretic, Esidrix)
Methychlorothiazide (Enduron)
OTHER MEDICATIONS
Phenothiazines (Thorazine)—widely used tranquilizers
Psoralens—a group of dermal pigmenting agents
Sulfonylureas (Dymelor, Diabinese)
Diphenhydramine (Benadryl)—an antihistamine
MISCELLANEOUS
Sunscreens
Tar
Oral contraceptives
Certain cosmetics[5,13,14]

TANNING. Tanning is the increase of pigmentation within the skin and is a protective mechanism activated by UVR exposure. An increase of **melanin,** the pigment responsible for darkening, within the skin causes the tan (see Fig. 8-1). The melanin functions as a biologic filter of UVR by scattering the radiation, by absorbing the UVR, and by dissipating the absorbed energy as heat.[19] The process of tanning is divided into two phases: immediate tanning and delayed tanning.

Immediate tanning appears most often in darkly pigmented individuals and occurs immediately following UVR exposure. Immediate tanning represents the darkening of melanosomes already present in the skin; it begins to fade 1 hour after exposure and is hardly noticeable 3 to 8 hours later.[14,19] Delayed tanning is the result of the formation of new pigment (melanin) through the process of melanogenesis. The process is initiated by production of erythema (sunburn) within the skin. Melanogenesis occurs within the melanocytes of the basal layer of the epidermis (Fig. 8-1), and the end products of this process are melanosomes, new pigment granules. These melanosomes are transferred from the melanocytes via nerve cells to nearby keratinocytes. As the keratinocytes gradually move outward to the skin's surface, the new pigment also migrates to the periphery. Delayed tanning usually becomes apparent 72 hours after UVR exposure.

Human skin color is a baseline that is influenced by various environmental factors (exposure to solar radiation, occupation, leisure activities) and the genetically determined level of melanin within the skin.[5,20] Individuals of all races have the same number of melanocytes per unit area, but darker individuals are able to produce greater amounts of melanin.[4]

Artificial Tanning Devices

In the past decade, artificial tanning devices have become popular in the spa and health club industry. These tanning salons, beds, and booths usually consist of an array of long tubes positioned in a frame that allows for exposure of the entire body. The manufacturers claim that these devices produce only UVR in the UV-A spectrum and therefore are safe. However, the production of this type of UV-A generator is largely unregulated and the effects of long-term exposure to UV-A are unknown. There is no standard of training required for the owners of these machines, and their knowledge of the tanning process and the dangers of UVR might be nil. Caution should be exercised before allowing anyone to be overexposed to UVR, either from sunlight or from an artificial source.

Long-Term Effect on Skin

The most serious effects of long-term UVR exposure are premature aging of the skin and skin cancer.[10,16,17] Lightly pigmented individuals are more susceptible to these maladies. Premature aging of the skin is characterized by dryness, cracking, and a decrease in the elasticity of the skin, and it results from a change in the epidermis called solar elastosis. An alteration in the skin's elastic fibers causes solar elastosis and has been tentatively linked to UVR-induced DNA damage.[14]

Skin cancer is the most common malignant tumor found in humans and has been epidemiologically and clinically associated with solar UVR.[14,16,20] Damage to DNA is suspected as the cause of skin cancer, but the exact cause is yet unknown. The major types of skin cancer are basal cell carcinoma, which rarely metastasizes (spreads to other areas), squamous cell carcinoma, which metastasizes in 5% of all cases, and malignant melanoma, which metastasizes in a majority of cases.[14,16] Fortunately the rate of cure exceeds 95% with early detection and treatment.

EFFECT ON EYES

For centuries it has been known that sunlight can have an adverse effect on vision. Snow blindness, the result of solar UVR being reflected from the snow to the unprotected eyes of winter outdoor enthusiasts, was first described in 375 BC.[19] UVR exposure of the eyes causes an acute inflammation called **photokeratitis.** It is a delayed reaction occurring from 6 to 24 hours after exposure, but occasionally it develops within 30 minutes. Conjunctivitis (inflammation of the mucous membrane that lines the inside of the eyelid) develops, accompanied by erythema of adjacent facial skin, and the injured person reports the sensation of a foreign body on the eye. Photophobia, increased tear production, and spasm of the ocular muscles may occur.[14,20] The acute reaction lasts from 6 to 24 hours, and all symptoms will generally clear by 48 hours with few residual effects. The eye, unlike the skin, does not develop a tolerance to UVR. The development of cataracts has been attributed to UVR, especially in wavelengths of greater than 2900 A.[18-20]

SYSTEMIC EFFECTS

The only systemic effect that can be objectively attributed to UVR (the only positive effect in general for that matter) is the photosynthesis of vitamin D following irradiation of the skin by UVR in the UV-B range.[18] The process is activated when the skin is irradiated by UVR at approximately 300 A wavelength. This activates a complicated biochemical pathway that travels from the skin to the liver and kidney and results in vitamin D being delivered to bones, to the intestines, to various organs, and to muscles. Vitamin D is responsible for regulating calcium and phosphorus, and after UVR exposure the absorption of these elements increases within the intestines and results in increased amounts of calcium and phosphorus within the blood. Consequently UVR can be used as a treatment for disorders of calcium and phosphorus metabolism, such as rickets and tetany. Presently the treatment of choice for such problems is dietary supplementation; however, if this is not effective, UVR is an acceptable alternative.

Although no other systemic effects can be objectively attributed to UVR exposure, there are several psychologic benefits and problems that may result from exposure. Many people relish the immediate sensation of warmth and relaxation that results from resting in the sun on a nice summer day; a general sense of well-being and good health surrounds the individual. Ideally this happy experience is not overindulged, resulting in a painful sunburn. Moderation is the key to preventing damage to the skin; this includes gradually increasing exposure to the sun and prudent use of sunscreens.

Europeans, especially those living in northern latitudes, are probably the world's most active sunbathers. During the spring and summer months, they will congregate in sunny areas and feed on the sunlight that is so unavailable during their dark winters. The use of artificial UVR for tanning purposes is great in these areas, certainly for the sense of well-being that follows brief UVR exposure and also for questionable medical reasons. The use of artificial UVR to pre-serve the summer's tan is also on the increase in the United States and can be witnessed in the rapidly increasing number of tanning salons and spas. The apparatus most likely to be employed in one of these establishments will produce UVR in the UV-A wavelength, and the management of the salon will be quick to point out that this is a safe alternative to natural sunlight. An individual can certainly achieve tanning from these devices, although not as effectively as from UV-B exposure, but the research is still cloudy on the safety of long-term exposure to UV-A.

Needless to say, the psychologic effect from the extreme skin damage from long-term exposure to UVR can be devastating. The peaches-and-cream complexion of a 20-year-old beauty queen can turn to withered leather at 40 if caution is not used out of doors and in the tanning salon. A diagnosis of skin cancer will surely throw a person's psychologic health into a downward spiral.

APPARATUS

Since the beginning of this century many types of UVR generators have been developed, including the carbon arc lamp, the fluorescent lamp, the xenon compact arc lamp, and the mercury arc lamps. Of these, the mercury arc lamps are the most common and they have been found to be safe, effective, and easy to operate.

The carbon arc lamp is composed of two carbon electrodes that consist of carbon and certain inorganic salts and metals. Initially the two electrodes are in contact when the current is applied and then are moved slightly apart, causing the current to arc across this small gap. As the salts and metals within the electrodes become heated, UVR is emitted, the majority between 3500 and 4000 A. The electrode gradually burns, and so the lamp will deteriorate and the electrodes must be replaced. This burning is noisy and causes an unpleasant odor, and the device requires a high electrical input.

The xenon compact arc lamp is composed of xenon gas enclosed in a vessel in which it is compressed to 20 times atmospheric pressure. An electric arc is passed through the gas, causing increased temperature. When the gas is heated to 6000° C (10,832° F), the atoms become incandescent and emit infrared, visible, and ultraviolet light waves. Most of the UVR is in the range of 3200 to 4000 A. Caution must be exercised when using a device with gas under such high pressure because rupture of the containing vessel could endanger the patient and operator.

The mercury arc lamps are divided into two categories, low-pressure and high-pressure mercury arcs. Both consist of mercury (a heavy metal in a liquid state) contained in a quartz envelope. When an electric arc is passed through the envelope, the mercury becomes vaporized and at 8000° C (14,432° F) the atoms become incandescent and emit ultraviolet, infrared, and visible light. In the low-pressure lamp, also called the cold quartz lamp, the temperature of the mercury electrons is greater than the mercury vapor and the temperature of the quartz envelope is about 60° C—hot, but not dangerous. The UVR spectrum produced by low-pressure lamps is limited to 1849 A and 2537 A. The 1849 A wavelength is blocked by the quartz envelope or it would combine with oxygen and produce ozone; 95% of the UVR produced by these lamps is the 2537 A wavelength, which is highly germicidal. The low-pressure mercury arc lamp does not require a warm up or cool down period, and it is used mainly where the bactericidal effect of UVR is desired.

A high-pressure mercury arc occurs when the mercury vapor temperature equals the mercury electron temperature and the pressure within the envelope reaches one atmosphere or more.[17] The quartz envelopes of these lamps becomes quite hot and may be cooled by a water jacket or circulating air; subsequently these are called hot quartz lamps. The UVR spectrum produced peaks at 2537, 2800, 2967, 3025, 3130, and 3660 A.[5,9,18,19] The 2537 A wavelength is absorbed by the increased density of the mercury vapor and does not pass from the lamp. Most of the UVR produced falls within the UV-B range. These lamps require a warm up period before reaching peak efficiency and a cool down period after the current is stopped before the lamp can be restarted. The high-pressure mercury arc lamps are mainly used to produce erythema and the accompanying photochemical reactions.

The fluorescent ultraviolet lamp or "blacklight" is actually a low-pressure mercury lamp. It consists of a tube of UV-transmitting glass that is coated with phosphors. The phosphors are fluorescing substances that absorb the UVR and then reemit it at a longer wavelength. Most of the UVR emitted ranges from 3000 to 4000 A, within the high UV-B and entire UV-A range.[18] These lamps are low-powered and generally used in multiples. These lamps are used where exposure of several people simultaneously is desired.

The mercury arc lamps are the most likely kind of UVR lamp to be used in a sports medicine setting, and generally the lamps will be either a standing model or a hand-held model. The standing model consists of a mercury arc lamp surrounded by a reflector. The opening below the lamp and reflector can be closed by the use of shutters. The lamp, reflector, and shutters are supported by a column and the height of the column is adjustable. At the base of the column is a housing that contains the electrical controls contained within the configuration of the unit (Fig. 8-2). The hand-held unit is used for very local treatments and produces the bactericidal spectral bond of 2536 A. It is very effective for treating local skin infections and, with the addition of a special lens, is used for diagnostic purposes.

TECHNIQUE OF APPLICATION

Before operation of any UVR generator, sports therapists must thoroughly familiarize themselves with the equipment; the operation manual must be understood and available if needed. Faulty operation of the equipment can endanger both the patient and the operator. The lamp and reflector must be kept clean by wiping with gauze and methyl alcohol or by following the manufacturer's instructions. The quality of UVR is greatly diminished by dirty lamps and reflectors. The entire device must be completely inspected prior to use to ensure safe operation.

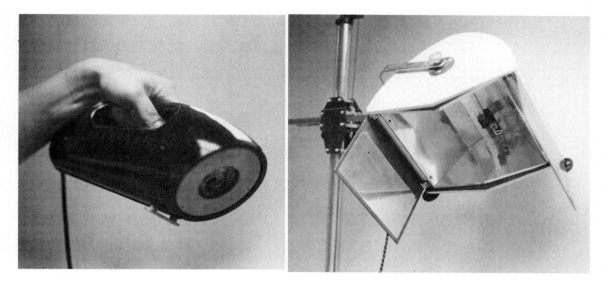

Figure 8-2. *(Left)* A hand-held cold quartz ultraviolet lamp. *(Right)* A standing hot quartz ultraviolet lamp. Note the open shutters.

The effectiveness of the apparatus must be determined before UVR therapy can begin. The lamps in these devices deteriorate over time and accumulation of dirt and other residues on the lamp and reflector can also alter the effect of the UVR. Two lamps of the same model may have two differing effects, depending on the age of the lamp and its condition. The effectiveness of the lamp is assessed by determining the skin sensitivity to UVR of the patient to be treated. This sensitivity is measured by the **minimal erythemal dose.** The minimal erythemal dose is the exposure time needed to produce a faint erythema of the skin 24 hours after exposure.[5,16] Prior to testing, the patient should be questioned regarding photosensitizing drugs and the area of skin to be tested should be cleaned. The area of the test should have pigmentation similar to the area to be treated. The forearm is a common choice for the test site.

For the skin test, the patient should be positioned comfortably and eye protection must be provided the patient and the operator. The goggles must fit snugly, since UVR can be reflected behind the lens of ordinary sunglasses. The patient may be instructed to close his eyes as an added precaution. The patient is draped except for the test site; a good quality bed sheet or bath towel provides an adequate barrier to UVR. A piece of typing paper with five cutouts 1 inch square and 1 inch apart is placed over the test site (Fig. 8-3). If necessary the lamp is warmed up with the protective shutters closed. The lamp is positioned over the patient with care being taken to adjust the height of the lamp from the patient to the same level as for treatment. With the lamp in position, the shutters are opened and the cutouts covered at 15-second intervals so that

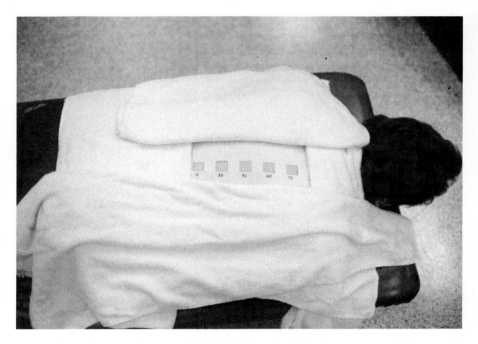

Figure 8-3. The skin test. The patient's back is draped and has been sequentially exposed to ultraviolet radiation for 15, 30, 45, 60, and 75 seconds.

the five portions of the skin will be exposed for 15, 30, 45, 60, and 75 seconds. The patient returns in 24 hours and a visual inspection determines the minimal erythemal dose. This information is used as the basis for determining treatment time.[3]

Areas tested that reveal no erythema 24 hours after testing have received a suberythemal dose, whereas those demonstrating erythema at 24 hours have received the minimal erythemal dose. At 48 hours if erythema is still present, a first-degree erythemal dose has been given, and a second-degree erythemal dose has been given if erythema persists from 48 to 72 hours. If the erythema lasts past 72 hours after testing, then a third-degree erythemal dose has been given. The third-degree erythemal dose is pathologic and causes destruction of the skin. Second-degree and third-degree doses are seldom used except in the case of stubborn skin infections, and when they are used, the skin surrounding the area of treatment should be well protected from exposure. First-degree and second-degree doses can be estimated; first-degree erythemal doses approximately correspond to 2.5 times the minimal erythemal dose and second-degree doses correspond to 5 times the minimal erythemal dose.[5]

Since human skin adapts to UVR exposure, the minimal erythemal dose will gradually increase with repeated treatments. Therefore it is necessary to gradually increase exposure time in order to achieve the same reaction. Once the treatment time has been determined, it is increased 5 seconds per treatment with the height of the lamp remaining constant. Conversely, treatment time should be reduced 5 seconds for each day missed or it should be set back to the original minimal erythemal dose.

In order to give consistent treatments, the operator needs to be aware of the two laws of physics that apply directly to UVR treatments, the **inverse square law** and the **cosine law.** The inverse square law states that the strength of radiation of light from a point source varies inversely with the square of the distance from the source.[5,18] Therefore if the lamp is set closer to the patient than during the skin test, a stronger dose is given; if it is set further away, a weaker dose is given. The distance of the lamp from the patient must be kept constant if the intensity of the treatments is to be equal. The height of the lamp is generally standardized at each clinic, usually ranging from 24 to 40 inches.[10] My preference is to set the height of the lamp at 30 inches.

The cosine law states that for maximum absorption of radiant energy, the source must be perpendicular to the absorbing surface (the patient being the absorbing surface).[5,18] A deviation of 10 degrees causes no major alteration in the amount of energy absorbed. Therefore care should be taken in positioning the lamp and patient during testing and treatment.

Once the minimal erythemal dose has been established, treatment can commence. As with the skin test, the treatment area should be warm and provided maximum privacy since the patient may be partially or fully disrobed. Goggles, stopwatch, measuring tape, and draping must be readily available. The patient should be carefully draped so that areas not to receive UVR exposure are protected. Besides the eyes, the nipples and genitalia should be protected. It should be taken into account that UVR can be reflected from white linen and shiny equipment surfaces. If needed, the UVR apparatus should be warmed up with the protective shutter in place. The patient and operator are ready to begin treatment when the patient is comfortable, properly draped, and has his or her eyes protected. The lamp is positioned at proper height and angle, and the operator has his or her goggles in place and stopwatch ready. Treatment commences when the operator simultaneously opens the shutters and activates the stopwatch. At the end of the predetermined treatment time, the shutters are closed, the lamp is extinguished, and the patient is allowed to remove the goggles and dress. Accurate records noting the height of the lamp, time of exposure, and condition of the area treated must be kept. Also, the same lamp should be used for subsequent treatments since lamp deterioration causes differing intensities from UVR sources of even the same manufacturer's model.

Consistency is crucial if safe and effective UVR treatments are to be given. The setup of the patient and equipment should not vary without adequate reason. Usually the only variable is the length of treatment (exposure) and that is determined by and based on the skin test, the treatment prescription, the lesion to be treated, and the progression of treatment. If the length of treatment is in doubt, it is always best to yield to brevity rather than to endanger a patient.

CLINICAL USE   UVR therapy is used to obtain one or more of the following effects: increased vitamin D production, stimulation of the skin, sterilization, tanning, hyperplasia, and exfoliation (peeling).[18] The use of UVR is indicated for treatment of infectious and noninfectious skin diseases and for the excitation of calcium metabolism.[5] The development of antibiotics and other medications has greatly reduced the clinical use of UVR since these drugs are very effective and simple to employ in the treatment of disease. Today the most common use of UVR is in the treatment of dermatologic conditions such as psoriasis and acne and hard to cure infectious skin conditions such as pressure sores. The protocol for treating certain maladies with UVR follows.

PSORIASIS. The Goekerman technique developed in 1925 is still widely used. This consists of applying a crude tar ointment (2% to 5%) over the patches of psoriasis the night prior to treatment. The next morning the tar is removed, except for a thin film, and the area is irradiated with a UV-B source at minimal erythemal dosage.[2,5] The exposure time is gradually increased and the treatment is usually carried out for several weeks. In the past decade, a UV-A source and the photosensitizing drug psoralen have been used to treat psoriasis. This technique is called PUVA therapy and is discussed below.

DISTURBANCES OF CALCIUM AND PHOSPHORUS ABSORPTION. Conditions such as osteomalacia (rickets) and tetany can be treated with irradiation by a UV-B source. These disturbances of absorption are caused by a vitamin D deficiency. As previously discussed, vitamin D is produced following irradiation of the skin. Whole body irradiation is indicated if diet and oral supplementation of calcium and phosphorus do not produce improvement.[18]

PRESSURE SORES. Unlike most infectious skin disorders, pressure sores do not respond readily to antibiotic therapy. Irradiation of the lesion by low-pressure mercury or cold quartz lamp, which produces UVR of the bactericidal 2537 A wavelength, can be an effective means of treating this problem. The hand-held lamps are most useful since they can be used to produce a very localized reaction. Exposure time should be sufficient to produce a second-degree or third-degree erythemal dose response.[5,18] Care must be taken to protect the surrounding skin.

PUVA THERAPY. A treatment for psoriasis that consists of ingestion of oral methoxsalen, a psoralen, and exposure of the affected site to a UV-A light source. The methoxsalen increases the patient's sensitivity to UVR, and in the presence of UV-A it binds with DNA and inhibits DNA synthesis.[6] Unfortunately, several studies point to an increased risk of developing skin cancer following PUVA therapy, and problems with the safety of the UV-A sources have been uncovered.[1,6,7,15] Still, in selected cases PUVA therapy is considered by the American Academy of Dermatology to be safe, but its use should be limited to physicians with training in photochemotherapy.[1]

STERILIZATION. Bacteria are destroyed when exposed to UVR in the range of 2500 to 2700 A. This technique has been used to sterilize the air in operating rooms and to sterilize water. The technique is quite safe if human exposure to the UVR source is kept to a minimum.

DIAGNOSIS. A UVR source fitted with a special filter, a Wood's filter, can be used to aid in the diagnosis of certain skin disorders. The filter blocks all the UVR except that in the range of 3600 to 3700 A. This wavelength is most effective in causing exposed areas to fluoresce. The test is performed in a darkened room, and since all animal tissues fluoresce, the exposure to the filtered UVR will cause the exposed tissue to appear a specific color.[18] However, if an infection is present, the color of the area will correspond to the fluorescence of the infecting organism rather than the expected normal color. This abnormal coloration can be evaluated and a tentative diagnosis made.

INDICATIONS

Acne. General body irradiation may help, minimal erythemal dose applied three times per week

Aseptic wounds. Suberythemal dose applied every 3 days[2,5,10,12,18]

Folliculitis. Suberythemal dose applied every 3 days until clear

Pityriasis rosea. General body irradiation, minimal erythemal dose applied three times per week

Tinea capitum. Local first-degree erythemal reaction, repeated when initial response clears

Septic wounds. Local second-degree erythemal response, repeated every 3 days

Sinusitis. General body irradiation

CONTRA-INDICATIONS

Porphyrias
Pellagra
Lupus erythematosus
Sarcoidosis
Xeroderma pigmentosum
Acute psoriasis
Acute eczema
Herpes simplex
Renal and hepatic insufficiencies
Diabetes
Hyperthyroidism
Generalized dermatitis
Advanced arteriosclerosis
Active and progressive pulmonary tuberculosis[2,5,10-12,18]

The use of UVR therapy in athletic medicine has been limited. Many indications for its use, such as acne, skin infections, and fungal infections, are adequately treated with medication. Other problems, such as pressure sores and vitamin D deficiency, are seldom found among an athletic population. This does not mean that UVR should be excluded from the clinic; it most certainly has beneficial effects that could be used by sports therapists. But considering the small number of potential patients and the limited budgetary resources most sports therapists have available, UVR equipment will remain a low-priority item.

However, the population of the United States is gradually growing older and more active. Sports medicine is no longer limited to the college football star or the Olympic hopeful. Today sports medicine clinics are treating patients ranging from prepubescent marathoners to 70-year-old triathletes. As the number and age of active persons increase, so will the variety of problems to be treated. At present there is some inconclusive evidence that UVR can aid in the reduction of blood pressure, help to relieve asthma, cause a reduction in blood cholesterol, and aid in reducing the severity of upper respiratory infections.[18] The average patient being seen in a sports medicine clinic is generally not a world class athlete, but might be a 50-year-old executive who is emerging from 25 years of sedentary living. UVR might be a helpful part of this patient's treatment; as research continues, UVR may become a favored and useful treatment just as it was earlier in this century.

SUMMARY

1. UVR is that portion of the electromagnetic spectrum that ranges from 2000 to 4000 A.
2. Exposure to UVR causes a photochemical reaction within living cells and can cause alterations of DNA and cell proteins.
3. The irradiation of human skin causes an acute inflammation that is characterized by an erythema, increased pigmentation, and hyperplasia.
4. The effects of long-term exposure to UVR are premature aging of the skin and skin cancer.
5. The eye is extremely sensitive to UVR and will develop photokeratitis following exposure.
6. Many types of equipment are manufactured that produce UVR but the majority used clinically are of the low- and high-pressure mercury lamp variety.

GLOSSARY

DNA Deoxyribonucleic acid; the substance found in the chromosomes of the cell nucleus that carries the genetic code of the cell.

erythema A redness of the skin caused by capillary dilation.

fluorescence The capacity of certain substances to radiate when illuminated by a source of a given wavelength, a light of a different wavelength (color) than that of the irradiating source when illuminated by a given wavelength.

hyperplasia An increase in the size of a tissue; in the skin, an increased thickness of the epidermis.

keratin The fibrous protein that forms the chemical basis of the epidermis.

keratinocytes A cell that produces keratin.

melanin A group of dark brown or black pigments that occur naturally in the eye, skin, hair, and other animal tissues.

minimal erythemal dose The amount of time of exposure to UVR necessary to cause a faint erythema 24 hours after exposure.

photokeratitis An inflammation of the eyes caused by exposure to UVR.

RNA Ribonucleic acid; an acid found in the cell cytoplasm and nucleolus. It is intimately involved in protein synthesis.

REFERENCES

1 Bickford, E., et al.: Risks associated with the use of UV-A irradiators, Photochem. Photobiol. **30**(2):199-202, 1979.

2 Burdick Corp.: Burdick syllabus, ed. 7, Milton, Wisconsin, 1969.

3 Downer, A.: Physical therapy procedures, ed. 3, Springfield, 1981, Charles C Thomas, Publisher.

4 Goldman, L.: Introduction to modern phototherapy, Springfield, 1978, Charles C Thomas, Publisher.

5 Griffin, J., et al.: Physical agents for physical therapists, ed. 2, Springfield, 1982, Charles C Thomas, Publisher.

6 Hall, L.: Current status of oral PUVA therapy for psoriasis, J. Am. Acad. Dermatol. **1**(2):106-107, 1979.

7 Harbor, L.: PUVA therapy status, J. Am. Acad. Dermatol. **1**(2):150, 1979.

8 Kottke, F., et al.: Krusen's handbook of physical medicine and rehabilitation, ed. 3, Philadelphia, 1983, W.B. Saunders Co.

9 Kovacs, R.: Light therapy, Springfield, 1950, Charles C Thomas, Publishers.

10 Lewis, G.: Practical dermatology, Philadelphia, 1967, W.B. Saunders Co.

11 Mayer, E.: Clinical application of sunlight and artificial radiation, Baltimore, 1926, Williams & Wilkins.

12 Mayer, E.: The curative value of light, New York, 1932, D. Appleton Co.

13 Parish, P.: The doctors and patients handbook of medicines and drugs, New York, 1980, Alfred A. Knopf, Inc.

14 Parrish, J., et al.: UV-A biological effects of ultraviolet radiation, New York, 1979, Plenum Publishing Corp.

15 Pittekow, M., et al.: Skin cancer in patients with psoriasis treated with coal tar, Arch. Dermatol. **117**:465-468, 1981.

16 Rook, A., et al.: Textbook of dermatology, Oxford, 1979, Blackwell Scientific Publishers, Inc.

17 Stewart, W.: Dermatology: diagnosis and treatment of cutaneous disorders, St. Louis, 1978, The C.V. Mosby Co.

18 Stillwell, G.: Therapeutic electricity and ultraviolet radiation, Baltimore, 1983, Williams & Wilkins.

19 Urbach, F.: The biologic effects of ultraviolet radiation, London, 1969, Pergamon Press, Ltd.

20 U.S. Dept. of HEW, Public Health Service: Occupational exposure to ultraviolet radiation, Washington, D.C., 1972, National Institute for Occupational Safety and Health, HSM73-11009.

SUGGESTED READINGS

Bryant, B.G.: Treatment of psoriasis, Am. J. Hosp. Pharm. **37**:814-820, 1980.

Challner, A.V.J., Corless, D., Davis, A., Deane, G.H.W., Diffey, D., Gupta, S.P., and Magnus, I.A.: Personnel monitoring exposure to UV radiation, Clin. Exp. Dermatol. **1**:175-179, 1976.

Challner, A.V.J., and Duffey, B.L.: Problems associated with ultraviolet dosimetry in the photochemotherapy of psoriasis, Br. J. Dermatol. **97**:643-648, 1977.

Corless, D., and Gupta, S.P.: Response of plasma 25-hydroxyvitamin D to ultraviolet irradiation in long stay geriatric patients, Lancet 2 **23**:649-651, 1978.

Dietzel, F.: Effects of non-ionizing electromagnetic radiation on the development and intrauterine implantation of the rat. In Tyler, A.E., editor: Biological effects of nonionizing radiation, Ann. N.Y. Acad. Sci. **247**:367, 1975.

Everett, M.A., Olson, R.L., and Sayer, R.M.: Ultraviolet erythema, Arch. Dermatol. **92**:713, 1975.

Fischer, T.: Comparative treatment of psoriasis with UV-light, trioxsalen plus UV-light and coal tar plus UV-light, Acta. Derm. Venereol. **57**:345-350, 1977.

Fitzpatrick, T.B., Pathak, A., Magnus, I.A., and Curran, W.L.: Abnormal reactions of man to light, Ann. Rev. Med. **14**:195, 1963.

Giese, A., editor: Photophysiology, Volume IV, New York, 1968, Academic Press, Chapter II.

Giese, A., editor: Photophysiology, Volume V, New York, 1970, Academic Press, Chapters VI and VII.

Giese, A., editor: Photophysiology, Volume VI, New York, 1971, Academic Press, Chapter III.

Giese, A., editor: Photophysiology, Volume VII. New York, 1972, Academic Press, Chapters V and IX.

Gordon, M., editor: Pigment cell biology, New York, 1959, Academic Press, pp. 107-109, 127-137.

Grynbaum, B., et al.: Prevention of ultraviolet induced erythema, Arch. Phys. Med. Rehabil. **31**:587-592, 1950.

Hardie, R.A., and Hunter, J.A.A.: Psoriasis, Br. J. Hosp. Med. **20**:13-23, 1978.

Holick, M.F., and Clark, M.B.: The photogenesis and metabolism of vitamin D, Fed. Proc. 37 # **12**:2567-2574, 1978.

Hollaender, A., editor: Radiation biology, Volume II, New York, 1955, McGraw-Hill.

Holti, G.: Measurements of the vascular responses in skin at various time intervals after damage with histamine and ultraviolet radiation, Clin. Sci. **14**:143-155, 1955.

Jarratt, M., and Knox, J.M.: Photodynamic action: theory and applications, Prog. Dermatol. **8**:1, 1974.

Kelner, A.: Photoreactivation of ultraviolet irradiated escherichicoli, with special reference to the dose reduction principal and to ultraviolet induced mutation, J. Bacteriol. **58**:11-22, 1949.

Licht, S., editor: Therapeutic electricity and ultraviolet radiation, ed. 2, New Haven, 1967, Licht, p. 271.

Lynch, W.S., et al.: Clinical results of photochemotherapy, Cutis, **20**:477-480, 1977.

Macleod, M.A., and Blacklock, N.J.: UVL induced changes in calcium absorption and excretion and in serum vitamin D_3 levels measured in black skinned and caucasian males, J. R. Nav. Med. Serv. **65**:75-78, 1979.

Marisco, A.R., et al.: Ultraviolet light and tar in the Goeckermann treatment of psoriasis, Arch. Dermatol. **112:**1249-1250, 1976.

Montagna, W., and Labitz, W., editors: The epidermis, New York, 1964, Academic Press, p. 408.

Morison, W.L., et al.: Controlled study of PUVA and adjunctive therapy in the management of psoriasis, Br. J. Dermatol. **98:**125-132, 1978.

Ohayashi, T., Yoshimoto, S., and Yasamura, M.: Effect of wavelength on the photochemical reaction of ergocalciferol (vitamin D_2) irradiated by monochromatic ultraviolet light, J. Nutr. Sci. Vitaminol. **23:**281-290, 1977 (in English).

Parrish, J.A., et al.: Photochemotherapy of psoriasis with oral methoxsalen and longwave ultraviolet light, N. Engl. J. Med. **291:**1207-1222, 1974.

Pathak, M.A., Harber, J.C., Seiji, M., et al., editors: Sunlight and man, Tokyo, 1974, U. of Tokyo Press, pp. 335-368.

Peak, M., et al.: Inactivation of transforming DNA by ultraviolet light. II. Protection by histadine, Mutat. Res. **20:**137-141, 1973.

Roenig, H.H.: Comparison of phototherapy systems for photochemotherapy, Cutis **20:**485-489, 1977.

Rogers, S., et al.: Effect of PUVA on serum 25-OH vitamin D in psoriatics, Br. Med. J. **833:**34, 1979.

Salem, L.: Theory of photochemical reactions, Science **191:**822, 1976.

Sams, W., and Winkleman, R.: The effect of ultraviolet light on isolated cutaneous blood vessels, J. Invest. Dermatol. **53:**79-83, 1969.

Sauer, G., editor: Manual of skin diseases, ed. 3, Philadelphia, 1973, J.B. Lippincott.

Segal, S.A.: PUVA: a caution, Pediatrics **62:**253, 1978.

Sulzberger, W., Wolf, J., and Witten, V.: Dermatology: diagnosis and treatment, ed. 2, Chicago, 1961, Year Book, pp. 85-96.

Task Force Committee on Photobiology of the National Program for Dermatology, L.C. Harber, Chairman. Arch. Dermatol. **109:**833-839, 1974.

Taylor, R.L.: Clinical study of ultraviolet in various skin conditions, Phys. Ther. **52:**279-282, 1972.

Telles, Coakley, and Kluger. Bureau of Radiological Health. Food and Drug Administration: Possible hazards from high intensity discharge mercury vapor and metal halide lamps, Nov., 1977.

Thomsen, D. E.: Phototherapy: treatment with light, Science News **105:**404, 1974.

Tronnier, H.: Zur Bedeutung der Hornschicht für die Lichtreaktionen der menschlichen Haut, Strahlentherapie **132:**128-133, 1967.

Urbach, F., editor: Biological effects of ultraviolet radiation, New York, 1969, Pergamon.

Van Der Leun, J.C.: Theory of ultraviolet erythema, Photochem. Photobiol. **4:**453-458, 1965.

Van Pelt, W.F., Payne, W.R., and Peterson, R.W.: A review of selected bioeffects thresholds for various spectral ranges of light, DHEW Publ. no. (FDA) 74-8010.

Weber, G.: Combined 8-methoxypsoralen and black light therapy of psoriasis: technique and results, Br. J. Dermatol. **90:**317-323, 1974.

Wurtman, R.J.: The effects of light on the human body, Sci. Am. **233:**69, 1975.

Young, P.: Turning on light turns off disease, National Observer, May 29, 1976.

Low-Power Lasers

Ethan N. Saliba and Susan H. Foreman

9

OBJECTIVES

Following completion of this chapter, the student will be able to:

- Describe the different types of lasers.

- Understand the physical principles used to produce laser light.

- Describe the characteristics of the helium neon and gallium arsenide low-power lasers.

- Describe the therapeutic applications of lasers in wound and soft tissue healing, edema reduction, inflammation, and pain.

- Understand the techniques for application of low-power lasers.

- Describe the classifications of lasers.

- Describe the safety considerations in the use of lasers.

- Describe the precautions and contraindications for low-power lasers.

Laser is an acronym for *l*ight *a*mplification by *s*timulated *e*mission of *r*adiation. Despite the image presented in science-fiction movies, lasers offer valuable applications in the industrial, military, scientific, and medical environments. Einstein in 1916 was the first to postulate the theorems that conceptualized the development of lasers. The first work with amplified electromagnetic radiation dealt with *masers*—*m*icrowave *a*mplification by *s*timulated *e*mission of *r*adiation. In 1955 Townes and Schawlow showed it is possible to produce stimulated emission of microwaves beyond the optical region of the electromagnetic spectrum. This work soon extended into the optical region of the electromagnetic spectrum, resulting in the development of devices called *optical masers.* The first working optical maser, the synthetic ruby laser, was constructed in 1960 by Theodore Maiman. Other types of lasers were devised shortly afterward. It was not until 1965 that the term laser was substituted for optical masers.[27]

Although lasers are relatively new, they have gone through extensive advances and refinements in a very short time. Lasers have been incorporated into numerous everyday applications that range from audio discs and supermarket scanning devices to communication and medical uses. This chapter will deal principally with the application of low-power lasers in the conservative management of medical conditions.

PHYSICS

Light is a form of electromagnetic energy that has **wavelengths** between 100 and 10,000 nanometers (nm = 10^{-9}) within the electromagnetic spectrum.[27] Visible light ranges from 400 nm (violet) to 700 nm (red). Beyond the red portion of the visual range are the **infrared** and microwave regions, and below the violet end are the ultraviolet, x-ray, gamma, and cosmic ray regions. Light energy is transmitted through space as waves that contain tiny "energy packets" called **photons.** Each photon contains a definite amount of energy depending on its wavelength (color).

Basic elements of the atomic theory are used to explain the principles of laser generation. The atom is the smallest particle of an element that retains all the properties of that element. The atom is divisible into fundamental particles called *neutrons, protons,* and *electrons.* Neutrons and positively charged protons are contained in the nucleus of the atom. **Electrons,** which are negatively charged, are equal in number to the protons and orbit the nucleus at distinct energy levels.

If an atom gains or loses an electron, it will become a negatively or positively charged ion, respectively. The polarity difference between the positively charged nucleus and the negatively charged electrons keeps the electrons orbiting the nucleus at these distinct energy levels. Electrons neither absorb nor radiate energy as long as they are maintained in their distinct orbit. An electron will stay in its lowest energy level (**ground state**) unless it absorbs an amount of energy adequate to move it to one of its higher orbital levels (Fig. 9-1). If an

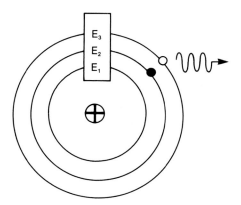

Figure 9-1. When energy is absorbed by an atom, an orbiting electron can become excited to a higher orbit. As the electron drops back to its original level, energy (photon) is released.

electron changes orbit, it will either gain or lose a distinct amount (quantum) of energy; it cannot exist between orbits.

If a photon of adequate energy level collides with an electron of an atom, it will cause the electron to change levels. When this occurs, the atom is said to be in an **excited state.** The atom stays in this excited state only momentarily and releases a photon (energy level) identical to the one it absorbed, which returns it to a ground state. This process is called **spontaneous emission** (Fig. 9-2). Energy levels are peculiar to the type of atom; therefore, an electron accepts only the precise amount of energy that will move it from one energy level to another. Another means of exciting atoms, other than photon collision, is an electrical discharge. The energy is generated by collision of electrons that are accelerated in an electrical field.[17]

Stimulated Emissions

The concept of **stimulated emission** was postulated by Einstein and is essential to the working principle of lasers. It states that a photon released from an excited atom stimulates another similarly excited atom to deexcite itself by releasing an identical photon.[27] The triggering photon continues on its way unchanged, and the subsequent photon released is identical in frequency, direction, and phase. These two photons promote the release of additional identical photons as long as other excited atoms are present. A critical factor for this occurrence is an environment with unlimited excited atoms, which is termed **population inversion.** Population inversion occurs when more atoms are in an excited state than in a ground state. It is caused by the application of an external power source to the lasing medium. The released photons are identical in phase, direction, and frequency. To contain them and to generate more photons, mirrors are placed at both ends of the chamber. One mirror is totally reflective, while the other is semipermeable. The photons are reflected within the chamber, which amplifies the light and stimulates the emission of other photons from excited atoms. Eventually, so many photons are stimulated that the

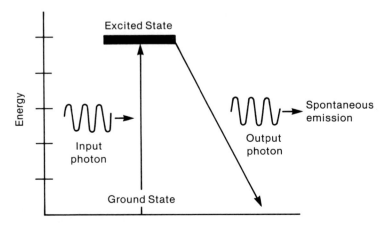

Figure 9-2. Spontaneous emission occurs when a photon changes energy levels.

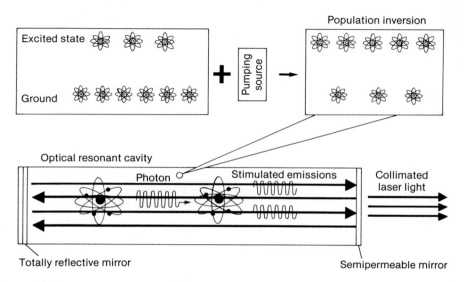

Figure 9-3. Pumping is a process of elevating an orbiting electron to a higher energy level, thus creating population diversion that is essential for laser operation.

chamber cannot contain the energy. When a specific level of energy is attained, photons of a particular wavelength are ejected through the semipermeable mirror. Thus, amplified light through stimulated emissions (LASER) is produced (Fig. 9-3).

The laser light is emitted in an organized pattern rather than in a random manner (as from a light bulb). Three properties distinguish the laser from incandescent and fluorescent light sources: **coherence, monochromaticity,** and **collimation.**[27]

Coherence means that all photons of light emitted from individual gas molecules are the same wavelength, and that the individual light waves are in phase with one another. Normal light, on the other hand, is composed of many wavelengths that superimpose their phases on one another.

Monochromaticity refers to the specificity of light in a single, defined wavelength; if the specificity is in the visible light spectrum, it is only one color. The laser is one of the few light sources that produces a specific wavelength.

The laser beam is well-collimated; that is, there is minimal divergence of the photons.[1] The photons move in a parallel fashion, thus concentrating the beam of light (Fig. 9-4).

TYPES OF LASERS

Lasers are classified according to the nature of the material placed between two reflecting surfaces. There are potentially thousands of different types of lasers, each with specific wavelengths and unique characteristics, depending on the lasing medium utilized. The lasing mediums used to create lasers include

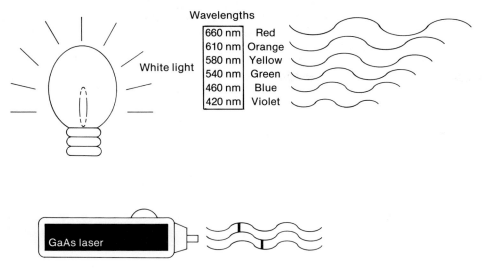

Figure 9-4. *(Top)*, White light contains electromagnetic energy of all wavelengths (colors) that are superimposed on each other. *(Bottom)*, Laser light is monochromatic (single wavelength), coherent (in phase), and collimated (minimal divergence).

the following categories: crystal and glass (solid-state), gas and excimer, semiconductor, liquid dye, and chemical.

- Crystal lasers include the synthetic ruby (aluminum oxide and chromium) and the neodymium, yttrium, aluminum, garnet (Nd:YAG) lasers, among others. Synthetic rather than natural materials are used to ensure purity of the medium, which is necessary for the physical characteristics of lasers to occur.[12]
- Gas lasers were developed in 1961, shortly after the first ruby laser. Gas lasers include the helium neon (HeNe), argon, and carbon dioxide (CO_2) lasers, along with numerous others. The HeNe laser is one type of low-power device under investigation in the United States for application in physical medicine.
- Semiconductor or diode lasers were developed in 1962 after the production of gas (HeNe) lasers. The gallium arsenide (GaAs) laser was the first diode laser developed; this low-power laser also is under investigation in the United States for application in physical medicine.
- Liquid lasers are also known as *dye lasers,* because they use organic dyes as the lasing medium. By varying the mixture of the dyes, the wavelengths of the laser can be varied.
- Chemical lasers usually are extremely high-power and are frequently used for military purposes.[17]

Lasers can be categorized as either high- or low-power, depending on the intensity of energy that they deliver. High-power lasers are also known as "hot" lasers because of the thermal responses they generate. These are used in the medical realm in numerous areas including surgical incision and coagulation and in ophthalmologic, dermatologic, oncologic, and vascular specialties. The use of low-power lasers (also known as "cold" or "soft" lasers) for wound healing and pain management is a relatively new area of application. These lasers produce a maximal output of less than 1 milliwatt (1 mW = $\frac{1}{1000}$ watt) in the United States and work by causing photochemical rather than thermal effects. No tissue warming occurs. The exact distinction of the power output that delineates a low- versus a high-power laser varies. Any laser that does not generate an appreciable thermal response is considered low-power. This category can include lasers capable of producing up to 500 mW of power (up to Class IV lasers).[5]

Low-power lasers, which have been studied and used in Europe for the past 20 to 25 years, have been investigated in the United States for the past decade. The potential applications for low-power lasers include treatment of tendon and ligament injury, arthritis, edema reduction, soft tissue injury, ulcer and burn care, scar tissue inhibition, and acutherapy.

EQUIPMENT

Lasers require the following components in order to operate:[17]

1. *Power supply.* Lasers use an electrical power supply that potentially can deliver up to 10,000 volts and hundreds of amps.
2. *Lasing medium.* This is the material that generates the laser light. It can include any type of matter—gas, solid, or liquid.
3. *Pumping device. Pumping* is the term used to describe the process of elevating an orbiting electron to a higher, "excited" energy level (see Fig. 9-4). This creates the population inversion that is essential for laser operation. The pumping device may be high voltage photoflash lamps, radio frequency oscillators, or other lasers. The pumping device is very specific to the type of lasing medium being used.
4. *Optical resonant cavity.* This contains the lasing medium. Once population inversion has occurred, this cavity, which contains the reflecting surfaces, directs the beam propagation.

The helium neon (HeNe) and gallium arsenide (GaAs) lasers are the two principal lasers currently under investigation in the United States for conservative management of medical conditions. The discussion will concentrate on these two types.

Helium Neon Laser

The HeNe laser uses a gas mixture of primarily helium with neon in a pressurized tube. This creates a laser in the red portion of the electromagnetic spectrum, with a wavelength of 632.8 nm. The power output of the HeNe laser can vary but typically ranges from 1.0 to 10.0 mW, depending on the gas density used. Larger tubes are necessary for higher power outputs, and each requires a precise power drive to operate.[5] Laser output can decrease depending on the care of the equipment, the number of operating hours, and whether fiberoptics are used. For example, rough handling can jar the reflecting surfaces, and a high number of hours in operation or poor fiberoptic quality can diminish the laser output. The HeNe laser in the United States delivers a power output of 1 mW through a fiberoptic tube in a continuous mode. Although the HeNe laser light is well-collimated, the utilization of fiberoptics causes a divergence of the beam from 18 to 21 degrees.[5] Fiberoptics can decrease the output delivery by 50% or more as the light travels from the lasing medium to the tip of the applicator. Fiberoptics make the delivery more convenient, because the size of the gas tube would make direct application difficult. HeNe lasers up to 6 mW have been manufactured for clinical use in Canada, which has fewer governmental restrictions. These higher-output lasers, although still considered low-power, allow delivery of desired dosages in reduced time.[6]

Gallium-Arsenide Laser

The GaAs laser utilizes a diode to produce an infrared (invisible) laser at a wavelength of 904 nm. Diode lasers are composed of semiconductor silicone materials that are precisely cut and layered. An electrical source is applied to each side, and lasing action is produced at the junction of the two materials. The cleaved surfaces function as partially reflecting surfaces that ultimately produce coherent light (Fig. 9-5).[12]

Diode lasers produce a beam that is elliptically shaped so that the lasers have a 10- to 35-degree divergence, despite the fact that no fiberoptics are used.[17] The 904-nm laser is delivered in a pulsed mode because of the heat produced at the junction of the diode chips. The GaAs laser manufactured in the United States has a peak power of 2 watts but delivers energy in a pulsed mode, which decreases the average power to 0.4 mW output if delivered at 1000 hertz (see the calculations in the Dosage section).

The application of additional layers of materials to other types of diodes

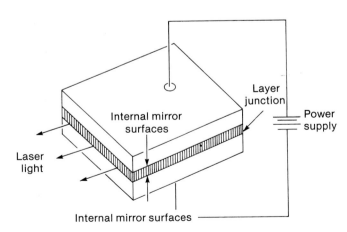

Figure 9-5. A diode is composed of silicone material that is cleaved and layered. The lasing action occurs at the junction of the layers when an electrical source is applied.

allows their operation in a continuous mode at room temperature.[17] The continuous mode results in higher average power outputs from the lasers. Higher-output diode lasers are manufactured for clinical applications in Canada and include the following:

780-nm wavelength with 5-mW output—continuous mode delivery
810-nm wavelength with 20-mW output—continuous mode delivery
830-nm wavelength with 30-mW output—continuous mode delivery

These diodes are interchangeable in a single base unit.[6]

The laser units available in the United States have the ability to deliver both HeNe and GaAs lasers. The same device can both measure electrical impedance and deliver electrical point stimulation. The impedance detector allows hypersensitive or acupuncture points to be located. The point stimulator can be combined with laser application when treating pain. The electrical stimulation is believed to provide spontaneous pain relief, while the laser provides more latent tissue responses.[7]

THERAPEUTIC APPLICATIONS OF LASERS

Because the production of lasers is a relatively new field, the biologic and physiologic effects of this concentrated light energy are still being explored. The effects of low-power lasers are subtle, primarily occurring at a cellular level. Various in vitro and animal studies have attempted to elucidate the interaction of photons with biologic structures. Although few controlled clinical studies have been reported in the literature, documented case studies and empirical evidence indicate that lasers are effective in reducing pain and aiding wound healing. The exact mechanisms for action are still uncertain, although proposed physiologic effects include acceleration in collagen synthesis, decrease in microorganisms, increase in vascularization, reduction of pain, and antiinflammatory action.[6]

Low-power lasers are best recognized for increasing the rate of wound and ulcer healing by enhancing cellular metabolism. Results from animal studies vary as to the benefits for wound healing, perhaps owing to the fact that the types of lasers, dosages, and protocols used have been inconsistent. In humans, improvement of nonhealing wounds indicates promising possibilities for treatment with lasers.

Wound Healing

Early investigations of the effects of low-power lasers on biologic tissues were limited to in vitro experimentation. Although it was known that high-power lasers could damage and vaporize tissues, little was known about the effect of small dosages on the viability and stability of cellular structures. It was found that low dosages (less than 10 joules (J) per cm^2) of radiation from low-output lasers had a stimulating action on metabolic processes and cell proliferation compared with incandescent or tungsten light.[2]

Mester and colleagues conducted numerous in vitro experiments with two lasers in the red portion of the visual spectrum—the ruby laser with a wavelength of 694.3 nm and the HeNe laser with a wavelength of 632.8 nm. Human tissue cultures showed significant increases in fibroblastic proliferation following stimulation by either laser tested.[18] Fibroblasts are the precursor cells to connective tissue structures, such as collagen, epithelial cells, and chondrocytes. When the production of fibroblasts is stimulated, one should expect a subsequent increase in the production of connective tissue. Abergel and associates documented that certain dosages of HeNe and GaAs lasers with a wavelength of 904 nm caused in vitro human skin fibroblasts to have a threefold increase in procollagen production.[2] This effect was most marked when low-level stimulation (1.94×10^{-7} to 5.84×10^{-6} J per cm^2 of GaAs and dosages of 0.053 to 1.589 J per cm^2 of HeNe) was given over a period of 3 to 4 days rather than given in a single exposure. Samples of tissue showed increases in fibroblasts and collagenous structures as well as increases in the intracellular material and swollen mitochondria of cells.[18] Furthermore, cells were undamaged with regard to their morphology and structure after exposure to low-power lasers.[3]

Analysis of the cellular metabolism with attention to the activity of DNA and RNA has been made.[2,18,25] Through radioactive markers, it was suggested that laser stimulation enhances the synthesis of nucleic acids and cell division.[8,18] Abergel[1] reported that laser-treated cells had significantly greater amounts of procollagen messenger RNA, further confirming that increased collagen production occurs due to modifications at the transcriptional level.

Low-power lasers were used further in animal studies to delineate both the beneficial applications of laser light and its potential harm. In an early study by Mester and associates, mechanical and burn wounds were made on the backs of mice.[19] Similar wounds on the same animals served as the controls, with the experimental wounds subjected to various doses of ruby laser. Although there were no histologic differences among the wounds, the lased wounds healed significantly faster, especially at a dosage of 1 J per cm^2. It also was demonstrated that repeated laser treatments were more effective than a single exposure.

Other researchers investigated the rate of healing and tensile strength of full thickness wounds when exposed to laser irradiation.[2,13-16,24] There were conflicting reports regarding rates of healing, with some studies showing no change in the rate of wound closure[13,16,24] and others showing significantly faster wound healing.[2,14,15] Although the experimental results were conflicting, an explanation for the discrepancy may be an indirect systemic effect of laser energy. Mester and colleagues[18] showed that it was not necessary to irradiate an entire wound to achieve beneficial results, because stimulation of remote areas had similar results. Kana and associates[14] described an increase in the rate of healing of both the irradiated and nonirradiated wounds on the same animal, compared with nonirradiated animals. This systemic effect was most marked with the argon laser. Several studies that investigated the rate of healing on living animal tissue used a second, nontreated control wound on the same animal. The rate of healing may have been confounded by this systemic effect. Whether the systemic effect involves a humoral component—a circulating element—producing immunologic effects has yet to be determined. A bactericidal effect and lymphocyte stimulation are proposed mechanisms for this phenomenon.

Tensile Strength

The increased tensile strength of lased wounds was confirmed more of-ten.[2,13,14,16,19,24] Wound contraction, collagen synthesis, and increases in tensile strength are fibroblast-mediated functions and were demonstrated most mark-edly in the early phase of wound healing. Wounds were tested at various stages of healing to determine their breaking point, compared with a control or nonlased wound. Laser-treated wounds had significantly greater tensile strengths, most commonly in the first 10 to 14 days after injury, although they approached the values of the control after that time.[1,16,24] Hypertrophic scars did not result as tissue responses normalized after a 14-day period. Treatment with HeNe laser in doses ranging from 1.1 to 2.2 J per cm^2 elicited positive re-sults when performed either twice a day or on alternate days. The increased tensile strength corresponds to higher levels of collagen.

Immunologic Responses

These early studies led to the hypothesis that laser exposure could enhance healing of skin and connective tissue lesions, but the mechanism was still un-clear. Biochemical analysis and radioactive tracers were used to delineate the immunologic effects of laser light on human tissue cultures. The laser irradia-tion caused increased phagocytosis by leukocytes with dosages of .05 J per cm^2.[18] This led to the possibility of a bactericidal effect, which was further dem-onstrated with laser exposures on cell cultures containing *Escherichia coli,* a common intestinal bacteria in humans. The ruby laser had an increased effect both on cell replication and on the destruction of bacteria via the phagocytosis of leukocytes.[18,19] Mester and coworkers also concluded that there were immu-nologic effects with the ruby, HeNe, and argon lasers. Specifically, there was a direct stimulatory influence on the T- and B-lymphocyte activity, a phenomenon that is specific to laser output and wavelength. HeNe and Argon lasers gave the best results with dosages ranging from 0.5 to 1 J per cm^2.[18] Trelles did sim-ilar investigations in vitro and in vivo and reported that lasers did not have bac-tericidal effects alone, but when used in conjunction with antibiotics there were significantly higher bactericidal effects compared with controls.[25]

With the confidence that they would cause little or no harm and that they could serve a therapeutic purpose, low-power lasers have been used clinically on human subjects since the 1960s. In Hungary, Mester and associates treated nonhealing ulcers that did not respond to traditional therapy with HeNe and Argon lasers with wavelengths of 632.8 and 488 nm, respectively.[18] The dos-ages varied but had a maximum of 4 J per cm^2. By the time of Mester's publica-tion 1120 patients had been treated, of whom 875 healed, 160 improved, and 85 did not respond. The wounds, which were categorized by cause, took an aver-age of 12 to 16 weeks to heal. Trelles also showed promising results clinically using the infrared GaAs and HeNe lasers on the healing of ulcers, nonunion fractures, and herpetic lesions.[25]

Gogia and colleagues in the United States treated nonhealing wounds with GaAs lasers, pulsed at a frequency of 1000 Hz for 10 seconds per cm^2 and used with a sweeping technique, held about 5 mm from the wound surface.[11] This protocol was used in conjunction with daily or twice daily sterile whirlpool treatments and produced satisfactory results, although statistical information was not reported. Empirical evidence by these authors suggested faster healing and cleaner wounds when subjected to GaAs laser treatment three times per week.

Inflammation

Biopsies of experimental wounds were examined for prostaglandin activity to delineate the effect of laser stimulation on the inflammatory process. A decrease in prostaglandin E (PGE_2) is a proposed mechanism by which laser therapy promotes the reduction of edema. During inflammation, prostaglandins cause vasodilation, which contributes to the flow of plasma into the interstitial tissue. By reducing prostaglandins, the driving force behind edema production is reduced.[6] The prostaglandin E and F contents were examined after treatment with HeNe laser at 1 J per cm^2.[18] In 4 days, both types of prostaglandins accumulated more than the controls. However, at 8 days, the PGE_2 levels decreased, while $PGE_{2\alpha}$ increased. There was also an increased capillarization during this phase. These data indicate that prostaglandin production is affected by laser stimulation, and these changes possibly reflect an accelerated resolution of the acute inflammatory process.[18]

Scar Tissue

Macroscopic examination of healed wounds was subjectively described after the laser experiments in most studies. In general, the wounds exposed to laser irradiation had less scar tissue and a better cosmetic appearance. Histologic examination showed greater epithelialization and less exudative material.[15]

Studies that utilized burn wounds showed more regular alignment of collagen and smaller scars. Trelles lased third-degree burns on the backs of hairless mice with GaAs and HeNe lasers and showed significantly faster healing in the lased animals.[25] The best results were obtained with the GaAs laser because of its greater penetration. Trelles found increased circulation with the production of new blood vessels in the center of the wounds compared with the controls. Edges of the wounds maintained viability and contributed to the epithelialization and closure of the burn. Since there is less contracture associated with irradiated wounds, laser treatment has been suggested for burns and wounds on the hands and neck, where contractures and scarring can severely limit function.

Pain

Lasers also have been effective in reducing pain and have been shown to effect peripheral nerve activity.[20] Rochkind and others produced crush injuries in rats and treated experimental animals with 10 J per cm^2 of HeNe laser energy applied transcutaneously along the sciatic nerve projection.[20] The amplitude of electrically stimulated action potentials was measured along the injured nerve and compared with controls up to 1 year later. The amplitude of the action potentials was 43% greater after 20 days, which was the duration of laser treatment. By 1 year, all lased nerves demonstrated equal or higher amplitudes than before injury. The controls followed an expected course of recovery and did not reach normal levels even after a year.

The effect of HeNe irradiation on peripheral sensory nerve latency has been investigated in humans by Snyder-Mackler and Bork.[23] This double-blind study showed that exposure of the superficial radial nerve to low dosages of laser resulted in a significantly decreased sensory nerve conduction velocity, which may provide information about the pain-relieving mechanism of lasers. Other explanations for pain relief may be hastened healing, antiinflammatory action, autonomic nerve influence, and neurohumoral responses (serotonin, norepinephrine) from descending tract inhibition.[6,7]

Chronic pain has been treated with GaAs and HeNe lasers, and positive results have been observed empirically and through clinical research. Walker conducted a double-blind study to document analgesia after exposure to HeNe irradiation in chronic pain patients compared with sham treatments.[28] When the superficial sites of the radial, median, and saphenous nerves as well as painful areas were exposed to laser irradiation, there were significant decreases in pain and less reliance on medication for pain control. These preliminary studies suggest positive results, although pain modulation is difficult to measure objectively.

Bone Response

Future uses of laser irradiation include the treatment of other connective tissue structures such as bone and articular cartilage.[21] Schultz and coworkers studied various intensities of the Nd:YAG laser on the healing of partial thickness articular cartilage lesions in guinea pigs.[21] During the surgical procedure, the lesions were irradiated for 5 seconds with intensities ranging from 25 to 125 J. After 4 weeks the low-dosage group (25 J) had chondral proliferation, and by 6 weeks the defect had reconstituted to the level of the surface cartilage. Normal basophilic cells were present with staining, indicating normal cellular structures. The higher-dosage groups and controls had little or no evidence of restoration of the lesion with cartilage. Bone healing and fracture consolidation have been investigated by Trelles and Mayayo.[26] An adapter was attached to an intramuscular needle so that the laser energy could be directed deeper to the periosteum. Rabbit tibial fractures showed faster consolidation with HeNe treatment of 2.4 J per cm^2 on alternate days. Histologic examination indicated more mature haversian canals with detached osteocytes in the laser-treated bone. There was also a remodeling of the articular line, which is impossible with traditional therapy.[25,26] The use of lasers for the treatment of nonunion fractures has begun in Europe.

Clinical Considerations

There have been no ill effects reported from laser treatments for wound healing.[4] More controlled clinical data are needed to determine efficacy and to establish dosimetry that elicits reproducible responses. The impressions of low-power lasers are that they have a biostimulative effect on impaired tissues unless higher dosages—in excess of 8 to 10 J per cm^2—are administered.[1] This effect does not influence normal tissue. Beyond these ranges, a bioinhibitive effect may occur.

The applications of the low-power laser in an athletic training environment are potentially unlimited. Its applications can include wound healing in lacerations, abrasions, or infections. Clean procedures should be maintained to prevent cross-contamination of the laser tip. Because the depth of penetration of the infrared laser is about 5 cm, other soft tissue injuries can be treated effectively by laser irradiation. Sprains, strains, and contusions have been observed by the authors to have faster healing rates with less pain. Acupuncture and superficial nerve sites also can be lased, or lasers can be combined with electrical stimulation to treat painful conditions.

TECHNIQUES OF APPLICATION

Application of laser therapy is relatively simple, but certain principles of dosimetry should be discussed so that the sports therapist can accurately determine the amount of laser energy delivered to the tissues. For general application, only the treatment time and the pulse rate vary. For research purposes, the sports therapist should measure the exact energy density emitted from the applicator before the treatments. Dosage is the most important variable in laser therapy and may be difficult to determine because of the variables mentioned previously (e.g., hours of operation or condition of the unit).

The laser energy is emitted from a handheld remote applicator. The GaAs laser houses the semiconductor elements in the tip of the applicator, whereas the HeNe laser contains its components inside the unit and delivers the laser light to the target area via a fiberoptic tube. The fiberoptic assembly is fragile and should not be crimped or twisted excessively. The fiberoptics used with the HeNe laser and the elliptical shape of the GaAs laser create beam divergence with both devices. This divergence causes the beam's energy to spread out over a given area, so that as the distance from the source increases the intensity of the beam lessens.

To administer a laser treatment, the tip should be in light contact with the skin and directed perpendicularly to the target tissue while the laser is engaged for the designated time. Commonly, a treatment area is divided into a grid of square centimeters, with each square centimeter stimulated for the specified time. This gridding technique is the most frequently utilized method of application and should be used whenever possible. Lines and points should not be drawn on the patient's skin because they may absorb some of the light energy (Fig. 9-6). If open areas are to be treated, a sterilized clear plastic sheet can be placed over the wound to allow surface contact.

An alternative is a scanning technique, in which there is no contact between the laser tip and the skin. With this technique the applicator tip should be held 5 to 10 mm from the wound. Because beam divergence occurs, there is a decrease in the amount of energy as the distance from the target increases. The amount of energy lost becomes difficult to quantify accurately if the distance from the target is variable. Therefore, it is not recommended to use this technique at distances greater than 1 cm. When using a laser tip of 1 mm with 30 degrees of divergence, the red laser beam of the HeNe should fill an area the size of 1 cm^2 (Fig. 9-7). Although the infrared laser is invisible, the same consideration should be given when using the scanning technique. If the laser tip comes into contact with an open wound, the tip should be cleaned thoroughly

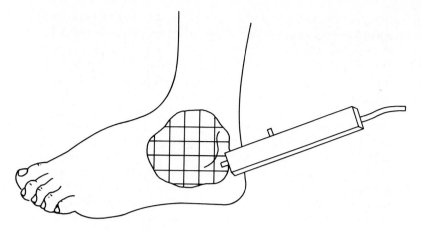

Figure 9-6. Grid application of laser. Laser aperture should be perpendicular to surface. Lase each square centimeter of the injured area for the specified time. The aperture should be in light contact with the skin.

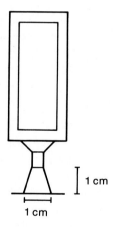

1 cm

1 cm

Figure 9-7. Scanning technique. When skin contact cannot be maintained, the remote should be held still in the center of the square centimeter grid at a distance of less than one centimeter. If using the HeNe laser, the red beam should fill a one square centimeter grid.

with a small amount of bleach or other antiseptic agents to prevent cross-contamination.

The scanning technique should be differentiated from the wanding technique, in which a grid area is bathed with the laser in an oscillating fashion for the designated time. As in the scanning technique, the dosimetry is difficult to calculate if a distance of less than 1 cm cannot be maintained. The wanding technique is not recommended because of irregularities in the dosages.

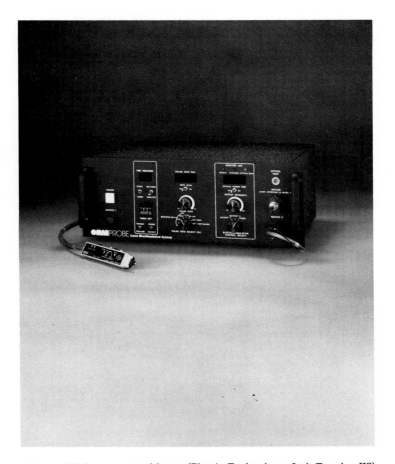

Figure 9-8. Low-powered laser. (Physio Technology, Ltd. Topeka, KS)

DOSAGE

Physio Technology, LD. (Topeka, KS) is the only manufacturer in the United States that currently produces low-power HeNe and GaAs lasers (Fig. 9-8). Table 9-1 describes the contrasting specifications of these lasers. The HeNe laser has a 1.0-milliwatt (mW) average power output at the fiber tip and is delivered in the continuous wave mode. The GaAs laser has an output of 2 watts (W) but has an average power of only 0.4 mW when pulsed at its maximum rate of 1000 Hz. The frequency of the GaAs is variable, and the sports therapist may choose a pulse rate of 1 to 1000 Hz, each with a pulse width of 200 nanoseconds (nsec $= 10^{-9}$) (Fig. 9-9).

The pulsed modes drastically reduce the amount of energy emitted from the laser. For example, for 2-W laser pulsed at 100 Hz:

$$
\begin{aligned}
\text{Average power} &= \text{pulse rate} \times \text{peak power} \times \text{pulse width}\\
&= 100\ \text{Hz} \times 2\ \text{W} \times (2 \times 10^{-7}\ \text{sec})\\
&= 0.04\ \text{mW}
\end{aligned}
$$

TABLE 9-1   **Parameters of Low-Output Lasers**

	Helium Neon (HeNe)	Gallium Arsenide
Laser type	Gas	Semiconductor
Wavelength	632.8 nanometers	904 nm
Pulse rate	Continuous wave	1−1000 Hz
Pulse width	Continuous wave	200 nanoseconds
Peak power	3 milliwatts	2 watts
Average power	1.0 milliwatts	.04−0.4 milliwatts
Beam area	0.01 centimeters	0.07 centimeters
FDA class	Class II laser	Class I laser

Copied with permission from Physio Technology

This contrasts the power output of 0.4 mW with 1000 Hz. Therefore, it can be seen that adjustment of the pulse rate alters the average power, which significantly affects the treatment time if a specified amount of energy is required. In the past it was thought that altering the frequency of the laser would increase its benefits. Recent evidence indicates that the total number of joules is more important; therefore, higher pulse rates are recommended to decrease the treatment time required for each stimulation point.[6]

The dosage or energy density of laser is reported in the literature as joules per square centimeter (J per cm^2). One J is equal to 1 watt per second (W/s). Therefore, dosage is dependent on the following factors:

1. The output of the laser in mW
2. The time of exposure in seconds
3. The beam surface area of the laser in cm^2

Dosage should be accurately calculated to standardize treatments and to establish treatment guidelines for specific injuries. The intention is to deliver a specific number of J per cm^2 or mJ per cm^2. After setting the pulse rate, which

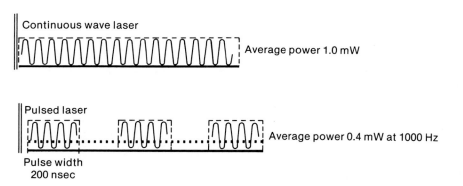

Figure 9-9. Continuous Wave versus Pulsed Energies.

determines the average power of the laser, only the treatment time per cm^2 needs to be calculated:[6]

$$T_A = (E/Pav) \times A$$

T_A = treatment time for a given area
E = millijoules of energy per cm^2
Pav = average laser power in milliwatts
A = beam area in cm^2

For example: To deliver 1 J per cm^2 with a 0.4-mW average power GaAs laser with a 0.07 cm^2 beam area:

$$T_A = (1 \text{ J per cm}^2/.0004 \text{ W}) \times 0.07 \text{ cm}^2$$
$$= 175 \text{ seconds or } 2:55 \text{ minutes}$$

To deliver 50 mJ per cm^2 with the same laser, it would only take 8.75 seconds of stimulation. Charts are available to assist the sports therapist in calculating the treatment times for a variety of pulse rates. The GaAs laser can only be pulsed up to 1000 Hz, resulting in an average energy of 0.4 mW. Therefore, the treatment times may be exceedingly long to deliver the same energy density with a continuous wave laser (Table 9-2).

Depth of Penetration

Any energy applied to the body can be absorbed, reflected, transmitted, and refracted. Biologic effects result only from the absorption of energy; as more energy is absorbed, less is available for the deeper and adjacent tissues.

    The depth of penetration of laser light depends on the type of laser energy delivered. Absorption of HeNe laser energy occurs rapidly in the superficial structures, especially in the first 2 to 5 mm of soft tissue. The response that occurs from absorption is termed the *direct effect*. The *indirect effect* is a lessened response that occurs deeper in the tissues. The normal metabolic processes in the deeper tissues are catalyzed from the energy absorption in the superficial structures to produce the indirect effect. HeNe laser has an indirect effect on tissues up to 8 to 10 mm deep.[6]

    The GaAs laser, which has a longer wavelength, is directly absorbed in tissues at depths of 1 to 2 cm and has an indirect effect up to 5 cm (Fig. 9-10). Therefore, this laser has better potential for the treatment of deeper soft tissue injuries such as strains, sprains, and contusions. The radius of the energy field expands as the nonabsorbed light is reflected, refracted, and transmitted to ad-

TABLE 9-2   **Treatment Times for Low-Output Lasers**

Laser Type	Average Power (mW)	Joules per Centimeter Squared (J/cm^2)						
		0.05	0.1	0.5	1	2	3	4
HeNe (632.8 nm) Continuous wave	1.0	0.5	1.0	5.0	10.0	20.0	30.0	40.0
GaAs (904 nm) Pulsed @ 1000 Hz	0.4	8.8	17.7	88.4	176.7	353.4	530.1	706.9

Treatment Time in seconds/cm^2

Copied with permission from Physio Technology.

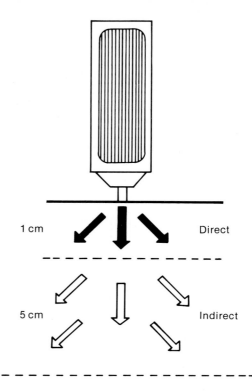

Figure 9-10. Depth of penetration with the GaAs laser. Direct penetration is up to 1 cm with the GaAs laser. The stimulation causes an indirect effect up to 5 cms. Penetration is greatest with skin contact.

jacent cells as the energy penetrates. The sports therapist should stimulate each square centimeter of a grid, although there will be an overlap of areas receiving indirect exposure.

Treatment Protocols

Research suggests some laser densities for treating several clinical models. These average from 0.05 to 0.5 J per cm^2 for acute conditions and from 0.5 to 3.0 J per cm^2 for more chronic conditions.[6] The responses of the tissues depend on the dosage delivered, although the type of laser used can also influence the effect. The response obtained with different dosages and with different lasers varies considerably among studies, leaving treatment parameters to be determined largely empirically. In the literature, there seems to be little differentiation when comparing the dosages of HeNe and GaAs lasers, although their depths of penetration differ significantly. The laser units produced in the United States have relatively low average power, so the tendency is to administer dosages in millijoules rather than joules. Three to six treatments may be required before the effectiveness of laser therapy can be determined.

Although higher laser output is recommended to reduce treatment times, overstimulation should be avoided. The Arndt-Schultz principle, which states that more is not necessarily better, is applicable with laser therapy. For this reason, laser therapy should be administered at a maximum of one application daily per treatment area. When using large dosages, treatment is recommended on alternate days. If the effects of laser therapy reach a plateau, the frequency of treatments should be reduced or the treatments discontinued for 1 week, at which time the treatment can be reinstated if needed.[25]

SUGGESTED TREATMENT PROTOCOLS
Pain

The use of low-power lasers in the treatment of acute and chronic pain can be implemented in various ways. After proper diagnosis of the pain's cause, the site to be treated can be gridded. The entire area of injury should be lased as described previously. Table 9-3 lists some suggested treatment protocols for various clinical conditions. When trigger points are being treated, the probe should be held perpendicular to the skin with light contact. If a specific structure such as a ligament is the target tissue, the laser probe should be held in contact with the skin and perpendicular to that structure. When a joint is being treated, the patient should be positioned so that the joint is open, to allow penetration of the energy to the intraarticular areas.

The treatment of acupuncture and trigger points with laser can be augmented with electrical stimulation for pain management. Charts can be used for reference to determine appropriate acupuncture points. The impedance detector in the laser remote enhances the ability to locate these sites. Points should be treated distally to proximally for best results.

Occasionally patients may experience an increase in pain after a laser

TABLE 9-3   **Suggested Treatment Applications**

Application	Laser Type	Energy Density
Trigger point		
Superficial	Helium Neon	$1-3$ J/cm^2
Deep	Gallium Arsenide	$1-2$ J/cm^2
Edema reduction		
Acute	Gallium Arsenide	$0.1-0.2$ J/cm^2
Subacute	Gallium Arsenide	$0.2-0.5$ J/cm^2
Wound healing (superficial tissues)		
Acute	Helium Neon	$0.5-1$ J/cm^2
Chronic	Helium Neon	4 J/cm^2
Wound healing (deep tissues)		
Acute	Gallium Arsenide	$0.05-0.1$ J/cm^2
Chronic	Gallium Arsenide	$0.5-1$ J/cm^2
Scar tissue	Gallium Arsenide	$0.5-1$ J/cm^2

Copied with permission from Physio Technology.

treatment. This phenomenon is believed to reflect the initiation of the body's normal responses to pain that have become dormant.[5] Laser therapy has been found to help resolve the condition by enhancing normal physiologic processes. As stated previously, several treatments should be administered before deeming the modality ineffective in pain management.

Wound Healing

Although ulcerations and open wounds are uncommon in an athletic training environment, contusions, abrasions, and lacerations can be treated with laser therapy to hasten healing time and decrease infection. The wound should be cleaned appropriately and all debris and eschar removed. Heavy exudate that covers the wound will diminish the laser's penetration; therefore, lasing around the periphery of the wound is recommended. The scanning technique should be utilized over open wounds unless a clear plastic sheet is placed over the wound to allow direct contact. Opaque materials can absorb some of the laser energy and are not recommended. Facial lacerations can be treated with the laser, although care should be taken not to direct the beam into the patient's eyes. The risk of retinal damage from the low-power lasers used in the United States is slight.

Scar Tissue

Laser energy affects only what is metabolically diminished and does not change normal tissue. Hypertrophic scars can be treated with lasers owing to their bioinhibitive effects. Bioinhibition requires prolonged treatment times and may be clinically impractical because of the low power output of the lasers used in the United States. Pain and edema associated with pathologic scars have been effectively treated with low-power lasers. Thick scars have varied vascularity, which makes laser transmission irregular; therefore, it often is recommended to treat the periphery of the scar rather than the center.

Edema and Inflammation

The primary action of laser application for control of edema and inflammation is through the interruption of the formation of intermediate substrates necessary for the production of inflammatory chemical mediators—kinins, histamines, and prostaglandins. Without these chemical mediators, the disruption of the body's homeostatic state is minimized and the extent of pain and edema is diminished. It is also believed that laser energy can optimize cell membrane permeability, which regulates interstitial osmotic-hydrostatic pressures. Therefore, during tissue trauma, the flux of fluid into the intracellular spaces would be reduced. Laser treatment is usually applied by gridding over the involved areas or by treating related acupuncture points if the area of involvement is generalized.

SAFETY

Few safety considerations are necessary with the low-power laser. However, as the varieties of lasers evolved and their uses increased in the United States, it became necessary to develop national guidelines not only for safety but for therapeutic efficacy. The Center for Devices and Radiological Health of the Food and Drug Administration (FDA) now regulates the manufacture and sale of lasers in the United States. Laser equipment commonly is grouped into four FDA classes with simplified and well-differentiated safety procedures for each.[22]

1. Class I or "exempt" lasers are considered nonhazardous to the body. All invisible lasers with average power outputs of 1 mW or less are Class I devices. These include the GaAs lasers with wavelengths of 820 to 910 nm.[17] The invisible infrared lasers should contain an indicator light to identify when the laser is engaged.

2. Class II or "low-power" lasers are hazardous only if a viewer stares continuously into the source. This class includes visible lasers that emit up to 1 mW average power, such as the HeNe laser.

3. Class III or "moderate-risk" lasers can cause retinal injury within the natural reaction time. The operator and patient are required to wear protective eyewear. However, under normal use these lasers cannot cause serious skin injury or produce hazardous diffuse reflections from metals or other surfaces.[22]

4. Class IV or "high-power" lasers present a high risk of injury and can cause combustion of flammable materials. Other dangers are diffuse reflections that may harm the eyes and cause serious skin injury from direct exposure. These high-power lasers seldom are used outside research laboratories and restricted industrial environments.[22]

The low-power lasers used in treating sports injuries are categorized as Class I and II laser devices and Class III medical devices. Class III medical devices include new or modified devices not equivalent to any marketed before May 28, 1976.[9] To use a low-power laser in the United States on human subjects, a research proposal must be approved by an Institutional Review Board (IRB). The IRB can be established through a manufacturer, university, or hospital to obtain an Investigational Device Exemption (IDE). By requiring documentation of the results and side effects of lasers, the FDA regulations serve to generate scientific data to determine the safety and efficacy of the device in question.

Lasers deliver nonionizing radiation; thus, no mutagenic effects on DNA and no damage to the cells or cell membranes have been found.[6] No deleterious effects—including carcinogenic responses—have been reported after low-power laser exposure, unless the laser is applied to already cancerous cells. Tumor cells may proliferate when stimulated.[10]

Precautions and Contraindications

Some suggestions for laser use include the following.

1. Laser therapy should not be used over cancerous growths.

2. It is better to underexpose than to overexpose. If clinical results reach a plateau, a reduction in dosage or in treatment frequency may improve results.

3. Avoid direct exposure into the eyes because of possible retinal burns. If lasing for extended periods, as for wound healing, safety glasses are recommended to avoid exposure from reflection.

4. Although no adverse reactions have been documented, the use of laser therapy during the first trimester of pregnancy is not recommended.

5. A low percentage of patients, especially those with chronic pain, may experience an episode of syncope during the laser treatment. Symptoms usually subside within minutes. If symptoms last longer than 5 minutes, no further treatments should be given.

CONCLUSION The use of low-power lasers appears to have only positive effects; this in itself should induce professional caution in deeming it a panacea. Currently, with these power outputs, lasers are recognized as non−significant risk devices. However, low-power lasers have not been granted recognition by the FDA as a safe or effective modality. Although many empirical and clinical findings show promising results, more controlled studies are essential to determine the types of lasers and dosages that are required to attain reproducible results.

SUMMARY

1. The first working laser, the ruby laser, was developed in 1960 and initially was called an optical maser.
2. Visible light wavelengths range from 400 to 700 nanometers. Light is transmitted through space in waves and is composed of photons emitted at distinct energy levels.
3. An atom is excited when energy is applied and raises an orbiting electron to a higher orbit. When the electron returns to its original orbit, it releases energy in the form of a photon—a process called spontaneous emission.
4. Stimulated emission occurs when the photon is released from an excited atom and promotes the release of an identical photon from a similarly excited atom.
5. For lasers to operate, a medium of excited atoms must be generated. This is termed population inversion and results when an external energy source (pumping device) is applied to the medium.
6. Characteristics of laser light vary from those of conventional light sources in three ways: laser light is monochromic (single color or wavelength), coherent (in phase), and collimated (has minimal divergence).
7. Laser can be thermal (hot) or nonthermal (low-power, soft, or cold). The categories of lasers include solid state (crystal or glass), gas, semiconductor, dye, and chemical.
8. Helium-neon, HeNe (gas) and gallium-arsenide, GaAs (semiconductor) lasers are two low-power lasers being investigated by the FDA for application in physical medicine. These low-power lasers currently are being used in the United States and in other countries for wound and soft tissue healing and pain relief.
9. HeNe lasers deliver a characteristic red beam with a wavelength of 632.8 nm. The laser is delivered in a continuous wave and has a direct penetration of 2 to 5 mm and an indirect penetration of 10 to 15 mm.
10. GaAs lasers are invisible and have a wavelength of 904 nm. They are delivered in a pulse mode and have an average power output of 0.4 milliwatts.

This laser has a direct penetration of 1 to 2 cm and an indirect penetration of 5 cm.

11. The proposed therapeutic applications of lasers in physical medicine include acceleration of collagen synthesis, decrease in microorganisms, increase in vascularization, and reduction of pain and inflammation.

12. The ideal technique of laser application consists of gentle contact with the skin surface with the applicator held perpendicular to the target surface. Dosage appears to be the critical factor in eliciting the desired response, but exact dosimetry has not been determined. Dosage can be fluctuated by varying the pulse frequency and the treatment times.

13. The laser is applied by developing an imaginary grid over the target area. The grid is composed of 1-cm squares; the laser is applied to each square for a predetermined time. Trigger or acupuncture points also are treated for painful conditions.

14. The FDA considers low-power lasers as low-risk investigational devices. Their use in the United States requires an IRB approval and informed consent prior to treatment.

15. Although no deleterious effects have been reported, certain precautions and contraindications exist. Contraindications include lasing over cancerous tissue, directly into the eyes, and during the first trimester of pregnancy. Occasionally pain may increase initially when laser treatments begin, but this does not indicate cessation of treatment. A low percentage of patients have experienced syncope episodes during laser treatment, but this is usually self-resolving. If symptoms persist for longer than 5 minutes, future laser treatments are not advised.

16. Future research for determining efficacy and treatment parameters is needed to substantiate the application of low-power lasers in physical medicine.

GLOSSARY

coherence Property of identical phase and time relationship. All photons of laser light are the same wavelength.

collimation A state of being parallel.

continuous wave An uninterrupted beam of laser light (as opposed to a pulsed beam).

diode laser A solid-state semiconductor used as a lasing medium.

divergence The bending of light rays away from one another; the spreading of light.

electron A fundamental particle of matter possessing a negative electrical charge and very small mass.

excited state State of an atom that occurs when outside energy causes the atom to contain more energy than is normal.

fiberoptic A solid glass or plastic tube that conducts light along its length.

frequency The number of cycles or pulses per second.

ground state The normal, unexcited state of an atom.

infrared A portion of the electromagnetic spectrum between the visible and microwave regions. Infrared wavelengths range from 780 to 100,000 nm.

laser A device that concentrates high energies into a narrow beam of coherent, monochromatic light.

monochromaticity Production of a single color or wavelength by light source.

photon The basic unit of light; a packet or quantum of light energy.

population inversion A condition in which more atoms exist in a high-energy, excited state than in a normal ground state. This is required for lasing to occur.

spontaneous emission When an atom in a high-energy state emits a photon and drops to a more stable ground state.

stimulated emission Release of two photons owing to

interaction of a photon with an atom already in a high-energy state and consequent decay of the atomic system.

wavelength The distance from a peak to the same point on the next peak of an electromagnetic or acoustic wave.

REFERENCES

1 Abergel, R.P.: Biochemical mechanisms of wound and tissue healing with lasers, Second Canadian low power medical laser conference, March 1987.
2 Abergel, R.P., Lyons, R.F., Castel, J.C., et al.: Biostimulation of wound healing by lasers: experimental approaches in animal models and in fibroblast cultures, J. Dermatol. Surg. Oncol. **13**:127-133, 1987.
3 Bostara, M., Jucca, A., Olliaro, P., et al.: In vitro fibroblast and dermis fibroblast activation by laser irradiation at low energy, Dermatologica **168**:157-162, 1984.
4 Castel, J.C.: Laser biophysics, Second Canadian low power medical laser conference, Ontario, Canada, March 1987.
5 Castel, M.F.: Personal communication, Medelco, Ontario, Canada, March 1989.
6 Castel, M.F.: A clinical guide to low power laser therapy, Downsview, Ontario, 1985, Physio Technology Ltd.
7 Cheng, R.: Combination laser/electrotherapy in pain management, Second Canadian low power medical laser conference, Ontario, Canada, March 1987.
8 Enwemeka, C.S.: Laser biostimulation of healing wounds: specific effects and mechanisms of action, J. Ortho Sp. Phys. Ther. **9**:333-338, 1988.
9 Fact sheet: laser biostimulation, Rockville, Md., Food and Drug Administration, Center of Devices and Radiological Health, 1984.
10 Farnham, J.: Personal communication, March 1989.
11 Gogia, P.P., Hurt, B.S., and Zirn, T.T.: Wound management with whirlpool and infrared cold laser treatment, Phys. Ther. **68**:1239-1242, 1988.
12 Hallmark, C.L., and Horn, D.T.: Lasers—the light fantastic, ed. 2, Blue Ridge Summit, Pa., 1987, TAB Books Inc.
13 Hunter, J., Leonard, L., Wilson R., et al.: Effects of low energy laser on wound healing in a porcine model, Lasers Surg. Med. **3**:285-290, 1984.
14 Kana, J.S., Hutschenreiter, G., Haina, D., and Waidelich, W.: Effect of low power density laser radiation on healing of open skin wounds in rats, Arch. Surg. **116**:293-296, 1981.
15 Longo, L., Evangelista, S., Tinacci, G., et al.: Effect of di-ode-laser silver arsenide-aluminum (Ga-Al-As) 904 nm on healing of experimental wounds, Lasers Surg. Med. **7**:444-447, 1987.
16 Lyons, R.F., Abergel, R.P., White, R.A., et al.: Biostimulation of wound healing in vivo by a helium neon laser, Ann. Plast. Surg. **18**:47-77, 1987.
17 McComb, G.: The Laser cookbook: 88 practical projects, Blue Ridge Summit, Pa., 1988, TAB Books Inc.
18 Mester, E., Mester, A.F., and Mester, A.: Biomedical effects of laser application, Lasers Surg. Med. **5**:31-39, 1985.
19 Mester, E., Spiry, T., Szende, B., et al.: Effect of laser rays on wound healing, Am. J. Surg. **122**:532-535, 1971.
20 Rochkind, S., Nissan, M., Barr-Nea, L., et al.: Response of peripheral nerve to HeNe laser: experimental studies, Lasers Surg. Med. **7**:441-443, 1987.
21 Schultz, R.J., Krishnamurthy, S., Thelmo, W., et al.: Effects of varying intensities of laser energy on articular cartilage: a preliminary study, Lasers Surg. Med. **5**:577-588, 1985.
22 Sliney, D., and Wolkarsht, M.: Safety with lasers and other optical sources: a comprehensive handbook, New York, 1980, Plenum Press.
23 Snyder-Mackler, L., and Bork, C.E.: Effect of helium neon laser irradiation on peripheral nerve sensory latency, Phys. Ther. **68**:223-225, 1988.
24 Surinchak, J.S., Alago, M.L., Bellamy, R.F., et al.: Effects of low-level energy lasers on the healing of full-thickness skin defects, Lasers Surg. Med. **2**:267-274, 1983.
25 Trelles, M.: Medical applications of laser biostimulation, Second Canadian low power medical laser conference, Ontario, Canada, March 1987.
26 Trelles, M.A., and Mayayo, E.: Bone fracture consolidates faster with low power laser, Lasers Surg. Med. **7**:36-45, 1987.
27 Van Pelt, W.F., Stewart, H.F., Peterson, R.W., et al.: Laser fundamentals and experiments, Rockville, Md., 1970, U.S. Department of Health, Education and Welfare.
28 Walker, J.: Relief from chronic pain by low power laser irradiation, Neurosci. Lett. **43**:339-344, 1983.

SUGGESTED READINGS

Bloom, A.L.: Gas lasers, New York, 1971, John Wiley & Sons, pp 1-24.
Caspers, K.: Laser stimulation therapy, Phys. Med. Rehabil. **18**:426, 1977.
Gamaleya, N.F.: Laser biomedical research in Tae-USSR. In Wolbarsht, M.L., editor: Laser applications in medicine and biology, New York, 1977, Plenum Press.
Goldman, I.: Basic reactions in tissue. In Goldman, I. editor: The Biomedical laser: technology and clinical applications, New York, 1981, Springer-Verlag, pp 6-9.
Goldman, J.A., et al.: Laser therapy of rheumatoid arthritis, Lasers Surg. Med. **1**:1, 1980.
Goldman, L.: Biomedical aspects of the laser, New York, 1967, Springer-Verlag, pp 1-7.

Haina, D., et al.: Animal experiments on light-induced wound healing. In Wolbarght, M.L., editor: Laser in basic biomedical research (IV), New York, 1977, Plenum Press, pp 221-223.

Kana, J.S., et al.: Effect of low-power density laser radiation of healing of open skin wounds in rats, Arch. Surg. **116:**3, 1981.

Kleinkort, J.A., and Foley, R.A.: Laser acupuncture: its use in physical therapy, Am. J. Acupuncture **12:**51, 1984.

Kohtiao, A., et al.: Temperature rise and photocoagulation of rabbit retinas exposed to the CW laser, Am. J. Ophthalmol. **62:**3, 1966.

Kovacs, L.: Experimental investigation of photostimulation effect of low energy HeNe laser radiation. In Wolbarght, M.L., editor: Laser in basic biomedical research (IV), New York, 1977, Plenum Press.

Kovacs, I.B., Mester, E., and Gorog, P.: Laser-induced stimulation of the vascularization of the healing wound: an ear chamber experiment, Experientia **4:**341, 1974.

Kroetlinger, M.: On the use of laser in acupuncture, Int. J. Acupuncture Electrother. Res. **5:**297, 1980.

Lappin, P.W.: Ocular damage thresholds for the helium-neon laser, Arch. Environ. Health **20:**2, 1970.

Lengyell, B.A.: Lasers-generation of lightly stimulated emission, New York, 1962, John Wiley & Sons, pp 1-15, 22-23, 83-99.

Litwin, M.S., and Glew, D.H.: The biological effects of laser radiation, J.A.M.A. **187:**842, 1964.

MacMillan, J.D., Maxwell, W.A., and Chichester, C.O.: Lethal photosensitization of microorganisms with light from a continuous-wave gas laser, Photochem. Photobiol. **5:**555, 1966.

Moore, W.: Biological aspects of laser radiation. A review of hazards, Rockville, Md, 1969, U.S. Government Printing Office (DHEW Monograph).

Snyder-Mackler, L., and Bork, C.: The effect of cold laser on musculoskeletal trigger points: a double blind study, Poster-Presentation, National Convention, American Physical Therapy Association, Las Vegas, June, 1989.

Snyder-Mackler, L., Barry, A., Perkins, A., et al.: Effects of HeNe laser irradiation on skin resistance and pain in patients with trigger points in the neck and back, Physical Therapy **69**(5):336-341, 1989.

Yew, D.T., Ling Wong, S.L., and Chan, Y.: Stimulating effect of the low dose laser—a new hypothesis, Acta Anat. **112:**131, 1982.

Traction as a Specialized Modality

10

Daniel N. Hooker

OBJECTIVES

Following completion of this chapter, the student will be able to:

- Discuss the effect and therapeutic value of traction on bone, muscle, ligaments, joint structures, nerve, blood vessels, and intervertebral disk.

- Describe the parameters of traction.

- Discuss the effect that changing a parameter might have on treatment results.

- Outline the setup procedure for mechanical, positional, and manual traction to both the lumbar and the cervical spine.

In the care of the athletic population, **traction** has not traditionally been one of the more frequently used treatments. The age, vigor, and condition of the athletic population, along with the expense of the equipment, time-consuming setup, and lack of data supporting traction's effectiveness, all lead to the low use of and low interest in traction by the sports therapist. New equipment and the inversion fad have raised the interest and acceptance of the athletic population in the use of traction for both preventative and therapeutic treatment programs. Some of the concepts of traction discussed in this chapter are generalizable to the treatment of the extremities, but the discussion has been aimed specifically at cervical and lumbar spinal traction.

Traction has been used since ancient times in the treatment of painful spinal conditions, but the literature on traction and its clinical effectiveness is limited.[5-7,12,17,20] Most of the clinical studies go into great depth about the pathology being treated and give only a cursory description of the traction setup, making duplication of the traction method difficult.

Traction can be defined as a drawing tension applied to a body segment.[3]

EFFECTS ON SPINAL MOVEMENT

Traction encourages movement of the spine both overall and between each individual spinal segment.[1] Changes in overall spinal length and the amount of separation or space between each vertebra have been shown in studies of both the lumbar and the cervical spine[5,11-12,19-20] (Fig. 10-1).

The amount of movement varies according to the position of the spine, the amount of force, and the length of time the force is applied. Separations of 1 to 2 mm per intervertebral space have been reported. This change is very transient and the spine quickly returns to the previous intervertebral space relationships when traction is released and the erect posture is assumed.[6,11-12,17] Decreases in pain, paresthesia, or tingling while traction is applied may be caused by the physical separation of the vertebral segments and the resultant decrease in pressure on sensitive structures. If these changes occur while the patient is being treated with traction, the prognosis for the patient is good and traction should be continued as part of the treatment plan.[1,4] Any lasting therapeutic changes must be assumed to occur from adjustments or adaptations of the structures around the vertebrae in response to the traction.

EFFECTS ON BONE

Bone changes, according to **Wolff's law,** usually occur in response to compressive or distractive loads. Traction would place a distractive load on each of the vertebrae affected by the traction load. Although bone tissue adapts relatively quickly, bony changes do not occur fast enough to cause the symptom changes that occur with traction application. An intermittent traction with a rhythmic on and off load cycle not only provides distraction load but also promotes movement. The major effect of traction on the bone may come from the increase in spinal movement that reverses any immobilization-related bone weakness by increasing or maintaining bone density.

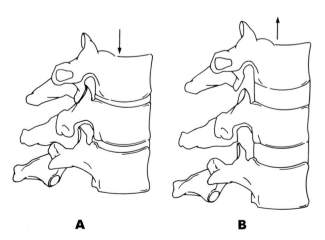

                    A   **B**

Figure 10-1. A, Spine in normal resting position. **B,** Spine under traction load with overall increase in length and overall increased separation between vertebrae.

The ligamentous structures of the spinal column will be stretched by traction. Structural changes of the ligaments occur relatively slowly in response to mechanical stresses because ligaments have **viscoelastic properties** that allow them to resist shear forces and to return to their original form following the removal of a deforming load.[1,4]

EFFECTS ON LIGAMENTS

With rapid loading, the ligaments become stiffer or resistant to changes in length and will be able to absorb a high load or force before failure occurs. With this type of loading, overstress could produce a significant injury.[4] The Wild West and the cervical traction of horse thieves gives us a great example of this type of loading. The sudden drop of body weight as the horse rides out and leaves the thief suspended by a rope around his neck places a rapid load on the ligaments and bones of the cervical spine. This overstress produces no adaptive change as it overwhelms the ligamentous and bony structures, causing a fracture dislocation of the upper cervical spine with spinal cord compression and resulting in the death of the thief.

Slow loading rates will allow the ligament to lengthen as it absorbs the force of the load. Overstress can still produce injury but it will not be as severe as in the high loading rates. The amount of **ligament deformation** accompanying a low rate of loading will be higher than in rapid loading situations. Loading should be applied slowly and comfortably.[4] The ligament deformation will allow the spinal vertebrae to move apart.

In ligaments shortened or contracted by an injury or a long-term postural problem, traction is important in restoring normal length. The traction force provides the stress that encourages the ligament to make adaptive changes in length and strength. The traction force in this instance would have to be heavy enough to stimulate adaptive changes but not heavy enough to overwhelm the ligament. In acute severely sprained ligaments, a traction force may overwhelm the ligament and have a negative effect on the healing process. Traction treatment should be a part of an overall treatment program that includes strengthening and flexibility exercises.[1]

When they are stretched, the ligaments put pressure on or move other structures within the ligamentous structure (**proprioceptive nerves**) and external to the ligament structure (**disk material, synovial fringes,** vascular structures, nerve roots). This pressure or movement can have a big impact on painful problems if pressure on a sensitive structure (nerve, vascular) is reduced. Activation of the proprioceptive system will also relieve pain by providing a gating effect similar to a transcutaneous electrical nerve stimulation treatment.[1,5]

The mechanical tension created by the traction has a good effect on **disk protrusions** and disk-related pain. Normally the disk helps to dissipate compressive forces while the spine is in an erect posture (Fig. 10-2).

EFFECTS ON THE DISK

In the normal disk, internal pressure increases but the nucleus pulposus (fluidlike center of the fibrocartilaginous vertebral disk) does not move with changes in the weight-bearing forces as the spine moves from flexion to extension.[18] When an injury occurs to the disk structures and the disk loses its nor-

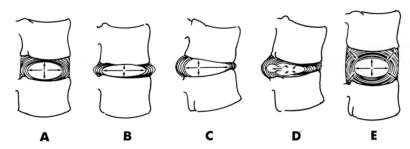

A   B   C   D   E

Figure 10-2. Fluid dynamics of the intervertebral disk. **A,** Normal disk in noncompressed position; internal pressure, indicated by arrows, is exerted relatively equally in all directions. The internal annular fibers contain the nuclear materials. **B,** Sitting or standing with compression of an injured disk causes the nucleus to become flatter. Pressure in this instance still remains relatively equal in all directions. **C,** In an injured disk, movement in the weight-bearing position causes a horizontal shift in the nuclear material. If this was forward bending, the bulge to the left would take place at the posterior annular fibers while the anterior annular fibers would be slackened and narrow. **D,** Weakness of the annular wall would allow the nuclear material to create a herniation and possibly put pressure on sensitive structures in the area. **E,** When placed under traction, the intervertebral space expands, lowering the disk pressure. The taut annulus creates a centripetally directed force. Both these factors encourage the nuclear material to move and decrease the herniation and its effects.

mal fullness, the vertebrae can move closer together. The annular fibers bulge just as an underinflated car tire bulges when compared with a normally inflated one[18] (Fig. 10-2, *B*).

If the disk is damaged and movement occurs in a weight-bearing position, the disk nucleus will shift according to fluid-dynamic principles. Pressure on one side squeezes the nucleus in the opposite direction (Fig. 10-2, *C*). If tears develop in the annular fibers, the nucleus will tend to take the path of least resistance and move in this direction (Fig. 10-2, *D*).

Traction that increases the separation of the vertebral bodies decreases the central pressure in the disk space and encourages the **disk nucleus** to return to a central position. The mechanical tension of the **annulus fibrosus** and ligaments surrounding the disk also tends to force the nuclear material and cartilage fragments toward the center.[1,5,7,10-12,17]

Movement of these materials relieves pain and symptoms if they are compressing nervous or vascular structures. Decreasing the compressive forces also allows for better fluid interchange within the disk and spinal canal.[1,5] The reduction in **disk herniation** is unstable and the herniation tends to return when compressive forces return[11,12] (Fig. 10-2, *D* and *E*).

The positive effect of traction in this instance may be destroyed by allowing the patient to sit after treatment. Minimizing compressive forces after treatment may be equally as important to the treatment's success as the traction.[1] The sitting posture increases the disk pressure, causing the nucleus to follow the path of least resistance and a return of the disk herniation.

The articular joints of the spine (**facet joints**) can be affected by traction, primarily through increased separation of the joint surfaces. **Meniscoid structures,** synovial fringes, or osteochondral fragments (calcified bone chips) impinged between joint surfaces are released and a dramatic reduction in symptoms is noticed when joint surfaces are separated. Increased joint separation decompresses the articular cartilage, allowing the synovial fluid exchange to nourish the cartilage. The separation may also decrease the rate of degenerative changes from osteoarthritis. Increased proprioceptive discharge from the facet joint structures provides some decrease in pain perception.[1,4-6,12]

EFFECTS ON ARTICULAR FACET JOINTS

The vertebral muscles can be effectively stretched by traction provided that the positions of the spine during traction are selected to optimize the stretch of particular muscle groups. The initial stretch should come from body positioning, and the addition of traction will then provide some additional stretch. The muscular stretch would lengthen tight muscle structures, allowing better muscular blood flow, and also activate muscle proprioceptors, providing even more of a gating influence on the pain. All these properties lead to a decrease in muscular irritation.[1,8,12]

EFFECTS ON THE MUSCULAR SYSTEM

The nerve is the structure at which traction's effects are most often directed. Pressure on nerves or roots from bulging disk material, irritated facet joints, bony spurs, or narrowed foramen size causes the neurologic malfunctioning often associated with spinal pain. Tingling is usually the first clinical sign indicating that there is pressure on a nerve structure. If the pressure is not relieved or if damage of the nerve as a result of trauma or **anoxia** has resulted in an inflammation, the tingling may not respond to traction.[6,7,17,19-22]

EFFECTS ON THE NERVES

Unrelieved pressure on a nerve will cause slowing and eventual loss of impulse conduction. The signs of motor weakness, numbness, and loss of reflex become progressively more apparent and are indicative of nerve degeneration. Pain, tenderness, and muscular spasm are also associated with continued pressure on the nerve.

Anything that decreases the pressure on the nerve increases the blood's circulation to the nerve, decreasing edema and allowing the nerve to return to normal functioning. Some degenerative changes are reversible depending on the amount of degeneration and the amount of **fibrosis** that occurs during the repair process.[1,5,19-21]

The previous discussion outlines the effect of traction on the major systems involved in spine-related pain and dysfunction. The complexity and interrelationships among these systems make determining specific causes of pain and dysfunction very difficult. Traction is not specific to one system but has an effect on each system, and collectively the effect can be very good. Traction can affect the pathologic process in any of the systems, and then all the structures in-

EFFECTS ON THE ENTIRE BODY PART

volved can begin to normalize. Traction should not stand alone as a treatment but should be considered as part of an overall treatment plan, and each component of any spine-related dysfunction should be treated with other appropriate modalities.[1,4,5,17,20]

CLINICAL APPLICATION

The discussion of specific traction setups is organized according to lumbar and cervical traction. Each of these areas will contain discussions of postural, manual, and machine-assisted traction. The traction setups mentioned in this chapter should be used as starting points in a treatment plan. The parameters of time, position, and traction force should be adapted to the patient, rather than forcing the patient to adapt to a predetermined traction setup.

The treatment plan should include the clinical criteria for judging the success and continued use of traction. Positive changes should occur within 5 to 8 treatment days if traction is going to be successful; for example, if an athlete has a positive straight leg raise sign (i.e., pain in the back with a passive straight leg raise). This is a measurable clinical criterion that can be used to judge the treatment's success. If the straight leg raise test is positive at 20 degrees of hip flexion before and after traction, and after successive treatments the straight leg raise test is positive at increasing degrees of hip flexion, then the treatment can be considered successful.

Lumbar Traction

Spinal **nerve root impingement,** from a variety of causes ranging from disk herniation or prolapse to **spondylolisthesis,** is the leading diagnosis for which traction is prescribed. Traction has also been used to treat joint hypomobility, arthritic conditions of the facet joints, mechanically produced muscle spasm, and joint pain.[1,7,12,17,20]

Lumbar Positional Traction

Normal spinal mechanics allow movements to occur that narrow or enlarge the intervertebral foramina. If the patient is placed in the backlying position with hips and knees flexed, the lumbar spine bends forward and the spinous processes separate. This movement increases the size of the intervertebral foramen bilaterally (Fig. 10-3). The flexed postures used to treat low-back pain are examples of this positional traction.

The greatest **unilateral foramen opening** occurs by positioning the patient sidelying with a pillow or blanket roll between the iliac crest and the lower border of the rib cage. The side on which increased foramen opening is desired should be superior. The roll should be close to the level of the spine where the traction separation is desired. The spine side bends around the roll (Fig. 10-4). The patient's hips and knees are then flexed until the lumbar spine is in a forward-bent position (Fig. 10-5, *A*). This accentuates the opening of a foramen. Maximal opening can be achieved by adding trunk rotation toward the side of the superior shoulder[16,19-21] (Fig. 10-5, *B*).

Positional traction is normally used when the patient is on a very restricted activity program because of low-back pain. The positions are used on a

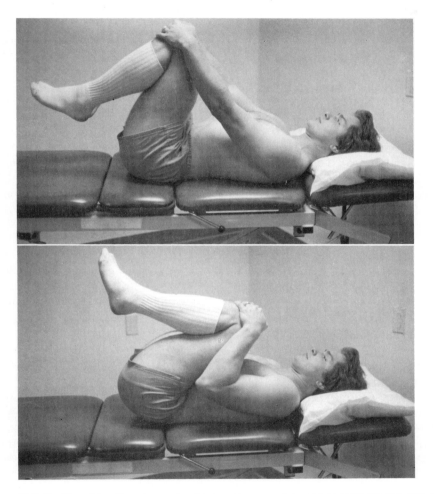

Figure 10-3. Positional traction; knees to chest posture can be used to increase the size of the lumbar intervertebral foramen bilaterally.

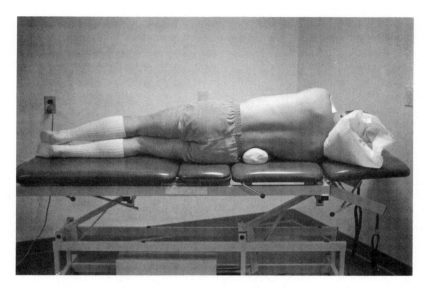

Figure 10-4. Positional traction; patient positioned sidelying with a blanket roll between iliac crest and rib cage. This increases the intervertebral foramen size of the left side of the lumbar spine.

trial and error basis to determine maximum comfort and to attempt to relieve pressure on nerve roots.

The results of the patient evaluation should be used to determine whether the painful side should be up or down when using the sidelying positional traction technique. Protective scoliosis is the most obvious sign that will help determine patient position: if the patient leans away from the painful side, the painful side should be up; if the patient leans toward the painful side, the painful side should be down (Fig. 10-6).

The first situation is most common and is attributed to a disk herniation lateral to the nerve root. The second situation is less common and is attributed to a disk herniation medial to the nerve root. If the herniation is lateral, sidebending the spine away from the pain should relieve the symptoms, whereas sidebending toward the pain should aggravate the symptoms. If the herniation is medial, sidebending the spine away from the pain should aggravate the symptoms, whereas sidebending toward the pain should relieve the symptoms. Patients with these symptoms may also be good candidates for unilateral traction[1,4,16-17,19-20] (Fig. 10-7). Facet irritation is capable of causing similar scoliotic curves; in most instances the scoliosis is convex toward the painful side.

Inversion Traction

Inversion traction, another positional traction, is the latest fad for prevention of back problems. Specialized equipment or simply hanging upside down from a chinning bar will place a person in the inverted position. The spinal column is lengthened because of the stretch provided by the weight of the trunk. The

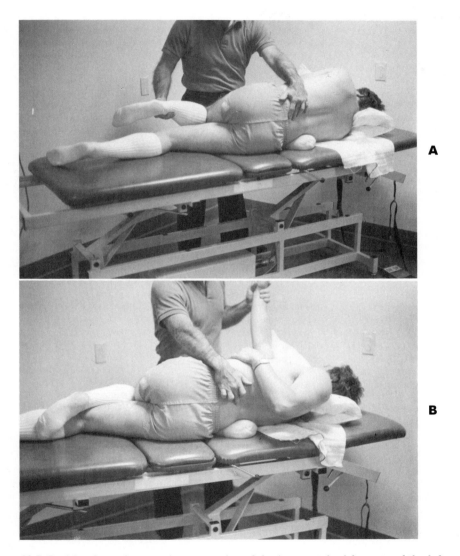

Figure 10-5. Positional traction; maximum opening of the intervertebral foramen of the left side of the patient's lumbar spine is achieved by flexing the upper hip and knee and rotating the patient's shoulders so he is looking over the left shoulder (left rotation).

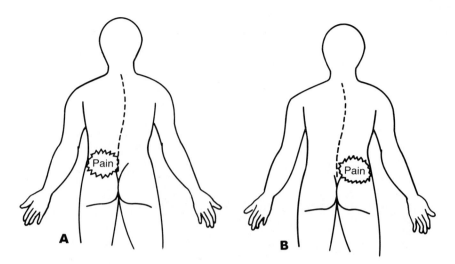

Figure 10-6. A, Patient leaning away from the painful side. The patient's left side should be placed up while sidelying over a blanket roll to open up the upper foramen or the nerve roots away from the lateral herniation or both. **B,** Patient leaning toward the painful side. The patient's left side should be placed up while sidelying over a blanket roll to pull the nerve roots away from a medial herniation.

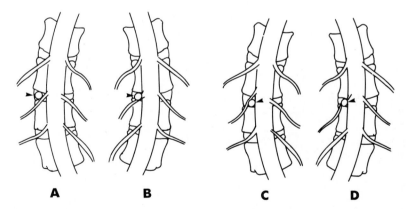

Figure 10-7. A, Herniation lateral to a nerve root with spine laterally bent to minimize nerve root pressure. **B,** If laterally flexed toward the herniation, the nerve root symptoms of tingling, pain, numbness, weakness, and loss of reflex may become more pronounced. **C,** Herniation medial to a nerve root with the spine laterally bent to minimize nerve root pressure. Note that *A* and *C* are laterally bent in opposite directions. **D,** If laterally flexed away from the herniation, the nerve root symptoms of tingling, pain, numbness, weakness, and loss of reflex may become more pronounced.

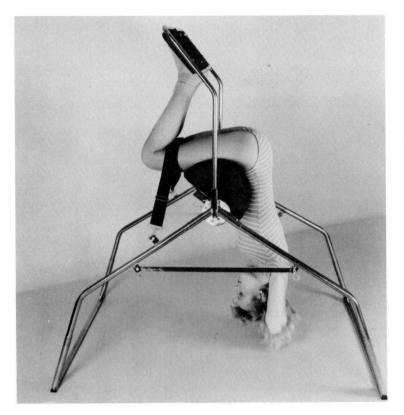

Figure 10-8. Inversion traction apparatus. (Courtesy Lossing Orthopaedic, Minneapolis, MN 55404.)

force of the trunk in this position is usually calculated to be approximately 40% of body weight (Fig. 10-8).

When the person is comfortable and able to relax, the length of the spinal column will increase. These length changes will coincide with decreases in spinal muscle activity.[1,13-14]

No research-supported protocols exist for this method of traction, although a slow progression of time in the inverted position seems to be best. One study suggests the electromyographic activity decreases after 70 seconds in the inverted position. If the patient is comfortable completely inverted, 70 seconds may be used as a minimum treatment time. The inverted position may be repeated 2 or 3 times at a treatment session, with a 2 to 3 minute rest between bouts. Longer treatment times may also enhance results. Maximum treatment times range from 10 to 30 minutes. Setup procedures are equipment-dependent and the manufacturer's protocols should be followed and modified as necessary to meet the needs of the patient.[1-2,13-14]

Blood pressure should be monitored while the patient is in the inverted position. If a rise of 20 mm of mercury above the resting diastolic pressure is found, the therapist should stop the treatment for that session.[1-2,13]

Contraindications include hypertensive (140/90) individuals and anyone with heart disease or glaucoma. Patients with sinus problems, diabetes, thyroid conditions, asthma, migraine headaches, detached retinas, or hiatal hernias should consult their physicians before treatment is initiated.

Recent surgery or musculoskeletal problems to the lower limb may require modification of the inversion apparatus. In addition, meals or snacks should not be eaten during the hour before treatment to keep the patient comfortable.

One method of testing the patient's tolerance to the inverted position is to have the patient assume the hand-knee position and put his or her head on the floor, holding that position for 60 seconds. Any vertigo, dizziness, or nausea may indicate that this patient is a poor candidate for inversion and that the treatment progression should be very slow[1-2,13] (Fig. 10-9).

Manual Lumbar Traction

Manual lumbar traction is used for lumbar spine problems to test the patient's tolerance to traction, to arrive at the most comfortable treatment setup, to make the traction as specific to one vertebral level as possible, and to provide the specificity needed for a traction manipulation of the spine. The disadvantage is that maintaining the large forces necessary for separation of the lumbar vertebrae for a period of time is difficult and energy consuming for the sports therapist.[1,19-20]

Having a split table will eliminate most of the friction between the patient's body segments and the treatment table and is essential for effective delivery of manual lumbar traction[1,4,19,21] (Fig. 10-10). The therapist's effort does not cause separation of the vertebral segments unless the frictional forces are overcome first.

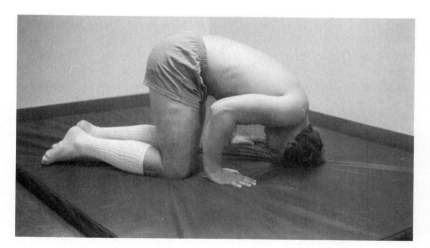

Figure 10-9. Inversion tolerance test position. Any vertigo, dizziness, or nausea may indicate that this patient is a poor candidate for inversion treatment.

To make the traction specific to a vertebral level, the patient is positioned side-lying on the split table. For traction specific to L3-4, L4-5, and L5-S1 levels, the patient's upper leg is used as a lever and the lumbar spine is flexed until motion of the spinous process just below that level is felt (Fig. 10-11). The patient's trunk is then rotated toward the upper shoulder until the spinous process just above the desired level is felt (Fig. 10-12).

If lumbar levels T12, L1, L1-2, and L2-3 are to be given specific traction, the patient is again positioned sidelying. These levels require positioning in reverse order from the lower levels. First the trunk is rotated (Fig. 10-12), then the lumbar spine is flexed[1,4] (Fig. 10-11).

In both instances the rotation and flexion tighten and lock joint structures in which these motions have taken place, leaving the desired segment with more movement available than the upper or lower levels. When traction is applied, greater movement of the desired level occurs while movement at other levels is minimized because of the joint locking created by the preliminary positioning.

The split table is then released and the sports therapist palpates the spinous processes of the selected intervertebral level, places his or her chest against the anterior superior iliac spine of the patient's upper hip, and leans toward the patient's feet. Enough force is used to cause a palpable separation of the spinous processes (Fig. 10-13). Intermittent movement is most easily accomplished, while sustained traction becomes physically more difficult.[1,4]

Unilateral leg pull traction has been used in the treatment of hip joint problems or difficult lateral shift corrections. A thoracic countertraction harness is used to secure the patient to the table. The sports therapist grabs the patient's ankle and brings the patient's hip into 30-degree flexion, 30-degree abduction, and full external rotation. A steady pull is applied until a noticeable distraction is felt[4] (Fig. 10-14).

Text continued on p. 226.

**Level Specific
Manual Traction**

**Unilateral Leg
Pull Manual
Traction**

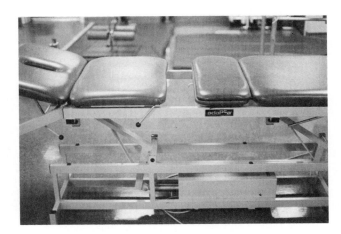

Figure 10-10. Split table with movable section to decrease frictional forces.

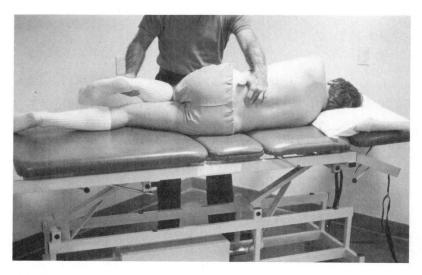

Figure 10-11. Positioning the patient for maximum effect at a specific level. The lumbar spine is flexed, using the patient's upper leg as a lever. The sports therapist palpates the interspinous area between two spinous processes. The upper spinous process is the one at which maximum effect is desired. When the lumbar spine flexes and the sports therapist feels the motion of the lower spinous process with the palpating hand, the foot is placed against the opposite leg so that further flexion is not allowed.

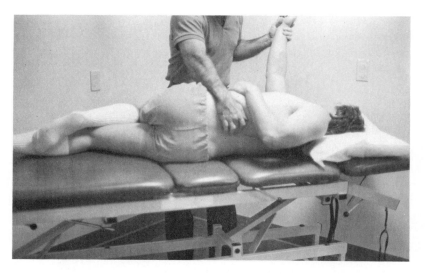

Figure 10-12. Positioning the patient for maximum effect at a specific level. The patient's trunk is rotated by the sports therapist until motion of the upper spinous process is felt by the sports therapist. Trunk rotation should be passively produced by the sports therapist, positioning the patient's upper arm with hand on the rib cage, and pulling on the patient's lower arm, creating trunk rotation toward the upper arm. In this case it is rotation to the left.

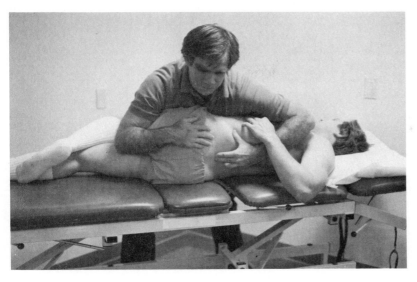

Figure 10-13. Manual lumbar traction with maximum effect at a specific level. The sports therapist has positioned the patient for maximum effect and is palpating the interspinous area between the two spinous processes where maximum traction effect is desired. The sports therapist then places his or her chest against the anterior superior iliac spine and the patient's upper hip. The split table is released and the sports therapist leans toward the patient's feet, using enough force to cause a palpable separation of the spinous processes at the desired level.

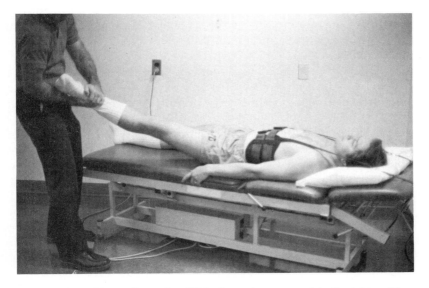

Figure 10-14. Unilateral leg pull traction. With the patient secured to the table with a thoracic countertraction harness, the sports therapist brings the patient's hip into 30-degree flexion, 30-degree abduction, and maximum external rotation. A steady pull is then applied.

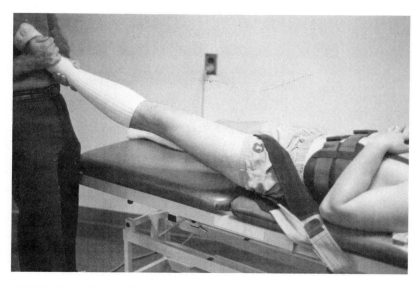

Figure 10-15. Unilateral leg pull traction for sacroiliac joint problems. A strap is placed through the groin and secured to the table. The sports therapist brings the patient's hip into 30-degree flexion and 15-degree abduction, and then applies a traction force to the leg.

In suspected sacroiliac joint problems, a similar setup can be used. A banana strap is placed through the groin on the side to be stretched. This strap will secure the patient in position. The sports therapist grabs the patient's ankle, brings his or her hip into 30-degree flexion and 15-degree abduction, and then applies a sustained or intermittent pull to create a mobilizing effect on the sacroiliac joint[4] (Fig. 10-15).

As a preliminary to mechanical traction, manual traction is helpful in determining what degree of lumbar flexion, extension, or sidebending is most comfortable and will also give an indication of the treatment's success. The most comfortable position is usually the best therapeutic position.[4,19,21]

Patient comfort may have a bigger impact on the traction's results than the angle of pull, the force used, the mode, or the duration of the treatment. The inability of the patient to relax in any traction setup will affect the traction's ability to cause a separation of the vertebrae. The lack of vertebral separation would minimize some of the traction's therapeutic benefits.[4,19,21]

Mechanical Lumbar Traction

When using mechanical traction, the sports therapist will have to select and adjust the following parameters of the traction equipment and patient position:

1. Body position: prone, supine, hip position, bilateral or unilateral direction of pull
2. Force used
3. Intermittent traction: traction time and rest time
4. Sustained traction

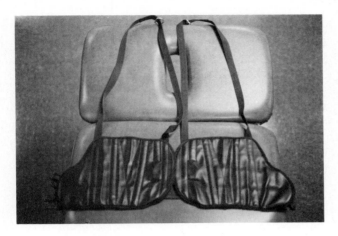

Figure 10-16. Vinyl-backed traction harness.

5. Duration of treatment
6. Progressive steps
7. Regressive steps

The research on mechanical lumbar traction gives us a strong protocol for using traction to decrease disk protrusion and nerve root symptoms. The protocols for use in other pathologies are not supported by research, but clinical empiricism and inference from some of the research give a good working protocol. The sports therapist will need to match his or her traction to the patient's symptoms and make adjustments based on the clinical results.[4,7,16,19]

Patient Setup and Equipment

A split table or other mechanism to eliminate friction between body segments and the table surface is a prerequisite to effective lumbar traction. Otherwise, most of the force applied would be spent overcoming the coefficient of friction[1,4,12,19,21] (Fig. 10-10).

A nonslip traction harness is needed to transfer the traction force comfortably to the patient and to stabilize the trunk while the lumbar spine is placed under traction. A harness lined with a vinyl material is best because it adheres to the patient's skin and does not slip like the cotton-lined harness. Clothing between the harness and the skin will also promote slipping. The vinyl-sided harness does not have to be as constricting as the cotton-backed harness to prevent slippage, thus increasing the patient's comfort[4,19,21] (Fig. 10-16).

The harness can be applied when the patient is standing next to the traction table prior to treatment. The pelvic harness is applied so the contact pads and upper belt are at or just above the level of the iliac crest (Fig. 10-17).

Shirts should never be tucked under the pelvic harness because some of the tractive force would be dissipated pulling on the shift material. The contact pads should be adjusted so that the harness loops will provide a posteriorly directed pull, encouraging lumbar flexion (Fig. 10-18). The harness firmly adheres to the patient's hips.[4,19,21]

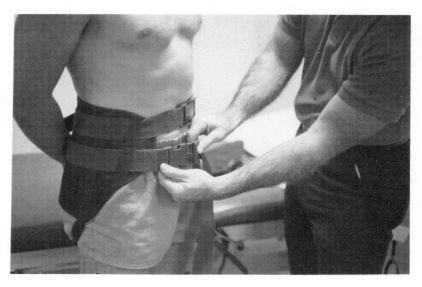

Figure 10-17. Pelvic harness for mechanical lumbar traction. The contact pads are applied so that the upper belt is at or just above the level of the iliac crest.

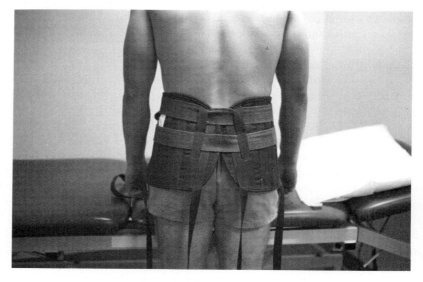

Figure 10-18. The traction straps from the pelvic harness should bracket the patient's buttocks if a lumbar flexion pull is desired. If a straight pull is desired, the pelvic harness should be adjusted so that the straps bracket the patient's lateral hip area.

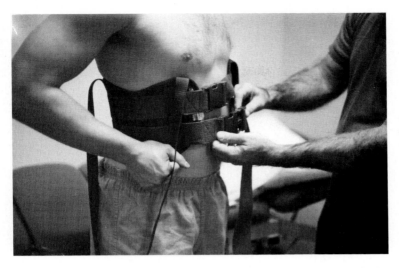

Figure 10-19. Thoracic countertraction harness. Rib pads are positioned over the lower rib cage.

The rib belt is then applied in a similar manner with the rib pads positioned over the lower rib cage in a comfortable manner. The rib belt is then snugged up and the patient is positioned on the table[4,19,21] (Fig. 10-19).

The standing application of the traction harness is easier and more effective if the patient is to be placed in prone position for treatment[4,19,21] (Fig. 10-20). The traction harness can also be applied by laying it out on the traction table and having the patient lie down on top of it. The pads are then adjusted and the belts snugged with the patient lying down.

Body Position

Body position has been reported to have a big impact on traction results, but this has been empirically derived rather than research supported. The sports therapist needs a good understanding of the mechanics of the lumbar spine to make decisions about position that will best affect a patient's symptoms.[1,4,12,17,19-21]

Generally, the neutral spinal position allows for the largest intervertebral foramen opening, and it is usually the position of choice whether the patient is prone or supine. Extension beyond neutral lumbar spine causes the bony elements of the foramen to create a narrower opening. Lumbar spinal flexion beyond neutral causes the ligamentum flavum and other soft tissues to constrict the foramen's opening[19,21] (Fig. 10-21).

Saunders[19,21] recommends the prone position with a normal to slightly flattened lumbar lordosis (an abnormal anterior curve) as the position of choice in disk protrusions. The amount of lordosis may be controlled by using pillows under the abdomen. The prone position also allows the easy application of other modalities to the pain area and an easier assessment of the amount of spinous process separation[4,19,21] (Fig. 10-22).

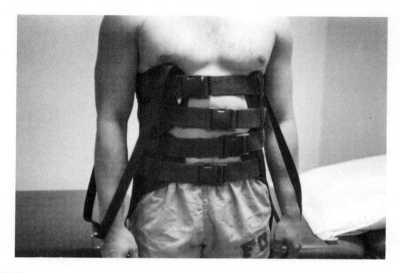

Figure 10-20. Applying the pelvic and thoracic harnesses may be easier if done while the patient is standing.

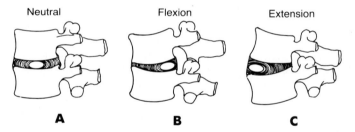

Neutral   Flexion   Extension

A   **B**   **C**

Figure 10-21. A, Neutral lumbar spine position allows for the largest intervertebral foramen opening before traction is applied. **B,** Flexion, while it may tend to increase the posterior opening, puts pressure on the disk nucleus to move posterior. Other soft tissue may also close the foramen opening. **C,** Extension beyond neutral tends to close the foramen down as the bony arches come closer together.

In traction applied to a patient in the supine position, hip position was found to affect vertebral separation. As hip flexion increased from 0 to 90 degrees, traction produced a greater posterior intervertebral space separation[17] (Fig. 10-23).

Unilateral pelvic traction has also been recommended when a stronger force is desired on one side of the spine. Patients with protective scoliosis, unilateral joint dysfunction, or unilateral lumbar muscle spasm with scoliosis may do quite well with this approach. Only one side of the pelvic harness is hooked to the traction device to accomplish this technique[20] (Fig. 10-24).

In patients with protective scoliosis, when the patient leans away from the painful side, the traction should be applied on the painful side. When the

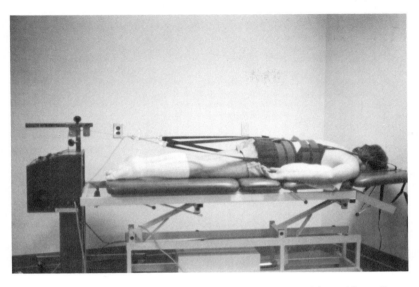

Figure 10-22. Mechanical lumbar traction; patient in the prone position with a pillow under the abdomen to help control lumbar spine extension.

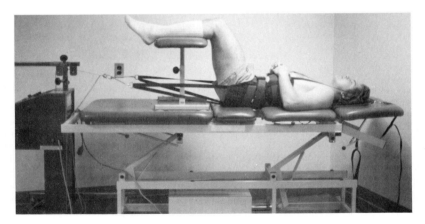

Figure 10-23. Mechanical lumbar traction; patient in the supine position with hips flexed to approximately 90 degrees.

patient leans toward the painful side, the traction should be applied on the nonpainful side (see Fig. 10-6).

In patients with scoliosis caused by muscle spasm, the traction force should be applied from the side with the muscle spasm (Fig. 10-25). In unilateral facet joint dysfunction, the traction should be applied from the side of most complaint.[19]

Overall, patient positioning for traction should be varied according to a pa-

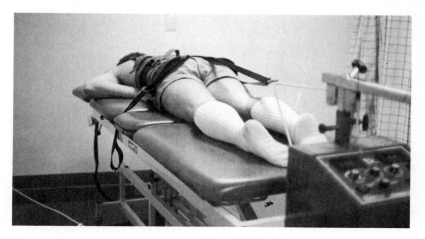

Figure 10-24. Mechanical lumbar traction with a unilateral pull; only one of the pelvic straps is hooked to the traction device.

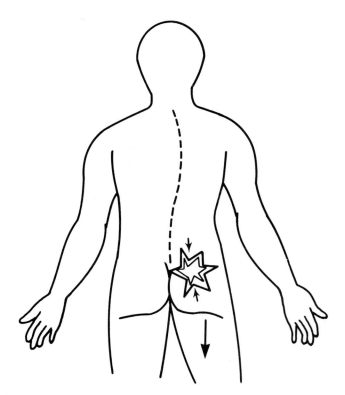

Figure 10-25. In a patient with scoliosis caused by muscle spasm *(right)*, the unilateral traction force should be applied using only the right pelvic strap.

tient's needs and comfort. Experimentation with positioning is encouraged so that the traction's effect on the patient will be maximized.

Patient comfort is far more important than relative position in making patient position decisions. If the patient cannot relax, the traction will not be successful in causing vertebral separation.[4,19,21]

Several researchers have indicated that no lumbar vertebral separation will occur with traction forces less than one quarter of the patient's body weight. The traction force necessary to cause effective vertebral separation will range between 65 and 200 pounds.[1,11-12,19,21] This force does not have to be used on the first treatment, and progressive steps both during and between treatments are often necessary to comfortably reach these therapeutic loads. A force equal to half the patient's body weight is a good guideline to use in selecting a force high enough to cause vertebral separation. These high weight levels pose no danger, as cadaver research indicates a force of 440 pounds or greater is necessary to cause damage to the lumbar spine components[11,12] (Fig. 10-26).

Caution must be used when using traction of the lumbar spine, because there is a tendency for the nucleus pulposus gel to imbibe fluid from the vertebral body, thus increasing pressure within the disk. This happens in a very short period of time. When pressure is released and weight is applied to the

Traction Force

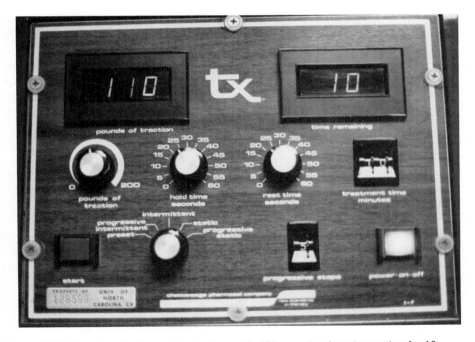

Figure 10-26. Traction device set for traction with 100 pounds of static traction for 10 minutes with 6 progressive steps.

disk, this excess fluid increases pressure on the annulus and exacerbates the patient's symptoms. Therefore, it is recommended that during an initial treatment with lumbar traction a maximum of 30 pounds be used to determine whether traction will have a negative effect on the symptoms.[5]

The research has been aimed at forces necessary to cause vertebral separation. Traction certainly has effects that are not associated with vertebral separation, and if these effects are desired, less force may be necessary to get them.

Intermittent versus Sustained

Good results have been reported with both intermittent and sustained traction. In most cases of lumbar disk problems, sustained traction seems to be the treatment of choice. Partial reduction in disk protrusions was observed in 4 minutes of sustained traction.[11-12,19,21] Good results were also reported using intermittent traction in the treatment of ruptured intervertebral disk.[7]

Separation of the posterior intervertebral space was noted with a 10-second-hold intermittent traction.[17] Posterior intervertebral separations using 100 pounds of force were similar when intermittent and sustained traction modes were compared.[12] The electromyographic activity of the sacrospinalis musculature showed similar patterns when sustained and intermittent traction were compared.[8]

Sustained traction is favored in treating intervertebral disk herniation because sustained traction allows more time with the disk uncompressed to cause the disk nuclear material to move centripetally and reduce the disk herniation's pressure on nerve structures. When used for this purpose, sustained traction may be superior to intermittent traction.[4,19,21]

In deciding on sustained versus intermittent traction, the sports therapist should follow the guidelines for treating diagnosed disk herniations with sustained traction, while most other traction-appropriate diagnoses may be treated with intermittent traction. Intermittent traction, in any case, is usually more comfortable when using higher forces, and increased comfort will be one of the primary considerations because there is no conclusive evidence supporting the choice of one method over the other.*

The timing of the traction and rest phases of intermittent traction has not been researched. Short (less than 10 seconds) traction phases will cause only minimal interspace separation but will activate joint and muscle receptors and create facet joint movements.[4,5] Longer (more than 10 seconds) traction phases will tend to stretch the ligamentous and muscular tissues long enough to overcome their resistance to movement and create a longer lasting mechanical separation. When using high traction forces, the comfort of the patient may dictate the adjustment of the traction time. Longer total treatment time will also be tolerated with intermittent traction.[4-6,12,19]

Rest phase times should be relatively short but should also be comfort oriented. The rest time should be adjusted to allow the patient to recover and feel relaxed before the next traction cycle. The sports therapist should monitor the

*References 1, 4, 7, 12, 17, 19, and 21.

traction patient frequently to adjust traction and rest time adjustments to maintain the patient in a relaxed comfortable state.

The total treatment times of sustained traction and intermittent traction are only partially research-based. With sustained traction, Mathews[11] found reduction in disk protrusion after 4 minutes with further reduction at 20 minutes. Complete reduction in protrusions was seen at 38 minutes. Other researchers found no difference in separation of the cervical spine when times of 7, 30, and 60 seconds were compared.[5,11,12]

Duration of Treatment

When dealing with suspected disk protrusions, the total treatment time should be relatively short. As the disk space widens, the pressure inside the disk decreases and the disk nucleus will move centripetally. The projected time for pressure within a disk to equalize is 8 to 10 minutes. At this point the nuclear material is no longer moving centripetally. With longer time in this position, osmotic forces will equalize the pressure within the disk with that of the surrounding tissue. When the pressure equalization occurs, the traction effect on the protrusion is lost. The intradiskal pressure may increase when the traction is released if the traction stays on too long. This increased pressure would result in increased symptoms. This situation has not been reported when treatment times are kept at 10 minutes or less.[19,21] If this reaction does occur, shorter treatment times or long-hold (60 seconds' traction, 10 to 20 seconds' rest) intermittent traction may be necessary to control the symptoms.

Some sources advocate traction times of up to 30 minutes.[4,11,12] The contradiction in philosophy may be because of pathology or the individual anatomy of each patient. However, an adverse reaction to traction (i.e., a dramatic increase in symptoms when the traction is released) is something the sports therapist should try to avoid.

Total treatment time for sustained traction when treating disk-related symptoms should start at less than 10 minutes. If the treatment is successful in reducing symptoms, the time should be left at 10 minutes or less. If the treatment is partially successful or unsuccessful in relieving symptoms, the sports therapist may increase the time gradually over several treatments to 30 minutes.

Some traction equipment is built with progressive and regressive modes. The machine will progressively increase the traction force in a preselected number of steps. A gradual increase in pressure lets patients accommodate slowly to the traction and helps them to stay relaxed. A gradual progression of force also allows the sports therapist to release the split table after the slack in the system has been taken up by several progressions[1,4] (Fig. 10-27).

Progressive and Regressive Steps

Regressive steps do just the opposite and allow the patient to come down gradually from the high loads. Again, patient comfort is the primary consideration because no research supports any protocol[1,4] (Fig. 10-28).

Some equipment has the capability to be programmed for progressive and regressive steps and also to have minimum traction forces allowing a sustained force with intermittent peaks[1,4] (Fig. 10-29). To achieve these kinds of traction

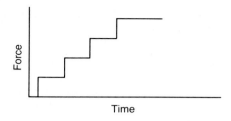

Figure 10-27. Progressive steps for lumbar traction of X pounds. Four steps are used: the first is ¼ X pounds, the second ¾ X, etc. Each lasts for an equal time.

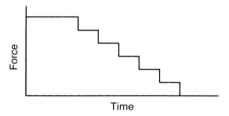

Figure 10-28. Regressive steps for lumbar traction of X pounds. Six equal regressive steps are used: the first drops the traction force from X to ⅚ X, the second to ⅘ X, etc. Each lasts for an equal time.

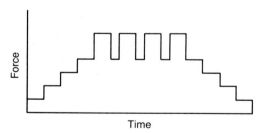

Figure 10-29. Progressive and regressive steps with a minimum sustained traction force.

setups with a machine that is not programmable, manual operation and timing will be necessary.

Throughout the discussion on lumbar traction, patient comfort comes up again and again in regard to the parameters of the treatment setup. One of the primary keys to successful traction treatment is the relaxation of the patient. The use of appropriate modalities before and during the traction treatment will add to the total effectiveness of the treatment plan. Bracing or appropriate exercise after traction may also enhance the results and prolong the benefits

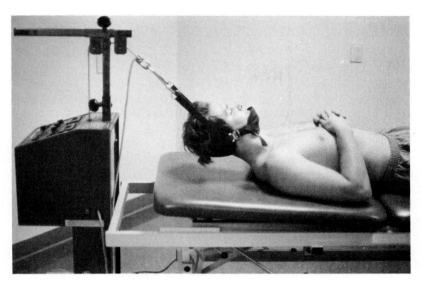

Figure 10-30. Mechanical cervical traction; patient in the supine position with traction harness placed so that maximum pull is exerted on the occiput and the patient is in a position of approximately 20 to 30 degrees of neck flexion.

gained. Better technology and more research will help refine the traction art and provide better results from this type of treatment.

The objectives for using traction in the cervical region do not vary much from the objectives for using traction in the lumbar region. Reasonable objectives for cervical traction include stretch of the muscles and joint structures of the vertebral column, enlargement of the intervertebral spaces and foramina, centripetally directed forces on the disk and soft tissue around the disk, mobilization of vertebral joints, increases and changes in joint proprioception, relief of compressive effects of normal posture, and improvement in arterial venous and lymphatic flow.[4-6,12,22-23] In athletics, diagnoses and symptoms requiring traction are found infrequently.[15] These diagnoses are usually found in older populations. The literature does provide a relatively clear protocol to use in trying to achieve vertebral separation using a mechanical traction apparatus.

The patient should be supine or long-sitting with the neck flexed between 20 and 30 degrees (Fig. 10-30). A sitting posture can be used, but this is clinically more cumbersome and is not supported by the research as an optimal position of cervical traction.

A traction force above 20 pounds, applied intermittently for a minimum of 7 seconds' traction time and with adequate rest time for recovery is recommended. This traction should be continued over 20 to 25 minutes. Higher forces up to 50 pounds may produce increased separation, but the other parameters

Cervical Traction

should remain the same. The average separation at the posterior vertebral area is 1 to 1.5 mm per space while the anterior vertebral area separates approximately 0.4 mm per space. Greater separations are expected in the younger population than in the older population. Within 20 to 25 minutes from the time traction is stopped and normal sitting or standing postures are resumed, the vertebral separation returns to its previous heights. The upper cervical segments do not separate as easily as lower cervical segments.[5-6,12] This traction force can be applied either manually or mechanically.

Mechanical Traction Protocol

The traction harness must be arranged comfortably so that the majority of pull is placed on the occiput rather than the chin (see Fig. 10-30). Some cervical traction harnesses do not have a chin-piece. These harnesses may have an advantage, provided that the traction force is effectively transferred to the structures of the cervical spine.[4-6]

For diagnoses or symptoms that require stretching the posterior neck and ligamentous structures, the following parameters should be used:

1. The neck-trunk angle should be positioned at less than 30 degrees. Various rotations and sidebendings can also be used.
2. Force should be 20 pounds or more applied intermittently with a 20-second traction time.
3. Treatment duration should be 10 minutes or longer.
4. The addition of pain-reducing and heating modalities will add to the benefits gained by the traction[1,4-6,12] (Fig. 10-31).

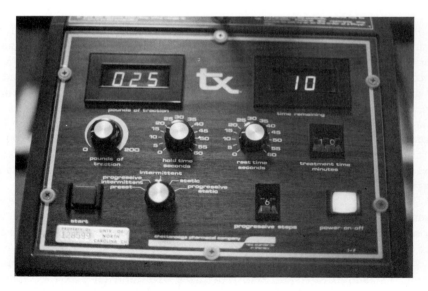

Figure 10-31. Control panel of traction machine with parameters adjusted for intermittent cervical traction.

In most cases in athletics (sprains and strains), simple manual traction used to produce a rhythmic longitudinal movement will be very successful in helping decrease pain, muscle spasm, stiffness, and inflammation and also in reducing joint compressive forces. Manual traction is infinitely more adaptable than mechanical traction, and changes in the direction, force, duration of the traction, and patient position can be made instantaneously as the sports therapist senses relaxation or resistance.[1,4-5,12]

The patient's head and neck are supported by the sports therapist. The hand should cradle the neck and provide adequate grip for the effective transfer of the traction force to the mastoid processes. One hand should be placed under the patient's neck with the thenar eminence (base of the thumb) in contact with one mastoid process and the fingers cradling the neck reaching across toward the other mastoid process[1] (Fig. 10-32, A).

The sports therapist then provides a gentle (less than 20 pounds) pull in a cephalic direction. Intervertebral separation is not desired because of the damage to the ligaments or capsule. A head halter or similar harness may be used to deliver the force also (Fig. 10-32, B).

The force should be intermittent, with the traction time between 3 and 10 seconds. The rest time may be very brief, but the tractive force should be released almost completely. The total treatment time should be between 3 and 10 minutes.[1,4-5]

When pain is limiting or affecting movement, a bout of traction should be followed by a reassessment of the painful motion to determine increases or decreases in pain or motion. Successive bouts of traction can be used as long as the symptoms are improving. When the symptoms stabilize or are worse on the reassessment, the traction should be discontinued.[4]

A variety of patient head and neck positions can be used in cervical traction. Different head and neck positions will place some vertebral structures under more tension than others. Good knowledge of cervical kinesiology and biomechanics and good knowledge and skill in joint mobilization are required before the sports therapist should experiment with extensive position changes[1,4,5] (Fig. 10-33).

At the completion of the traction treatment, in cases of strain or sprain, protection of the neck with a soft collar is often desirable to prevent extremes of motion, minimize compressive forces, and encourage muscle relaxation. Instructions in sleeping positions and regular support postures are also important in caring for athletes with cervical problems.[1,4]

A mechanical traction device can be very costly and is beyond the budgetary limitations of many institutions. Thus, knowledge of techniques of manual traction will be necessary. A third option is a wall-mounted traction device that can provide cervical traction. These units are relatively inexpensive and can be effective if used appropriately. Weight application can be accomplished using plates, sand bags, or water bags. The patient should be placed in a comfortable position (sitting, prone) with 10 to 20 pounds of traction applied for 20 to 25

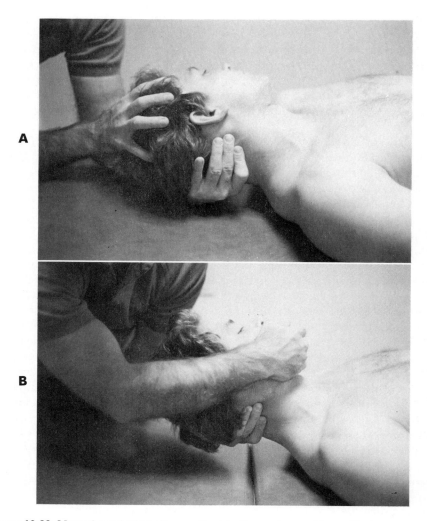

Figure 10-32. Manual cervical traction; patient in the supine position with the sports therapist's fingertips and thenar eminence contacting the mastoid process of the patient's skull.

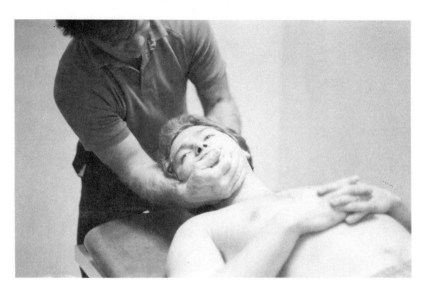

Figure 10-33. Manual cervical traction; patient is positioned with neck in flexion and with some neck rotation to the right. Laterally flexed positions may also be used.

minutes. Static traction is most easily employed although intermittent traction may also be used, if desired, by simply lifting the weight and releasing tension periodically (Fig. 10-34).

The Necktrac is another example of a fairly inexpensive home-use traction device (Fig. 10-35).

CONTRAINDICA-TIONS

Traction, except as a light mobilization, is contraindicated in acute sprains (first 3 to 5 days) or in any conditions in which movement is undesirable. In cases of vertebral joint instability, traction may perpetuate the instability or cause further strain. Certainly the serious problems associated with tumors, bone diseases, osteoporosis, and infections in bones or joints are also contraindications.

SUMMARY

1. Traction has been used to treat a variety of cervical and lumbar spine problems. The effect of traction on each system involved in the complex anatomic make-up of the spine needs to be considered when selecting traction as a part of a therapeutic treatment plan.
2. The traction protocol should be set up to manage a particular problem rather than applied in the same manner regardless of the patient or pathology. Traction is a flexible modality with an infinite number of variations available. This flexibility should allow sports therapists to adjust their protocols to match the patient's symptoms and diagnosis.

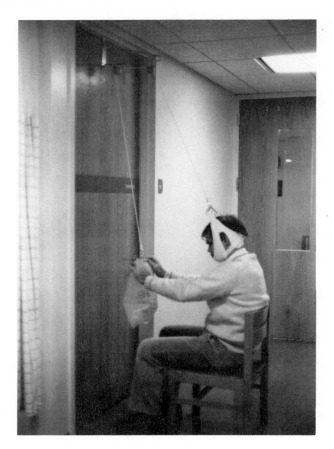

Figure 10-34. Cervical traction using a wall-mounted unit.

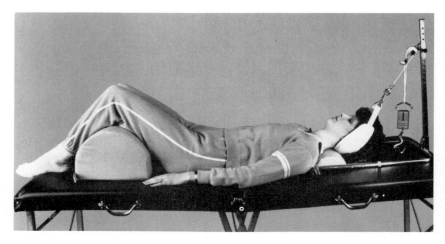

Figure 10-35. The Necktrac home-use traction device. (Courtesy Lossing Orthopedic 777 Harding St. NE Minneapolis, MN 55418)

3. Traction is capable of producing a separation of vertebral bodies; a centripetal force on the soft tissues surrounding the vertebrae; a mobilization of vertebral joints; a change in proprioceptive discharge of the spinal complex; a stretch of connective tissue; a stretch of muscle tissue; an improvement in arterial, venous, and lymphatic flow; and a lessening of the compressive effects of posture. Any of these effects can change the symptoms of the patient under treatment and help to normalize the patient's lumbar or cervical spine.

GLOSSARY

annulus fibrosus The interlacing cross-fibers of fibroelastic tissue that are attached to adjacent vertebral bodies that contain the nucleus pulposus.

anoxia Reduction of oxygen in body tissues below physiologic levels.

disk herniation The protrusion of the nucleus pulposus through a defect in the annulus fibrosus.

disk material Cartilaginous material from vertebral body surfaces, disk nucleus, or annulus fibrosus.

disk nucleus The protein polysaccharide gel that is contained between the cartilaginous end plates of the vertebrae and the annulus fibrosus.

disk protrusion The abnormal projection of the disk nucleus through some or all of the annular rings.

facet joints Articular joints of the spine.

fibrosis The formation of fibrous tissue in the injury repair process.

ligament deformation Lengthening distortion of ligament caused by traction loading.

meniscoid structures A cartilage tip found on the synovial fringes of some facet joints.

nerve root impingement Abnormal encroachment of some body tissue into the space occupied by the nerve root.

proprioceptive nervous system System of nerves that provide information on joint movement, pressure, and muscle tension.

spondylolisthesis Forward displacement of one vertebra over another.

synovial fringes Folds of synovial tissue that move in and out of the joint space.

traction Drawing tension applied to a body segment.

unilateral foramen opening Enlargement of the foramen on one side of a vertebral segment.

viscoelastic properties The property of a material to show sensitivity to rate of loading.

Wolff's law Bone remodels itself and provides increased strength along the lines of the mechanical forces placed on it.

REFERENCES

1 Burkhardt, S.: Course notes, cervical and lumbar traction seminar, Morgantown, W. Va., 1983.

2 Cooperman, J., and Scheid, D.: Guidelines for the use of inversion, Clin. Management **4**(1):6, 1984.

3 Dorland's illustrated medical dictionary, ed. 24, Philadelphia, 1965, W.B. Saunders Co.

4 Erhard, R.: Course notes, cervical and lumbar traction seminar, Morgantown, W. Va., 1983.

5 Grieve, G.P.: Neck traction, Physiotherapy **6**:260-265, 1982.

6 Harris, P.R.: Cervical traction: review of the literature and treatment guidelines, Phys. Ther. **57**:910-914, 1977.

7 Hood, L.D., and Chrisman, D.: Intermittent pelvic traction in the treatment of the ruptured intervertebral disk, Phys. Ther. **48**:21-30, 1968.

8 Hood, C.J., et al.: Comparison of EMG activity in normal lumbar sacrospinalis musculature during continuous and intermittent pelvic traction, J. Orthop. Sports Phys. Ther. **2**:137-141, 1981.

9 Kent, B.E.: Anatomy of the trunk, Part I, Phys. Ther. **54**:722-744, 1974.

10 Kent, B.E.: Anatomy of the trunk, Part II, Phys. Ther. **54**:850-859, 1974.

11 Mathews, J.A.: Dynamic discography: a study of lumbar traction, Ann. Phys. Med. **9**:275-279, 1968.

12 Mathews, J.A.: The effects of spinal traction, Physiotherapy **58**:64-66, 1972.

13 Nosse, L.J.: Inverted spinal traction, Arch. Phys. Med. Rehabil. **59**:367-370, 1978.

14 Qudenhoven, R.C.: Gravitational lumbar traction, Arch. Phys. Med. Rehabil. **59**:510-512, 1978.

15 O'Donoghue, D.H.: Treatment of injuries to athletes, ed. 3, Philadelphia, W.B. Saunders Co.

16 Paris, S.: Course notes, Basic course in spinal mobilization, Atlanta, Ga., 1977.

17 Reilly, J., et al.: Pelvic femoral position on vertebral separa-

tion produced by lumbar traction, Phys. Ther. **59**:282-286, 1979.

18 Roaf, R.: A study of the mechanics of spinal injuries, J. Bone Joint Surg. **42**B:810-819, 1960.

19 Saunders, H.D.: Lumbar traction, J. Orthop. Sports Phys. Ther. **1**:36-45, 1979.

20 Saunders, H.D.: Unilateral lumbar traction, Phys. Ther. **61**:221-225, 1981.

21 Saunders, H.D.: Use of spinal traction in the treatment of neck and back conditions, Clin. Orthop. **179**:31-38, 1983.

22 Stoddard, A.: Traction for cervical nerve root irritation, Physiotherapy **40**:48-49, 1954.

23 Varma, S.K., et al.: The role of traction in cervical spondylosis, Physiotherapy **59**:248-249, 1973.

Intermittent Compression Devices

11

Daniel N. Hooker

OBJECTIVES

Following completion of this chapter, the student will be able to:

- Discuss the effects of external compression on the accumulation and the reabsorption of edema following an athletic injury.
- Outline the setup procedure for intermittent external compression.
- Describe the effects that changing a parameter might have on edema reduction.
- Know when intermittent compression devices may best be used.

Edema accumulation following athletic trauma is one of the clinical signs at which considerable attention is directed in first aid and therapeutic rehabilitation programs. Edema is defined as the presence of abnormal amounts of fluid in the intercellular tissue spaces of the body. Intermittent pressure is one of the clinical modalities that is used to help reduce the accumulation of edema.

There are two distinct kinds of tissue swelling that are usually associated with athletic injuries. **Joint swelling,** marked by the presence of blood and joint fluid accumulated within the joint capsule, is one kind. This type of swelling occurs immediately following injury to a joint. Joint swelling is usually contained by the joint capsule and will have the appearance and feel of a water balloon. If pressure is placed on the swelling, the fluid moves but it immediately returns when the pressure is released.

Pitting edema is the other variety of swelling encountered in athletic injuries. This type of swelling leaves a pitlike depression when the skin is compressed. Pitting edema usually accumulates over several hours following the injury. Intermittent compression can be used with both varieties, but it is usually more successful with pitting edema.

**PHYSIOLOGIC
BASIS OF
EDEMA
ACCUMULATION
AND
MOVEMENT**

Plasma proteins, large diameter molecules, are normally contained within the vascular system. Less than 0.2% of the plasma proteins filter through the capillary walls in normal situations. Having the plasma proteins inside the vascular system helps maintain a relatively dry state in the intercellular spaces because the proteins create an imbalance in **osmotic pressure** and attract fluid to the intracapillary space (Fig. 11-1).

If plasma proteins leak into and accumulate in the intercellular spaces, more fluid would be attracted to the intercellular spaces and would alter fluid distribution, leading to excess fluid in these spaces. The lymphatic system usually removes the plasma proteins from the intercellular space, preventing this accumulation of intercellular fluid (see Fig. 11-1).

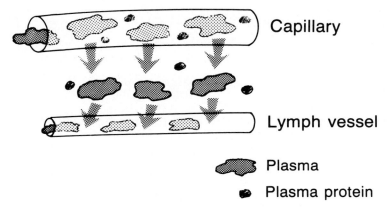

Figure 11-1. Plasma proteins outside the capillaries attract fluid to the intercellular space leading to an abnormal "wet state" in the intercellular spaces. Plasma is absorbed back into the lymphatic vessel and moves away from the injured area.

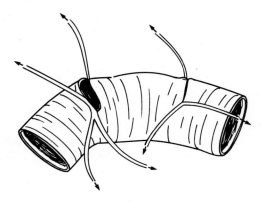

Figure 11-2. Lymphatic capillary with pore open to allow movement of plasma protein out of the intercellular space. As the intercellular fluid accumulates, the fibrils radiating from the seams in the lymphatic capillary pull the seam open to create a pore large enough for plasma proteins to enter.

The lymphatic capillaries are tubes of single layered **endothelial cells** with fibrils radiating from the junctions of the endothelial cells. These **fibrils** support the capillary and anchor them to the surrounding connective tissue (Fig. 11-2).

LYMPH AND THE LYMPHATIC SYSTEM

As fluid accumulates in the intercellular spaces it pulls on the fibrils, causing the endothelial cells in the lymphatic capillary to separate at their junctions. This separation forms a pore that allows the excess fluid and plasma proteins to enter the lymphatic capillaries from the intercellular spaces (see Fig. 11-2). This fluid and plasma protein comprise the **lymph** that is moved along the lymphatic system and reenters the blood stream. The lymphatic capillaries are the only routes available for the plasma protein to reenter the vascular system.

When a closed injury occurs capillaries are destroyed, causing the plasma proteins to be spilled into the intercellular spaces. The cells in the arterial capillary walls separate in response to hormones released by the injured tissues, and more plasma proteins escape from the vascular system and clog the intercellular spaces. This small increase in the plasma protein in the intercellular spaces causes an increase in the intercellular fluid volume by several hundred percent.

INJURY EDEMA

This fluid is trapped by the collagen fibers and proteoglycan molecules in the form of a gel. The gel prevents the free flow of fluid as seen in the joint fluid example. Clinically, this state is recognized as pitting edema. After finger pressure on the swollen part is released, a slight pit is left at the finger's previous location. Fluid seems to be squeezed out of the intercellular space and time is needed for the fluid to move slowly back into that space (Fig. 11-3).

As the intercellular fluid becomes greater, the lymph begins to flow. If the edema causes an overdistention of the lymph capillaries, the entry pores become ineffective and **lymphedema** results. Constriction of lymph capillaries or

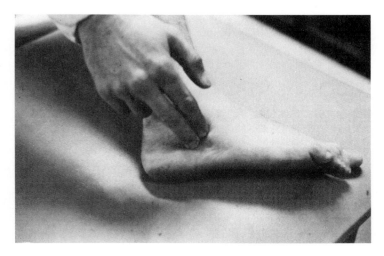

Figure 11-3. Ankle with pitting edema. Finger pressure squeezes fluid out of the intercellular space; an indentation is left when the pressure is removed.

larger lymphatic vessels from increased pressure will also discourage lymph flow and cause intercellular fluid to increase.[4]

TREATMENT OF EDEMA

Any treatment that encourages the lymph flow will decrease plasma protein content in the intercellular spaces and therefore decrease edema in the part. The standard methods of treatment in most sports therapy settings include elevation, compression, and muscular contraction[1,6,8,11,14] (Fig. 11-4).

The force of gravity can be used to augment normal lymph flow. The swollen part can be elevated so that gravity does not resist the flow of lymph but encourages its movement. Elevation of the injured swollen part above heart level is all that is necessary. The higher the elevation, the greater the effect on the lymph flow (see Fig. 11-4).

Rhythmic internal compression provided by muscle contraction will also squeeze the lymph through the lymph vessels, improving its flow back to the vascular system. This muscle contraction can be accomplished through isometric or active exercise or through electrically induced muscle contraction. When elevation is combined with muscular contraction, lymph flow is benefited.[1,6,7,14]

External pressure can also be used to increase lymph flow. Massage, elastic compression, and intermittent pressure devices are the most often used external pressure devices. This external compression not only moves the lymph along but also may spread the intercellular edema over a larger area, enabling more lymph capillaries to become involved in removing the plasma proteins and water.[1,6,8,14]

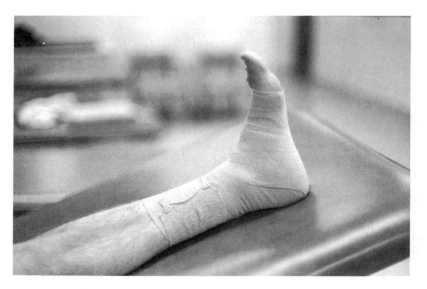

Figure 11-4. Ankle with elastic wrap compression in an elevated position.

The efficacy of using an intermittent compression device for the purpose of decreasing post acute edema has not been well documented in the literature. A recent study compared volumetric changes in post acute ankle sprains after treatment using a Jobst intermittent compression unit and elevation with the standard treatment protocol using compression with an elastic wrap and elevation. The Jobst intermittent compression device and the elastic wrap both created an increase in the volume of edema in the injured ankle following treatment. Elevation used alone without compression appeared to be superior in minimizing edema accumulation. A great need exists to pursue additional research to determine the value of compression in edema reduction in post acute injury.[9]

There are three parameters available for adjustment when using most intermittent pressure devices: inflation pressure, on-off time sequence, and total treatment time. Some very old intermittent pressure devices had a sequential pressure sleeve that could provide a distal to proximal milking action.[4] Reduction in edema does not require this milking action and most units manufactured today do not provide this action.[7]

CLINICAL PARAMETERS

None of the adjustments to parameters are backed by scientific data. Empiricism and clinical trials have been used to design the established protocols. Pressure settings have been loosely correlated with blood pressure and patient comfort to arrive at the therapeutic pressure. A pressure approximating the patient's diastolic blood pressure has been used in most treatment protocols. The arterial capillary pressures are approximately 30 mm Hg, and any pressure that exceeds this should encourage reabsorption of the edema and movement of the lymph. Maximum pressure should correspond to the systolic blood pressure. Higher pressure would shut off arterial blood flow and create a potentially uncomfortable tissue response as a result of low blood flow. Because of the difference in the size of the extremities, the pressures used in treating the lower extremities can be higher than pressures used in treating the upper extremities[3] (Fig. 11-5).

On and off time sequences are even more variable, with some protocols calling for a sequence of 1 minute on, 2 minutes off, while others reverse this to 2 minutes on, 1 minute off. Others use a 4 minutes on to 1 minute off ratio. These time periods are not research-based, and the sports therapist is left to his or her own empirical judgment as to the optimum time sequence for each patient. Patient comfort should be a primary deciding factor here.[1,3,7,10,13,15] Total treatment times have some basis in research, but again this is convenience or empirically based in many instances. Most of the protocols for primary lymphedema call for long 3- to 4-hour treatments. This time frame has been effective in many patients.

Researchers have shown a marked increase in lymph flow on initiation of massage; this flow decreases over a 10-minute period and stops when the massage is discontinued.[12,15] Clinical studies show significant gains in limb volume

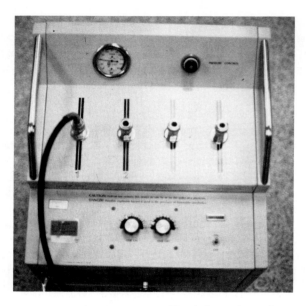

Figure 11-5. Pressure gauge and pressure control knob for an intermittent compression unit.

reduction after 30 minutes of compression.[13] In the athletic situation, a 10- to 30-minute treatment seems adequate unless the edema is overwhelming in volume or resistant to the treatment.

PATIENT SETUP AND INSTRUCTIONS

Patient setup using an intermittent compression device is relatively simple. The patient should have the appropriate-sized compression appliance fitted on the extremity in an elevated position (Fig. 11-6). The compression sleeves come as either half-leg, full-leg, full-arm, or half-arm. The deflated compression sleeve is connected to the compression unit via a rubber hose and connecting valve.

Once the machine has been turned on, three parameters may be adjusted: on/off time, inflation pressure, and treatment time. The on time should be adjusted between 60 and 120 seconds (Fig. 11-7). The off time is left at 0 until the sleeve is inflated and the treatment pressure is reached and then may be adjusted between 0 and 120 seconds (Fig. 11-8). When the unit cycles off, the patient should be instructed to move the extremity. A 60-seconds-on, 15-seconds-off setting seems to be both effective and comfortable for the patient.

The treatment should last between 20 and 30 minutes. Patients do not seem to tolerate comfortably treatments lasting longer than 30 minutes. On completion of the treatment time, the extremity should be measured to see if the desired results have been achieved. If the edema is reduced, the part should be wrapped with elastic compression wraps to help maintain the reduction. If the edema is not reduced, another treatment may be needed after a short recovery time.

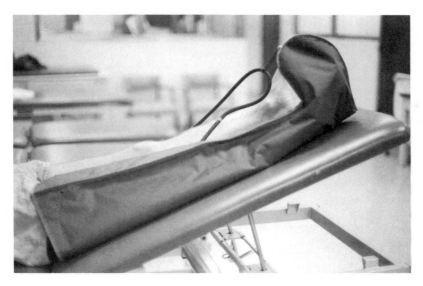

Figure 11-6. Uninflated compression appliance applied to patient's leg in an elevated position.

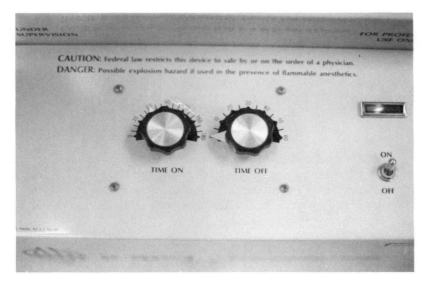

Figure 11-7. Time setting control knobs for on and off cycles of an intermittent compression unit. This illustrates the setting at the beginning of the treatment when the appliance is uninflated. The off time knob is increased when the proper inflation pressure is reached.

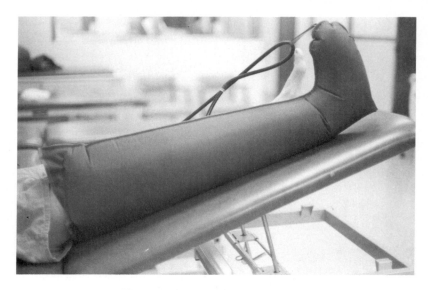

Figure 11-8. Inflated pressure sleeve.

Linear Compression Pumps

The most recent advance in compression devices is the development of the Wright Linear Pump (Fig. 11-9), a programmable gradient pneumatic pressure pump connected by three hoses to a three-celled sleeve. This design facilitates the movement of lymphedema from distal to proximal owing to a decreasing pressure gradient.[5]

The highest pressure is in the distal sleeve and, according to the manufacturer's recommendation, is determined by the mean value of systolic to diastolic pressure at the outset of a specifically determined 48-hour protocol whose purpose is to determine the effectiveness of the device in individual cases.[5] The middle cell is set at 20 mm lower than the distal cell, and the proximal cell pressure is reduced an additional 20 mm.

The length of each pressure cycle is 120 seconds. The distal cell is pressurized initially and continues pressurization for 90 seconds. Twenty seconds later the middle cell is inflated, and after another 20 seconds the proximal cell inflates. A final 30-second period allows pressure in all three cells to return to 0 after which the cycle repeats itself. Only a few studies have shown the efficacy of using decreasing pressure in a distal to proximal direction relative to previously existing compression sleeves.[4,5]

COLD AND COMPRESSION COMBINATION

Some manufacturers have coupled intermittent pressure with a coolant (either water or Freon). These devices have the advantage of cooling the injured part as well as compressing it. The Jobst Cryotemp is a controlled cold/compression unit that has a temperature adjustment ranging between 10° to 25°C. Cooling is accomplished by circulating cold water through the sleeve.

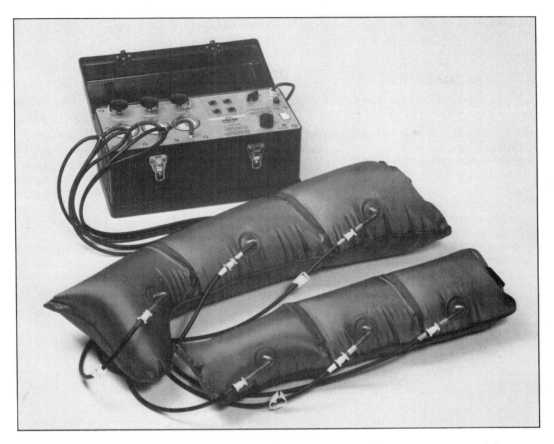

Figure 11-9. The Wright Linear Pump is a programmable gradient pressure sequential compression system.

The combination of cold and compression has been shown to be clinically effective in treating some conditions.[6,8] A study comparing a technique using an intermittent compression unit, cold, and elevation with one using an elastic wrap, cold, and elevation showed that the use of the compression device was more effective in edema reduction.[8]

Intermittent compression may also be used in conjunction with a low-frequency pulsed or surging electrical stimulating current setup to produce muscle pumping contractions.[2] The combination of these two modalities should facilitate resorption of injury byproducts by the lymphatic system (Fig. 11-10).

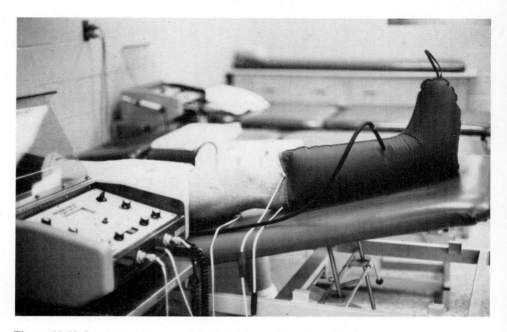

Figure 11-10. Intermittent compression used in combination with electrical stimulating currents to reduce edema.

SUMMARY

1. Edema following injury or surgery can be effectively managed using a compression pump program.
2. This treatment along with external elastic supports, elevation, and exercise will help reverse the edema and prevent its reaccumulation.
3. Treatment parameters are based on clinical studies rather than on research.

GLOSSARY

endothelial cells Cells that line the cavities of the vessels.

fibrils Connective tissue fibers supporting the lymphatic capillaries.

joint swelling Accumulation of fluid within the joint capsule.

lymph A transparent, slightly yellow liquid found in the lymphatic vessels.

lymphedema Swelling of subcutaneous tissues as a result of accumulation of excessive lymph fluid.

osmotic pressure The pressure that is necessary for movement of a solvent across a membrane that is permeable to that solvent.

pitting edema A type of swelling that leaves a pitlike depression on the skin when it is compressed.

REFERENCES

1 Brown, S.: Ankle edema and galvanic muscle stimulation, Phys. Sports Med. **9:** 137, 1981.

2 Elkins, E.C., Herrick, J.F., Grindley, J.H., et al.: Effect of various procedures on the flow of lymph, Arch. Phys. Med. Rehabil. **34:** 31-39, 1953.

3 Intermittent venous pressure devices, Class handout, Dou-

ley, P., West Chester State College, West Chester, Penn., 1971.

4 Kim-Sing, C., and Basco, V.: Postmastectomy lymphedema treated with the Wright Linear pump, Can. J. Surg. **30**(5):368-370, 1987.

5 Klein, M., Alexander, M., Wright, J., Redmond, C., and Le-Gasse, A.: Treatment of lower extremity lymphedema with the Wright Linear Pump: a statistical analysis of a clinical trial, Arch. Phys. Med. Rehabil. **69**: 202-206, 1988.

6 Kolb, P., and Denegar, C.: Traumatic edema and the lymphatic system, Athl. Train., Winter, **18**: 339-341, 1983.

7 Kruse, R., Kruse, A., and Britton, R.C.: Physical therapy for the patient with peripheral edema: procedures for management, Phys. Ther. Rev. **80**: 29-33, 1960.

8 Quillen, W.S., and Rouiller, L.: Initial management of acute ankle sprains with rapid pulsed pneumatic compression and cold, J. Orthop. Sports Phys. Ther. **4**: 39-43, 1982.

9 Rucinski, T.: The effects of intermittent compression on edema in post acute ankle sprains, Unpublished Master's thesis, University of North Carolina, 1989.

10 Sanderson, R., and Fletcher, W.: Conservative management of primary lymphedema, Northwest Med. **64**: 584-588, 1965.

11 Starkey, J.: Treatment of ankle sprains by simultaneous use of intermittent compression and ice packs, Am. J. Sports Med. **4**: 142-144, 1976.

12 Stillwell, G., et al.: Further studies on the treatment of lymphedema, Arch. Phys. Med. Rehabil. **38**: 435-441, 1957.

13 Wakim, K.G., et al.: Influence of centripetal rhythmic compression on localized edema of an extremity, Arch. Phys. Med. Rehabil. **36**: 98-103, 1955.

14 Wilkerson, J.: Contrast baths and pressure treatment for ankle sprains, Phys. Sports Med. **7**: 143, 1979.

15 Winsor, T., and Selle, W.: The effect of venous compression on the circulation of the extremities, Arch. Phys. Med. Rehabil. **34**: 559-565, 1953.

Massage

12

Clairbeth Lehn

OBJECTIVES

Following completion of this chapter, the student will be able to:

- Understand the effects of massage and the specific results of the procedures on the tissue and the muscular system of the body.

- Know and understand the signs of effective progress with the treatment, as well as recognize the dangers and know when to discontinue the procedures.

- Demonstrate knowledge and skills gained by application of massage techniques.

- Design a specific routine, selecting specific moves and strokes that are consistent with the goals set for the patient by the prescribing physician, and evaluate the results.

The earliest available medical records seem to indicate that massage has played an important role in the treatment of sick and injured people. A natural reaction when a part of the body hurts is to rub the injured area with a hand.

In early writings pertaining to medical treatments little difference is shown between massage, as we know it, and general exercise of the body. In fact, although there are very detailed descriptions of techniques, one has a great deal of difficulty in making a determination as to exactly what is meant because the terminology is unfamiliar. Language changes with time.

In Europe during the Middle Ages the influence of the Church of Rome and its religious teachings discouraged the use of massage as a healing practice. This brought the art to somewhat of a halt until enlightened individuals strove to bring medical knowledge into the forefront and scholars in the medical fields started to again delve into how and why the body functions as it does.

The word *massage* is derived from two sources. One is the Arabic verb *mass,* to touch, and the other is the Greek word *massein,* to knead. However, history shows that this was not an art exclusive to the Greeks and Arabs. The general knowledge of massage was also known and practiced by the Egyptians, Romans, Japanese, Persians, and Chinese.

In Sweden in the early part of the nineteenth century, Peter H. Ling (1776 to 1839), the acknowledged founder of curative gymnastics, used massage as a branch of gymnastics. He appears to be the founder of modern day massage techniques with some incorporation of French massage techniques into his system.[9]

Massage techniques have changed dramatically in the past 50 years. They are based on the research and teachings of Albert Hoffa (1859 to 1907), James B. Mennell (1880 to 1957), and Gertrude Beard (1887 to 1971). Medical practitioners of the twentieth century have added a scientific basis to massage along with additional techniques and terms. In modern day preventative and rehabilitative therapy, massage has earned a paramount place of honor.

PHYSIOLOGIC EFFECTS

Massage is a mechanical stimulation of the tissues by means of rhythmically applied pressure and stretching. The pressure compresses the soft tissues and distorts the nerve-ending networks of receptors. Stretching applies tension to soft tissues and it also distorts the nerve-ending plexuses of the receptors. The use of these two forces can, by changing the lumen of blood vessels and lymph vessel spaces, affect capillary, venous, arterial, and lymphatic circulation. We can demonstrate axon reflex. We can stimulate exteroceptors, both superficial and deep, in the skin; proprioceptors in the muscles—tendons; and interoceptors in the deep tissues of the body. We can loosen mucus and promote drainage of excess fluids from the lungs.[24]

How this is accomplished is determined by the massage techniques used and how they are applied. These effects probably result from physical, physiologic, and psychologic factors.

There are two mechanisms by which an effect ultimately occurs. The first mechanism is a reflex mechanism. If hands are passed lightly over the skin, a series of responses occur as a result of the sensory stimulus picked up by the proprioceptors. This reflex mechanism is believed to be an autonomic nervous system phenomenon. The reflex stimulus can occur alone (i.e., unaccompanied by the mechanical mechanism). Mennell[17] calls this the "reflex effect." In itself, it is not an effect but the cause of an effect (i.e., causes sedation, relieves tension, increases blood flow).

The second mechanism is mechanical in nature. When pressure of the massage is increased, a mechanical response occurs, namely, the pressure over the area actually forces blood and lymph to move into an "unpressured" area. As the mechanical stimulus becomes more effective, the reflex stimulus becomes less effective. The mechanical stimulus is always accompanied by some reflex stimulus. Deep veins, as well as superficial veins, are influenced by mechanical pressure. Mennell calls this the "mechanical mechanism." Again, pressure causes the effect, but it is not the effect itself.

The effect of massage on pain is probably regulated by both the gate control theory and the effect of neurotransmitters (see Chapter 1). With the gate theory of pain control, the massage may be causing presynaptic inhibition; with the neurotransmitters, endorphins may be stopping the release of a substance that is a pain transmitter.

Direct Effects

The effect of massage on the circulation of the blood, according to Pemberton,[18] takes place through a reflex influence on blood vessels from a sympathetic division in the nervous system. He believes that vessels in the muscular system are emptied during massage not only by being squeezed but also by this reflex action. Very light massage (**effleurage**) produces an almost instantaneous reaction through transient dilation of lymphatics and small capillaries. Heavier pressure brings about a more lasting dilation. Actual rate of flow remains the same. There is an increased number of red and white corpuscles in the blood and also an increased blood platelet count.

In the lymphatic system, movement of fluid depends on forces outside of the system. Such factors as gravity, muscle contraction, movement, and massage can affect the flow of lymph. When administering massage to an edematous part, elevation will also help to increase lymph flow.

The effect of massage on the nervous system will differ greatly according to the method employed, pressure exerted, and the duration of applications. Through the reflex mechanism, sedation is induced. Slow, gentle, rhythmical, and superficial effleurage may relieve tension and soothe, rendering the muscles more relaxed. This indicates an effect on sensory and motor nerves locally and some central nervous system response. The mechanical mechanism effect is stimulation. Faster and deeper massage—**pertrissage, friction,** and perhaps **tapotement**—may cause a feeling of well-being and a desire for activity.

The basic effect of massage on muscle tissue is to "maintain the muscle in the best possible state of nutrition, flexibility, and vitality so that after recovery from trauma or disease the muscle can function at its maximum."[24] Massage metabolically augments a chemical balance. The increased circulation means increased dispersion of waste products and an increase of fresh blood and oxygen. The mechanical movements assist in the removal and hasten the resynthesis of lactic acid. Massage does not increase strength, bulk, or muscle, nor does it increase muscle tone. There may be, however, a stretching of the intramuscular connective tissue mechanically.

Effects of massage on the skin include an increase in skin temperature, possibly as a result of direct mechanical effects, and indirect vasomotor action. It has also been found that increased sweating and decreased skin resistance to galvanic current resulted from massage.[2]

If skin becomes adherent to underlying tissues and scar tissue is formed, friction massage can usually be used to mechanically loosen the adhesions and to soften the scar. Massage toughens yet softens the skin. It acts directly on the surface of the skin to remove dead cells that result from prolonged casting of 6 to 8 weeks.

Massage does not alter general metabolism appreciably.[18] There is no change in acid-base equilibrium of blood. Massage does increase oxygen consumption and therefore will increase carbon dioxide production.

The effect of massage on scar tissue is that it stretches and breaks down the fibrous tissue. It can break down adhesions between skin and subcutaneous tissue and stretch contracted or adhered tissue.

Psychologic effects of massage can be as beneficial to some patients as the physiologic effects. The "hands on" effect helps patients feel as if someone is helping them. A general sedative effect can be most beneficial for the patient.

The major goal of massage is to assist in supporting the patient during the healing process. Physical changes that may be seen, felt, or reported by the patient are signs to which one has to pay close attention when giving a massage:

1. Relaxation is definitely desirable. The muscles will actually feel more pliable. The patient may appear lethargic; the facial expression or extremity position indicates a release of muscular tension.

2. The patient's skin becomes warm to the touch. Superficial tissue may take on a pink to red color. This depends on the amount of pressure and the pathology involved.

3. Relief of pain will be reported by the patient provided the treatment has been therapeutically valuable. Increased pain indicates that a change in treatment is in order. An interruption of the pain sensation cycle is quite possible following massage.

4. The sports therapist's approach should inspire a feeling of confidence in the patient, and the patient should respond with a feeling of well-being—a feeling of being helped.

PRINCIPLES OF TECHNIQUE

The sports therapist must have the basic essential knowledge of anatomy and of the particular area being treated. The physiology of the area to be treated and the total function of the patient must be considered. There should be an understanding of the existing pathology so that the process by which repair occurs is known. The sports therapist needs a thorough knowledge of massage principles and skillful techniques, as well as manual dexterity, coordination, and concentration in the use of massage techniques. The sports therapist also needs to exhibit such traits as patience, a sense of caring for the patient's welfare, and courteousness both in speech and manner.

The most important area that must be considered is the hands of the clinician. They must be clean, warm, dry, and soft. The nails must be short and smooth. Washing of the hands before and after treatment must take place for sanitary reasons. If the sports therapist's hands are cold, they should be placed in warm water for a short period. Rubbing them together briskly helps to warm them too.

Positioning is also important for the clinician. Correct positioning will allow relaxation, prevent fatigue, and permit free movement of arms, hands, and the body. Good posture will also help prevent fatigue and backache. The weight should rest evenly on both feet with the body in good postural align-

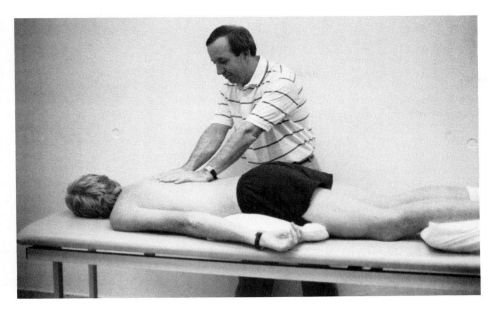

Figure 12-1. Position of sports therapist for stroking.

ment. When massaging a large area, the weight should shift from one foot to the other. You must be able to fit your hands to the contour of the area being treated. A good position is required to allow the correct application of pressure and rhythmic strokes during the procedure (Fig. 12-1).

EQUIPMENT

TABLE. A firm table, easily accessible from both sides, is most desirable. The height of the table should be reasonably comfortable for the sports therapist; leaning over or reaching up to perform the required movements should not be necessary. An adjustable table is almost a must in this situation. To facilitate cleaning and disinfecting, a washable plastic surface is much preferred. There should be a storage area close by for linens and lubricant. If the table is not padded, a mattress or foam pad should be used for the comfort of the patient.

LINENS AND PILLOWS. The patient should be draped with a sheet, so only that part to be massaged is uncovered (Fig. 12-2). Towels should be handy for removing the lubricant. A cotton sheet between the plastic surface of the table and the patient is required to absorb perspiration and for patient comfort. The surface of the plastic material is generally too cool for comfort. Pillows should be available to support the patient.

LUBRICANT. Some kind of lubricant should be used in almost all massage movements to overcome friction and avoid irritations by ensuring smooth contact of hands and skin. If the patient's skin is too oily, it may be desirable to wash the skin first.

The lubricant should be of a type that is absorbed slightly by the skin but

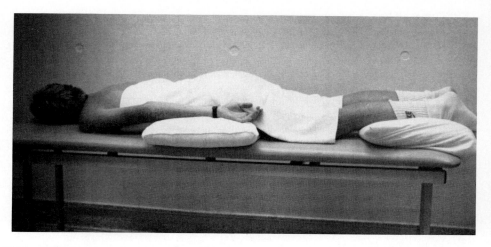

Figure 12-2. Draping of prone patient. Towels are used for removal of lubricant; sheets are used for draping. Pillows are placed under hips and ankles for patient comfort.

does not make it so slippery that the clinician finds it difficult to perform the required strokes. A light oil is recommended for lubrication. One that works well is a combination of one part beeswax to three parts coconut oil. These ingredients should be melted together and allowed to cool (Fig. 12-3). It is best to use oil in situations in which (1) the clinician's or patient's skin is too dry, (2) a cast has recently been removed, (3) scar tissue is present, (4) there is excess hair. Some types of oil that may be used are olive oil, mineral oil, cocoa butter, or hydrolanolin. The "warm creams" or analgesic creams are skin irritants and if used in conjunction with massage may cause a burn, depending on the skin type of the patient. These are also thought to cause blood to come to the surface of the skin, moving away from the muscles, which is exactly the opposite of what we are trying to accomplish through the massage techniques.

Alcohol may be used to remove the lubricant after massage. It is suggested that alcohol be placed in the clinician's hands before application to avoid the dramatic temperature drop that occurs when alcohol is applied directly to the patient.

Sometimes unscented powder should be used if the clinician's hands tend to perspire, or it may be used to prevent skin irritation.

Lubricant is not desired, nor should it be used, when applying friction movements since a firm contact between the skin and hands of clinician must take place.

PREPARATION OF THE PATIENT. The position of the patient is probably the most important aspect of ensuring a beneficial relaxation of the muscles from massage. The patient should be in a relaxed, comfortable position. Lying down, when possible, is most beneficial to the patient, and this also permits gravity to assist in the venous flow of the blood.

The part involved in the treatment must be adequately supported. It may

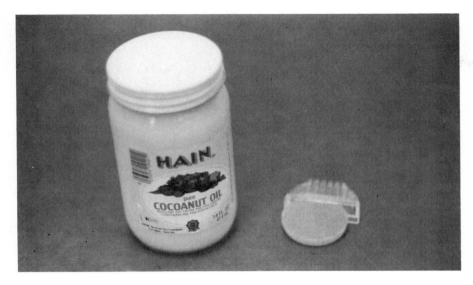

Figure 12-3. Example of lubricant to be used, beeswax and coconut oil.

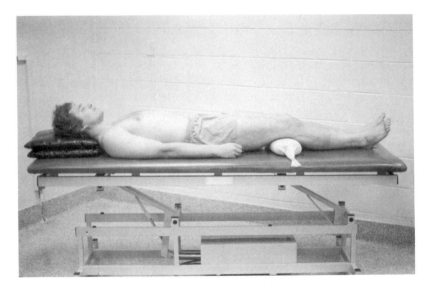

Figure 12-4. Patient supine with pillow under head and knees.

be elevated, depending on the pathology. When the patient is being treated in the prone position, for massage of the neck, shoulders, back, buttocks, or back of the legs, a pillow or a roll should be placed under the abdomen. Another pillow should be placed under the ankles so that the knees are slightly flexed (see Fig. 12-2). If the patient is in the supine position, small pillows should be placed under the head and under the knees (Fig. 12-4).

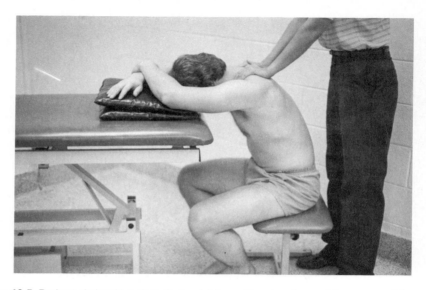

Figure 12-5. Patient sitting in a chair facing table and leaning forward is supported by pillows on the table with forearms and hands on the table for support. Sports therapist stands behind the patient.

Sometimes the prone position will be too painful for a patient to assume for massaging a shoulder, upper back, or neck. A position that may be more comfortable is sitting in a chair, facing the table, while leaning forward and supported by pillows on the table. Forearms and hands are on the table for additional support (Fig. 12-5). The sports therapist can administer the massage while standing behind the patient (Fig. 12-5).

The body areas not being treated should be covered to prevent the patient from being chilled (see Fig. 12-2). Clothing should be removed from the part being treated. Towels should cover any clothes near the area being treated to protect them from the lubricant (see Fig. 12-2).

APPLICATION   These points are important to consider when administering massage:

1. Pressure regulation should be determined by the type and amount of tissue present. It must also be governed by the patient's condition and which tissues are to be affected. The pressure must be delivered from the body, through the soft parts of the hands, and it is adjusted to contours of the patient's body parts.
2. Rhythm must be steady and even. The time for each stroke and time between successive strokes should be equal.
3. Duration depends on the pathology, size of the area being treated, speed of motion, age, size, and condition of the patient. One also should observe the response of the patient to determine duration of the procedure. Massage of the back or the neck area might take 15 to

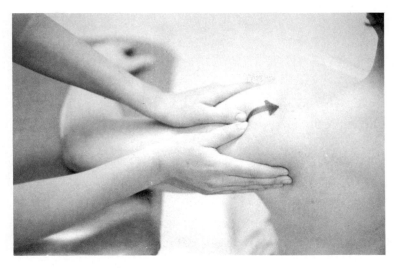

Figure 12-6. Forces should be applied in the direction of muscle fibers in the application of massage.

    30 minutes. Massage of a large joint (such as a hip or shoulder) may require less than 10 minutes.

4. If swelling is present in an extremity, treatment should begin with the proximal part. The purpose of this is to help facilitate the lymphatic flow proximally. The subsequent effects of distal massage in removing fluid or edema will be more efficient since the proximal resistance to lymphatic flow will be reduced. This technique has been referred to as the "uncorking effect."

5. Massage should never be painful, except possibly for friction massage, nor should it be given with such force that it causes ecchymosis (discoloration of the skin resulting from contusion).

6. In general, the direction of forces should be applied in the direction of the muscle fibers (Fig. 12-6).

7. During a session, one should begin and end with effleurage. The maneuvers should increase progressively to the greatest energy possible and end by decreasing energy maneuvers.

8. The sports therapist must consider the position in which massage can best be given and be sure the patient is warm and in a comfortable, relaxed position.

9. The body part may be elevated if this is necessary and possible (Fig. 12-7).

10. The sports therapist should be in a position in which the whole body, as well as hands and arms, can be relaxed and the procedure accomplished without strain (see Fig. 12-1).

11. Sufficient lubricant should be used so that the therapist's hands will

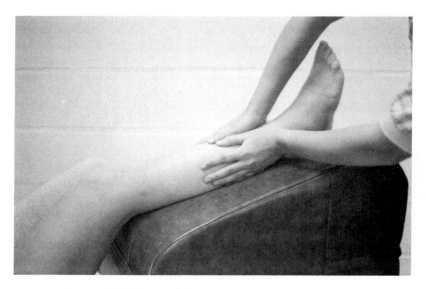

Figure 12-7. The part being massaged should be elevated.

move smoothly along the skin surface (except in friction). The use of too much lubricant should be guarded against.

12. Massage should begin with superficial stroking; this stroke is used to spread the lubricant over the part being treated.

13. Each stroke should start at the joint or just below the joint (unless massage over joints is contraindicated) and finish above the joint so that strokes will overlap.

14. The pressure should be in line with venous flow followed by a return stroke without pressure. The pressure should be in the centripetal direction (Fig. 12-8).

15. Care should be used over body areas. Hands should be relaxed and pressure adjusted to fit the contour of the area being treated.

16. Bony prominences and painful joints should be avoided if possible.

17. All strokes should be rhythmic. The pressure strokes should end with a swing off, in a small half circle, in order that the rhythm will not be broken by an abrupt reversal.

STROKES

EFFLEURAGE. This massage maneuver glides over the skin lightly without attempting to move the deep muscle masses. The main physiologic effect occurs when stroking is begun at the peripheral areas and moves toward the heart. The return flow of the venous and lymphatic systems is probably helped by this process. Circulation to the skin surface is also increased by stroking; the success is traced to the increased rate of metabolic exchange in the peripheral areas.

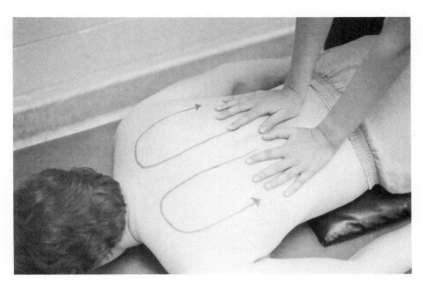

Figure 12-8. Massage pressure should be in line of venous flow followed by a return stroke without pressure.

The primary purpose of effleurage is to accustom the patient to the physical contact of the clinician. Initially effleurage serves to evenly distribute the lubricant. It also allows sensitive fingers to search for areas of muscle spasm or soreness and to locate trigger points and pressure points that can help in determining the type of procedures to be used during the massage.

At the start of the massage, the stroke should be performed with a light pressure, coming from the flat of the hand with fingers slightly bent and thumbs spread (Fig. 12-9). Once the unidirectional flow is established, going either centripetally or centrifugally, it should be continued throughout the treatment. Movement of the stroke should be toward the heart, and contact should be maintained with the patient at all times to enhance relaxation (Fig. 12-10).

Deep stroking massage is also a form of effleurage, except it is given with more pressure to produce a mechanical effect, as well as a reflex effect (Fig. 12-11).

Every massage begins and ends with effleurage. Stroking should also be used between other techniques. Stroking relaxes, decreases the defensive tension against harder massage techniques, and has a generally mentally soothing effect.

PETRISSAGE. Petrissage consists of kneading manipulations that press and roll the muscles under the fingers or hands. There is no gliding over the skin except between progressions from one area to another. The muscles are gently squeezed, lifted, and relaxed. The hands may remain stationary or may travel slowly along the length of the muscle or limb.

The purpose of petrissage is to increase venous and lymphatic return and
Text continued on p. 270.

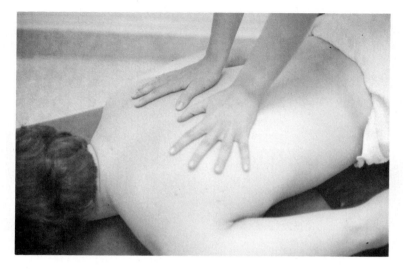

Figure 12-9. The stroke is performed with the heel of the hand, fingers slightly bent and thumbs spread.

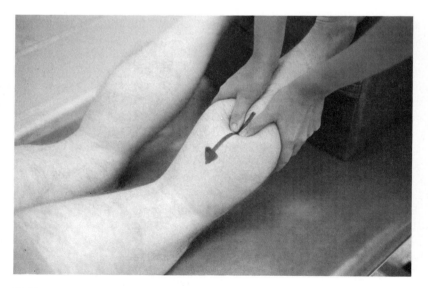

Figure 12-10. The kneading stroke is directed toward the heart and contact should be maintained with the patient.

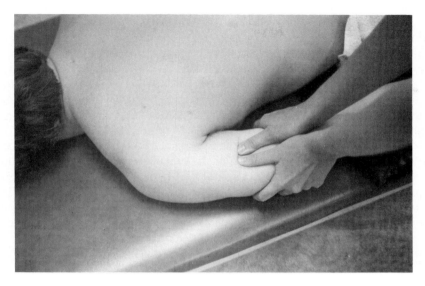

Figure 12-11. Deep stroking massage.

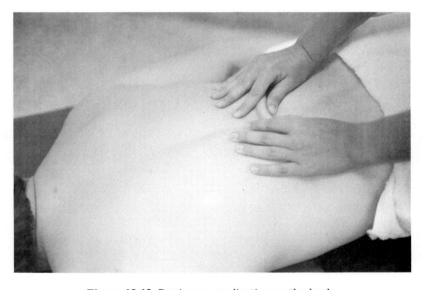

Figure 12-12. Petrissage application on the back.

to press metabolic waste products out of affected areas through intensive, vigorous action. This form of massage can also break up adhesions between the skin and underlying tissue, loosen adherent fibrous tissue, and increase elasticity of the skin.

Petrissage can be described as a kneading technique. It is the repeated grasping, application of pressure, releasing in a lifting or rolling motion, then moving an adjacent area (Fig. 12-12). Smaller muscles may be kneaded with one hand (Fig. 12-13). Larger muscles, such as the hamstrings or muscle groups, will require the use of both hands (Fig. 12-14). When kneading, the hands should move from the distal to the proximal point of the muscle insertion grasping parallel to or at right angles to the muscle fibers (see Fig. 12-10).

FRICTION. James Cyriax and Gillean Russell[6] have used a technique called deep-friction massage to affect musculoskeletal structures of ligament, tendon, and muscle to provide therapeutic movement over a small area. The purposes for friction movements are to loosen adherent fibrous tissue (scar), aid in the absorption of local edema or effusions, and reduce local muscular spasm. Inflammation around joints is softened and more readily broken down so that the formation of adhesions is prevented. Another purpose is to provide deep pressure over trigger points to produce reflex effects. This technique is performed by the tips of the fingers, the thumb, or the heel of the hand, according to the area to be covered, making small circular movements (Fig. 12-15). The superficial tissues are moved over the underlying structures by keeping the hand or fingers in firm contact with the skin (Fig. 12-16).

Transverse friction massage is a technique for treating chronic tendon in-

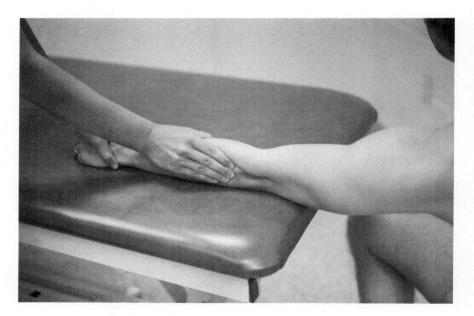

Figure 12-13. Petrissage kneading with one hand.

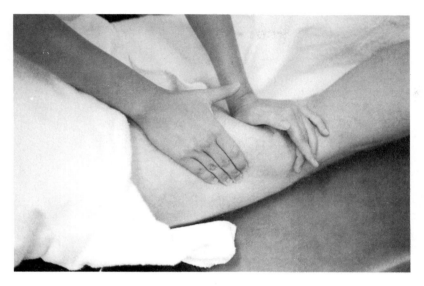

Figure 12-14. Petrissage kneading with both hands.

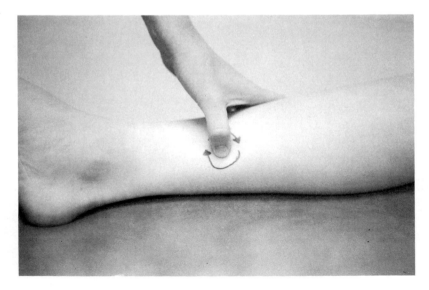

Figure 12-15. Thumb movement in a circle on acupressure point.

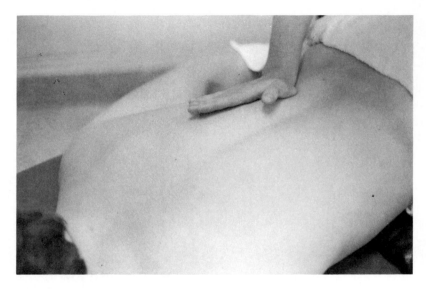

Figure 12-16. Superficial friction applied to the back by using the heel of the hand.

flammations.[6] Inflammation is an important part of the healing process. It must occur before the healing process can advance to the fibroblastic stage. In chronic inflammations, however, the inflammatory process "gets stuck" and never really accomplishes what it is supposed to. The purpose of transverse friction massage is to try and increase the inflammation to a point where the inflammatory process is complete and the injury can progress to the later stages of the healing process. This technique is used most often in chronic overuse problems such as lateral humeral epicondylitis, "jumper's knee," and rotator cuff tendinitis.

The technique involves placing the tendon on a slight stretch. Massage is done using the thumb or index finger to exert intense pressure in a direction perpendicular to the direction of the fibers being massaged (Fig. 12-17). The massage should last for 7 to 10 minutes and should be done every other day. Since transverse friction massage is a painful technique, it may help to apply ice to the treatment area prior to massage for analgesic purposes.

PERCUSSION OR TAPOTEMENT. Percussion movements are a series of brisk blows, administered with relaxed hands and following each other in rapid alternating movements. This technique has a penetrating effect that is used to stimulate subcutaneous structures. Percussion is often used to increase circulation or to get a more active flow of blood. Peripheral nerve endings are stimulated so that they convey impulses more strongly with the use of percussion techniques.

Types of percussion techniques are hacking—alternate striking of patient with the ulnar border of the hand (Fig. 12-18); slapping—alternate slapping with fingers (Fig. 12-19); beating—half-closed fist using the hypothenar eminence of the hand (Fig. 12-20); tapping with the tips of the fingers (Fig. 12-21);

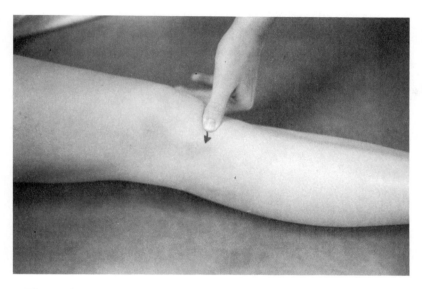

Figure 12-17. Transverse tendon friction massage on the patellar tendon.

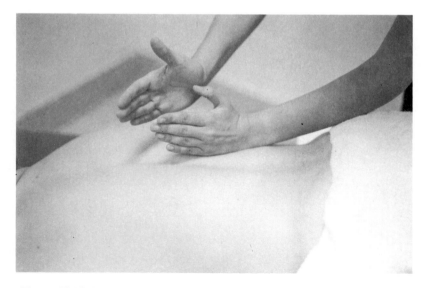

Figure 12-18. Percussion stroke of striking with the ulnar border of the hand.

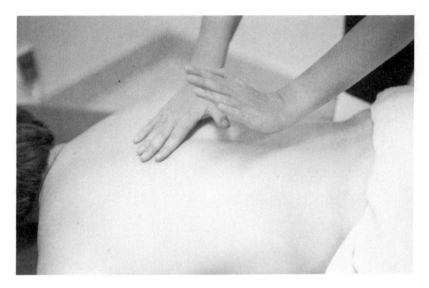

Figure 12-19. Percussion stroke of slapping with fingers.

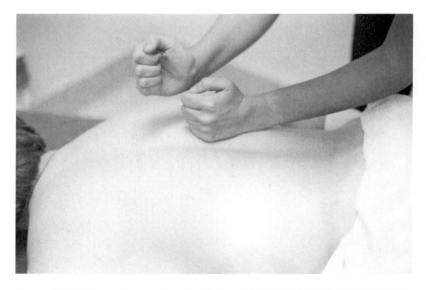

Figure 12-20. Percussion stroke of half-closed fist using hypothenar eminence.

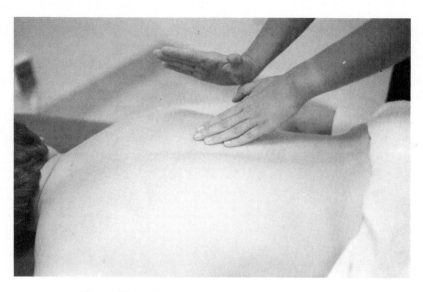

Figure 12-21. Percussion stroke using tips of fingers.

and clapping or cupping using fingers, thumb, and palm together to form a concave surface (Fig. 12-22). Clapping or cupping is used primarily in postural drainage.

VIBRATION. Vibration technique is a fine tremulous movement, made by the hand or fingers placed firmly against a part; this causes the part to vibrate. The hands should remain in contact with the patient and a rhythmical trembling movement will come from the whole forearm, through the elbow (Fig. 12-23).

ROUTINE. An example of a massage progression or routine would be:
1. Superficial stroking
2. Deep stroking
3. Kneading
4. Optional friction or tapotement
5. Deep stroking
6. Superficial stroking

The various individual classic massage techniques alone, however, do not make for a good massage. A proper program, intensity, tempo, and rhythm, as well as the proper starting, climax, and closing of the massage, are all important too. The form of the massage depends on the individual requirements of the patient.

INDICATIONS

The areas of treatment that we will most often see patients for are muscle, tendon, and joint conditions. Adhesions, muscle spasm, myositis, bursitis, fibrositis, tendinitis or tenosynovitis, and postural strain of the back all generally fall into this category.

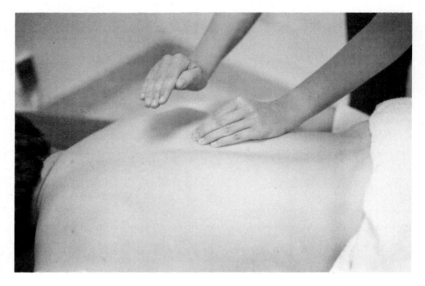

Figure 12-22. Percussion stroke of cupping using fingers, thumb, and palm together.

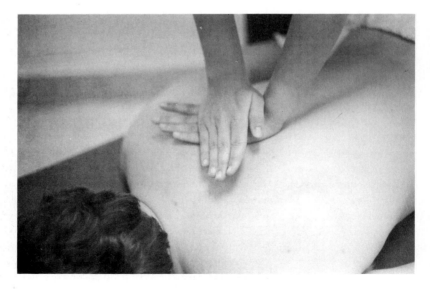

Figure 12-23. Vibration stroke.

Areas of concern that indicate that you should not treat a patient with massage include arteriosclerosis, thrombosis or embolism, severe varicose veins, acute phlebitis, cellulitis, synovitis, abscesses, skin injections, and cancers. Acute inflammatory conditions of the skin, soft tissues, or joints are also contraindications.

CONTRAINDICA-TIONS

Acupressure is a type of massage based on the ancient Chinese art of acupuncture. Acupuncture, along with herbal medicine, composes traditional Chinese medicine. Only recently has the amount of research, publication, and interest in acupuncture in Western medical literature increased dramatically.

ACUPRESSURE AND ACUPUNCTURE

The Chinese make no distinction between arteries, veins, or nerves when explaining the functions of the body.[15] They concentrate instead on an elaborate system of forces whose interplay is thought to regulate all bodily functions. The traditional, philosophical Chinese explanation has little correlation with the more scientifically oriented Western concepts of medicine, which rely heavily on anatomic and physiologic principles. Consequently, utilization of acupuncture as a therapeutic technique in Western medical practice has encountered considerable skepticism.

The Chinese believe that an essential life force known as *Chi* exists in everyone and controls all aspects of life. Chi is governed by the interplay of two opposing forces, the *yang* (positive) forces and the *yin* (negative) forces. Disease and pain result from some imbalance between the two.[14] The yin and yang flow through passageways or lines within the body called *jing* by the Chinese and known as meridians in the west. The twelve meridians within the body are named according to the part of the body with which they are associated. The meridians on one side of the body are duplicated by those on the other; however, two additional meridians exist that cannot be paired.[15]

1. Lung (L)
2. Large Intestine (LI)
3. Stomach (ST)
4. Spleen (SP)
5. Heart (H)
6. Small intestine (SI)
  *Not paired.

7. Urinary bladder (UB)
8. Kidney (K)
9. Pericardium (P)
10. Triple warmet (TW)
11. Gall bladder (GB)
12. Liver (LIV)
13. Governing Vessel (GV)*
14. Conception Vessel (CV)*

Along these meridians lie the acupuncture points that are associated with each particular meridian. These points are named according to the meridian on which they lie. Whenever there is pain or illness, certain points on the surface of the body become tender.[15] When pain is eliminated or the disease is cured, these tender points seem to disappear.[15] According to acupuncture theory, stimulation of specific points through needling can dramatically reduce pain in areas of the body known to be associated with a particular point. Thousands of acupuncture points have been identified by the Chinese. In the Nei Ching,[10] a classical text on Chinese medicine, 365 points that lie on the meridians have been enumerated. Additional acupuncture points have been identified on the auricle as well as the hand.

There is some evidence for the actual physical existence of these points.[23] The electrical resistance of the skin at certain points corresponding to the acupuncture points is lower than that of the surrounding skin, especially when a disease state is present. Examining acupuncture points by sectioning indicated increased nerve endings at these points. Russian investigators have reportedly discovered differences in skin temperature at these points. Despite this evidence, there is no definite physical attribute of all acupuncture points nor is there a thoroughly demonstrated mode of action for the technique. Whatever the explanation, it appears that the locations and effects of stimulating specific acupuncture points for the relief of pain were determined empirically.[16]

In Western medicine, the counterpart of the acupuncture point is the trigger point. Trigger points, like acupuncture points, are associated with visceral structures; stimulation of these points has also been demonstrated to result in a relief of pain.[8]

Acupuncture and trigger points are not necessarily one and the same. However, a study by Melzack, Fox, and Stillwell[16] attempted to develop a correlation coefficient between acupuncture and trigger points on the basis of two criteria: spatial distribution and associated pain patterns. They found a remarkably high correlation coefficient of .84, which suggested that acupuncture and trigger points used for pain relief, although discovered independently, labeled by totally different methods, and derived from such historically different concepts of medicine, represent a similar phenomenon and may be explained by the same underlying neural mechanisms.[16]

Physiologic explanations of the effectiveness of acupressure massage may likely be attributed to some interaction of the various mechanisms of pain modulation discussed in Chapter 1. There is considerable evidence that intense, low-frequency stimulation of these points triggers the release of β-endorphin.[19,20,21]

Acupressure Massage Techniques

By using acupuncture charts (Fig. 12-24) specific points are selected, which are described in the literature as having some relationship to the area of pain. The charts provide the sports therapist with a general idea of where these points are located. Two techniques may be used to specifically locate acupressure points. Since it is known that electrical impedance is reduced at acupuncture points, an ohmmeter may be used to locate the points. Perhaps the easiest technique is simply to palpate the area until either a small fibrous nodule or a strip of tense muscle tissue that is tender to the touch is felt.[3,4,5]

Once the point is located, massage is begun using the index or middle fingers, the thumb, or perhaps the elbow. Small friction-like circular motions are used on the point. The amount of pressure applied to these acupressure points should be determined by patient tolerance; however, it must be intense and will likely be painful to the patient. Generally, the more pressure the patient can tolerate, the more effective the treatment.

Text continued on p. 282.

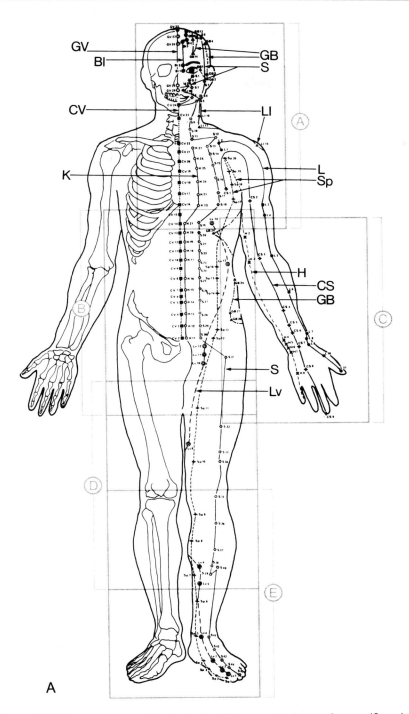

Figure 12-24. Acupuncture point charts should be used to locate the specific points.

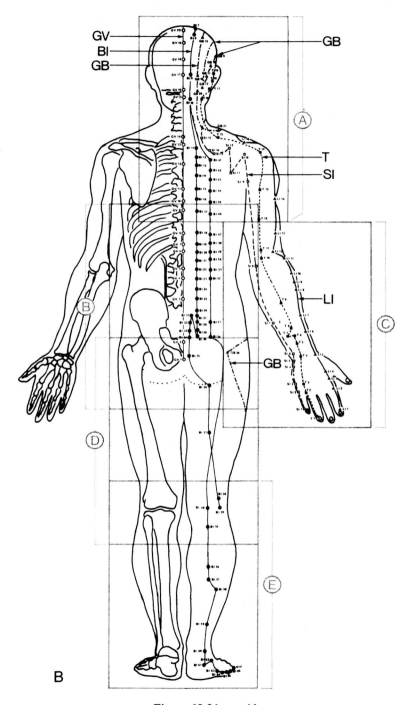

B

Figure 12-24, cont'd.

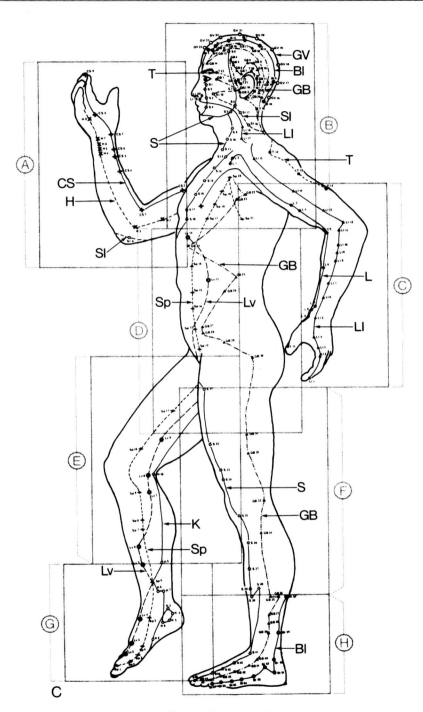

Figure 12-24, cont'd.

Effective treatment times range from 1 to 5 minutes at a single point per treatment. It may be necessary to massage several points during the treatment to obtain the greatest effects. If this is the case, it is best to work distal points first and to move proximally.

During the massage, the patient will report a dulling or numbing effect and will frequently indicate that the pain diminishes or subsides totally during the massage. The lingering effects of acupressure massage vary tremendously from patient to patient. The effects may last for only a few minutes in some but may persist in others for several hours.

CONNECTIVE TISSUE MASSAGE: BINDEGEWEBS-MASSAGE

Connective tissue massage (**Bindegewebsmassage**) was developed by Elizabeth Dicke, a German physical therapist who suffered from decreased circulation in her right lower extremity for which amputation was advised. In trying to relieve her lower back pain, she massaged the area with pulling strokes. She found that with the continued stroking there was a relaxation of the muscular tension and a prickling warmth in the area. She continued the technique on herself, and after 3 months, she had no low back pain and she had restored circulation to her right leg.

Connective tissue massage is a stroking technique carried out in the layers of connective tissue on the body surface. This stimulates the nerve endings of the autonomic nervous system. Afferent impulses travel to the spinal cord and the brain, and this causes a change in reaction susceptibility.[17]

Connective tissue is an organ of metabolism, therefore abnormal tension in one part of the tissue is reflected in other parts. All pathologic changes involve an inflammatory reaction in the affected part. One of the changes caused by inflammatory reaction is accumulation of fluid in the affected area. The area where these changes can most readily be detected is on the body surface. These changes are often seen as flattened areas or depressed bands that may be surrounded by elevated areas. The flat areas are the areas of main response and the connective tissue is tight, resisting pulling in any direction with movement.

The technique of connective tissue massage is not used as much in the United States as it is in European countries, especially Germany. As more results are seen, especially in the treatment of diseases associated with the pathology of circulation, this technique should become more widely accepted and used in this country.

General Principles of Connective Tissue Massage

POSITION OF THE PATIENT. The patient is usually in the sitting position for a connective tissue massage. Occasionally patients may be treated in a sidelying or prone position when they cannot be treated in a sitting position.

POSITION OF THE OPERATOR. The sports therapist should be in a position, seated or standing, that provides good body mechanics, is comfortable, and avoids fatigue.

APPLICATION TECHNIQUE. The basic stroke of pulling is performed with the tips, or pads, of the middle and ring fingers of either hand. Fingernails must be very short. The stroking technique is characterized by a tangential pull on the skin and subcutaneous tissues away from the fascia with the fingers. This technique should cause a sharp pain in the tissue. The stroke is a pull, not a push of the tissue. No lubricant is used. All treatments are started by the basic strokes from the coccyx to the first lumbar vertebra. Treatments last about 15 to 25 minutes. After 15 treatments, which are carried out two to three times per week, there should be a rest period of at least 4 weeks.

OTHER CONSIDERATIONS. Before any logical plan for treatment can be made, it is important to determine where any alterations in the optimum function of connective tissue have taken place, where the changes started, and if possible the cause of the alteration.

Evaluation is a most important part of an effective connective tissue massage program. The technique of stroking with two fingers of one hand along each side of the vertebral column will give much information about the sensory changes that are caused by alterations in the tension of surface tissues.

There are numerous arterial and venous disorders that may respond to connective tissue massage. Specific disabilities include: (1) scars on the skin; (2) fractures and arthritis in the bones and joints; (3) lower back pain, and torticollis in the muscles; (4) varicose symptoms, thrombophlebitis (subacute), hemorrhoids, and edema in the blood and lymph; (5) Raynaud's disease, intermittent claudication, frostbite, and trophic changes in the circulatory system. Connective tissue massage can also be used for myocardial dysfunctions, respiratory disturbances, intestinal disorders, ulcers, hepatitis, infections of the ovaries and uterus (subacute), amenorrhea, dysmenorrhea, genital infantilism, multiple sclerosis, Parkinson's disease, headaches, migraines, and allergies. Connective tissue massage is recommended to help in the process of revascularization following orthopedic complications such as fractures, dislocations, and sprains.

Contraindications to connective tissue massage include tuberculosis, tumors, and mental illnesses that result from psychologic dependence.

Connective tissue massage must be learned and performed initially under the direct supervision of someone who has been taught these highly specialized techniques. More detailed information about connective tissue massage can be found listed in the bibliography.[7,12,21]

MYOFASCIAL RELEASE

Myofascial release is a term that refers to a group of techniques used for the purpose of relieving soft tissue from the abnormal grip of tight fascia.[11] It is essentially a mild form of stretching that has been reported to have significant impact in treating a variety of conditions. Fascia is a type of connective tissue that surrounds muscles, tendons, nerves, bones, and organs. It is essentially continuous from head to toe and is interconnected in various sheaths or planes. During movement the fascia must stretch and move freely. If there is damage to the fascia owing to injury, disease, or inflammation, it will not only affect local adjacent structures but may also affect areas far removed from the site of the injury. Thus it may be necessary to release tightness in both the area of injury as well as in distant areas.[11]

Some specialized training is necessary for the sports therapist to understand specific techniques of myofascial release.[1] An in-depth understanding of the fascial system is essential. The type of technique used will depend on where the fascia is restricted. Generally release is accomplished by using an extremely mild combination of pressure and stretch. Fascia is composed primarily of collagen along with some elastic fibers. It will tend to soften and release in response to gentle pressure over a relatively long period of time.[11]

Acute cases tend to resolve in just a few treatments. The longer a condition has been present, the longer it will take to resolve. Occasionally dramatic results will occur immediately after treatment. It is usually recommended that treatment should be done at least three times per week.[11]

SUMMARY

1. Massage, as we know it today, is an improved and more scientific version of the various procedures that go back for thousands of years to the Greeks, Egyptians, and others.
2. Massage is the mechanical stimulation of tissue by means of rhythmically applied pressure and stretching. It allows the sports therapist, as a health care provider, to assist a patient to overcome pain and to relax through the application of the therapeutic massage techniques.
3. Massage has effects on the circulation, the lymphatic system, the nervous system, the muscles, the skin, scar tissue, psychologic responses, relaxation feelings, and pain.
4. The strokes used when giving a massage can include effleurage, petrissage, friction, percussion, or tapotement, and vibration.
5. Acupressure is increasing in use as sports therapists become more familiar with the location of the points and discover which points work best for a particular problem.
6. Connective tissue massage is a reflex zone massage. It is a relatively new form of treatment in this country and has its best effects on circulatory pathologies.
7. Myofascial release is a massage technique used for the purpose of relieving soft tissue from the abnormal grip of tight fascia.

GLOSSARY

acupressure The technique of using finger pressure over acupuncture points to decrease pain.

Bindegewebsmassage Reflex zone massage; uses a pulling stroke across connective tissue to effect change.

effleurage To stroke; any stroke that glides over the skin without attempting to move the deep muscle masses. The hand is molded to the part, stroking with more or less constant pressure, usually upward. Any degree of pressure may be applied, varying from the lightest possible touch to very deep pressure.

friction A technique that affects fibrositic adhesions in tendon, muscle, or ligament. It is performed by small circular movements that penetrate into the depth of a muscle, not by moving the finger on the skin, but by moving the tissues under the skin.

massage The act of rubbing, kneading, or stroking the superficial parts of the body with the hand or with an instrument for the purpose of modifying nutrition, restoring power of movement, or breaking up adhesions.

petrissage Massage technique that is a kneading manipulation. Consists of repeatedly grasping and releasing the tissue with one or both hands or parts thereof, in a lifting, rolling, or pressing movement. The outside characteristic of this movement as contrasted to stroking movements is that the pressure is applied intermittently.

tapotement A percussion massage; any series of brisk blows following each other in a rapid alternating fashion: hacking, cupping, slapping, beating, tapping, and pinchment. It is used when stimulation is the objective.

vibration A shaking massage technique; a fine tremulous movement made by the hand or fingers placed firmly against a part that will cause the part to vibrate. Often used for a soothing effect; may be stimulating when more energy is applied.

REFERENCES

1 Barnes, J.: Five years of myofascial release, Phys. Ther. Forum **6**(37):12-14, 1987.

2 Barr, J., and Taslitz, N.: Influence of back massage on autonomic functions, Phys. Ther. **50**:1679-1691, 1970.

3 Brickey, R., and Yao, J.: Acupuncture and transcutaneous electrical stimulation techniques, course manual in acutherapy post graduate seminars, Raleigh, N.C., 1978.

4 Castel, J.: Pain management with acupuncture and transcutaneous electrical nerve stimulation techniques and photo stimulation (Laser), course manual, 1982.

5 Cheng, R., and Pomerantz, B.: Electroacupuncture analgesia could be mediated by at least two pain relieving mechanisms: endorphin and non-endorphin systems, Life Sci. **25**:1957-1962, 1979.

6 Cyriax, J., and Russell, G.: Textbook of orthopedic medicine, vol. II., ed. 10, Baltimore, 1980, Williams & Wilkins.

7 Ebner, M.: Connective tissue massage: theory and therapeutic application, Huntington, N.Y. 1975, R.E. Krieger.

8 Fox, E., and Melzack, R.: Transcutaneous electrical stimulation and acupuncture: comparison of treatment for low back pain, Pain **2**:357-373, 1976.

9 Head, H.: Die Sensibilitätsstörungen der Haut bei viszeral Erkran Kungen, Berlin, 1898.

10 Hwang Ti Nei Ching (translation), Berkeley, 1973, University of California Press.

11 Juett, T.: Myofascial release—an introduction for the patient, Phys. Ther. Forum **7**(41):7-8, 1988.

12 Licht, S.: Massage, manipulation and traction, New Haven, 1960, Elizabeth Licht.

13 Man, P., and Chen, C.: Acupuncture aesthesia—a new theory and clinical study, Curr. Ther. Res. **14**:390-394, 1972.

14 Manaka, Y.: On certain electrical phenomena for the interpretation of Chi in Chinese literature, Am. J. Chin. Med. **3**:71-74, 1975.

15 Mann, F.: Acupuncture: the ancient Chinese art of healing and how it works scientifically, New York, 1973, Random House.

16 Melzack, R., Stillwell, D., and Fox, E.: Trigger points and acupuncture points for pain: correlations and implications, Pain **3**:3-23, 1977.

17 Mennell, J.B.: Physical treatment, ed. 5, Philadelphia, 1968, Blakiston Co.

18 Pemberton, R.: The physiologic influence of massage. In Mock, H.E., Pemberton, R., and Coulter, J.S. editors: Principles and practices of physical therapy, vol. I, Hagerstown, Md., 1939, W.F. Prior.

19 Prentice, W.: The use of electroacutherapy in the treatment of inversion ankle sprains, J. Nat. Athl. Train. Assoc. **17**(1):15-21, 1982.

20 Sjolund, B., and Eriksson, M.: Electroacupuncture and endogenous morphines, Lancet **2**:1085, 1976.

21 Tappan, F.: Healing massage techniques: a study of eastern and western methods, Reston, Va., 1978, Reston Publishing Co., Inc.

22 Wang, J.: Breaking out of the pain trap, Psychology Today **11**(2):78-82, 1977.

23 Wei, L.: Scientific advances in Chinese medicine, Am. J. Chin. Med. **7**:53-75, 1979.

24 Wood, E., and Becker, P.: Beard's massage, Philadelphia, 1981, W.B. Saunders Co.

SUGGESTED READINGS

Chamberlain, G.: Cyriax's friction massage: a review, J. Orthop. Sports Phys. Ther. **4**(1):16-22, 1982.

Cyriax, J.: Textbook of orthopedic medicine, vol. I, ed. 8, New York, 1982, Macmillan Publishing Co.

Ebner, M.: Connective tissue massage, Physiotherapy **64**:208-210, 1978.

Rogoff, J.: Manipulation, traction and massage, ed. 2, Baltimore, 1980, Williams & Wilkins.

Glossary

ablution Act of washing or bathing.

absolute refractory period Brief time period (.5 μsec) following membrane depolarization during which the membrane is incapable of depolarizing again.

absorption Energy that stimulates a particular tissue to perform its normal function.

accommodation Adaptation by the sensory receptors to various stimuli over an extended period of time.

acoustic spectrum The range of frequencies and wavelengths of sound waves.

ACTH Adrenocorticotropic hormone. This hormone has antiinflammatory actions.

action potential A recorded change in electrical potential between the inside and outside of a nerve cell, resulting in muscular contraction.

active electrode Electrode at which greatest current density occurs.

acupressure The technique of using finger pressure over acupuncture points to decrease pain.

adhesions Fibrous bands that hold together tissues that are normally separated.

afferent Conduction of a nerve impulse toward an organ.

air space plate A capacitor type electrode in which the plates are separated from the skin by the space in a glass case. Used with shortwave diathermy.

all or none response The depolarization of nerve or muscle membrane is the same once a depolarizing intensity threshold is reached: further increases in intensity do not increase the response. Stimuli at intensities less than threshold do not create a depolarizing effect.

alternating current Current that periodically changes its polarity or direction of flow.

ampere Unit of measure that indicates the rate at which electrical current is flowing.

amplitude The intensity of current flow as indicated by the height of the waveform from baseline.

analgesia Loss of sensibility to pain.

anesthesia Loss of sensation.

annulospiral endings One of two types of nerve endings associated with the muscle spindle and the stretch reflex.

annulus fibrosus The interlacing cross-fibers of fibroelastic tissue that are attached to adjacent vertebral bodies but contain the nucleus polposus.

anode Positively charged electrode in a direct current system.

anoxia Reduction of oxygen in body tissues below physiologic levels.

applicator The electrode used to transfer energy in microwave diathermy.

articular Dealing with two or more bones joining together to form a joint.

atonic Without tone.

avulsion fracture A fracture in which a small piece of bone is torn away by an attached tendon or ligament.

β-endorphin A neurohormone derived from β-lipotropin and containing enkephalin. It is similar in structure and properties to morphine. β-endorphin has a half-life of 4 hours.

β-lipotropin A pituitary hormone containing β-endorphin and enkephalin and having opiate activity.

bacteriostatic Inhibition of the growth of bacteria without destroying the bacteria.

Bindegewebsmassage Reflex zone massage; uses a pulling stroke across connective tissue to effect change.

bone density Amount of bone per unit of cubic space.

bradykinins A chemical formed in injured tissue as part of the inflammatory process that vasodilates small arterioles.

cable electrodes An inductance type electrode in which the electrodes are coiled around a body part creating an electromagnetic field.

calcific bursitis Hardening of the bursa sack.

calcification Hardening of tissue that results from deposits of lime salts.

capacitor setup A type of magnetic field heating that uses air space plates or pads.

cathode Negatively charged electrode in a direct current system.

central biasing The use of hyperstimulation analgesia to bias the central nervous system against transmitting painful stimuli to the sensory recognition area.

This occurs through hormonal influences created by brain stem stimulation.

cervical ganglia A mass of nerve cells located at the cervical portion of the sympathetic trunk.

chronaxie The duration of time necessary to cause observable tissue excitation, given a current intensity of 2 times rheobasic current.

circuit The path of current from a generating source through the various components back to the generating source.

clonus A forced series of alternating contractions and partial relaxations of muscle that occurs in some nervous diseases.

coaxial cable Heavy, well-insulated electrical wire.

coherence Property of identical phase and time relationship. All photons of laser light are the same wavelength.

cold-induced vasodilation Vasodilation following cold application.

collagen tissue Fibrous insoluble protein found in connective tissue, bone, ligaments, and cartilage.

collimation A state of being parallel.

colloid The fluid suspension of the body's intercellular fluid.

condenser electrodes An electrical current is conducted back and forth between the two electrodes. Highest concentration is under the electrodes, which may be pads or space plates. Highest concentration is also in fat tissue. Deeper absorption of current (deep heating effect) occurs between the electrodes.

conduction Heat loss or gain through direct contact.

congestion Presence of an abnormal amount of blood in the vessels as a result of an increase in blood flow or obstructed venous return.

consensual heat vasodilation Increased blood flow that spreads to a remote area of the body as a result of localized heating.

continuous wave An uninterrupted beam of laser light as opposed to a pulsed beam.

contraindication Special symptom or circumstance that renders the use of a remedy or procedure inadvisable.

contrast bath Hot (106° F) and cold (50° F) treatments in a combined sequence to stimulate superficial capillary vasodilation or vasoconstriction.

convection Heat loss or gain through the movement of air or water molecules across the skin.

conversion Changing of one energy into another.

cosine law Optimal radiation occurs when the source of radiation is at right angles to the center of the area being radiated.

coupling agent A substance used as a medium for the transfer of sound waves.

crossing patterns of disk herniation The protrusion of the nucleus pulposus through a defect in the annulus fibrosus.

cryokinetics The use of cold and exercise in the treatment of pathology or disease.

cryotherapy The use of cold in the treatment of pathology or disease.

crystal The part of the ultrasound head that vibrates and changes shape.

current The flow of electrons.

current density Amount of current flow per cubic area.

depolarization Process or act of neutralizing the cell membrane's resting potential.

diathermy The application of high-frequency electrical energy that is used to generate heat in body tissues as a result of the resistance of the tissue to the passage of energy.

diffusion Transfer of a substance from an area of greater to lesser concentration.

diode laser A solid-state semiconductor used as a lasing medium.

direct current Galvanic current that always flows in the same direction and may flow in either a positive or a negative direction.

disk herniation The protrusion of the nucleus pulposus through a defect in the annulus fibrosus.

disk material Cartilaginous material from vertebral body surfaces, disk nucleus, or annulus fibrosus.

disk nucleus The protein polysaccharide gel that is contained between the cartilaginous end plates of the vertebra and the annulus fibrosus.

disk protrusion The abnormal projection of the disk nucleus through some or all of the annular rings.

divergence The bending of light rays away from one another; the spreading of light.

DNA Deoxyribonucleic acid; the substance found in the chromosomes of the cell nucleus that carries the genetic code of the cell.

douche A current of water directed against the skin surface (e.g., scotch douche alternating hot and cold water).

duration Sometimes also referred to as pulse width. Indicates the length of time the current is flowing.

edema Excessive fluid in cells.

efferent Conduction of a nerve impulse away from an organ.

effleurage To stroke; any stroke that glides over the skin without attempting to move the deep muscle masses. The hand is molded to the part, stroking with more or less constant pressure, usually upward. Any degree of pressure may be applied, varying from the lightest possible touch to very deep pressure.

electrical field A technique of heating the tissues in shortwave diathermy in which the patient is part of the electrical circuit.

electrical potential The difference between charged particles at a higher and lower potential.

electrical stimulation The use of four or more electrodes. AA′ and BB′ arranged so the path of electric current A to A′ is crossed by the path of the electric current B to B′.

electromagnetic or induction field The patient is heated in a magnetic field and is not part of the circuit. Current flows through the tissues of least resistance.

electromagnetic spectrum The range of frequencies and wavelengths associated with radiant energy.

electromyography The pick-up and amplification of electrical signals generated by the muscle as it contracts.

electron Fundamental particle of matter possessing a negative electrical charge and very small mass.

electrostatic or condenser field The patient is placed between electrodes and becomes a part of a series circuit.

empirically Through observation or experience.

endogenous opiates Naturally occurring opiates.

endorphins Endogenous opiates whose actions have analgesic properties. They are neurohormones and not neurotransmitters (i.e., β-endorphins).

endothelial cells Cells that line the cavities of the vessels.

enkephalin Neurotransmitter proteins that are pain-relieving molecules. They block the passage of noxious stimuli by servicing descending neurons to counter ascending signals. They inhibit the release of substance P and are produced by enkephalinergic neurons.

enkephalinergic neurons Neurons with short axons that release enkephalin. They act as interneurons (internuncial neurons) and are found in the substantia gelatinosa, nucleus raphae magnus, and periaqueductal gray matter.

erythema Redness of the skin; inflammation. A redness of the skin caused by capillary dilation.

evaporation Loss of volume of liquid by changing into vapor; loss of heat by this process; heat transfer.

excited state State of an atom that occurs when outside energy causes the atom to contain more energy than is normal.

exostosis Bony growth that arises from the surface of a bone.

extracapsular ligament Ligament found outside of the joint capsule.

facet joints Articular joints of the spine.

Federal Communications Commission (FCC) Federal agency charged with assigning frequencies for all radio transmitters including diathermies.

fiberoptic A solid glass or plastic tube that conducts light along its length.

fibrils Connective tissue fibers supporting the lymphatic capillaries.

fibrosis The formation of fibrous tissue in the injury repair process.

flower spray endings One of two types of nerve endings associated with the muscle spindle and the stretch reflex.

fluidotherapy A modality of dry heat using a finely divided solid suspended in an air stream with the properties of liquid.

fluorescence The capacity of certain substances to radiate when illuminated by a source of a given wavelength, a light of a different wavelength (color) than that of the irradiating source.

focusing Narrowing attention to the appropriate stimuli in the environment.

frequency The number of cycles or pulses per second.

friction A technique that affects fibrositic adhesions in tendon, muscle, or ligament. It is performed by small circular movements that penetrate into the depth of a muscle, not by moving the finger on the skin, but by moving the tissues under the skin.

gamma system Nerve fibers that reset the muscle spindle to its adjusted length.

ground A wire that makes an electrical connection with the earth.

ground state The normal, unexcited state of an atom.

hematoma An area of swelling containing blood, usually clotted.

hertz A unit of frequency equal to one cycle per second.

high-voltage current Current in which the waveform has an amplitude of greater than 150 volts with a relatively short pulse duration of less than 100 μsec.

homeostatic A state of physiologic equilibrium, in this case a balance between the electrical composition of the tissue.

homogeneous Of like type.

Hubbard tank An immersion tank for the whole body, may have vertical depth for walking or supine treatment.

hybrid currents Currents that have waveforms containing parameters that are not classically alternating or direct.

hydrocollator A synthetic hot (170° F) or cold (0° F) gel used as an adjunctive modality to stimulate tissue temperature rise or tissue temperature lowering.

hydrocortisone An antiinflammatory steroid.

hydrogymnastics Exercises using the buoyant properties of immersion in water.

hydrostatic pressure The pressure exerted by a liquid at rest.

hydrotherapy Cryotherapy and thermotherapy techniques that use water as the medium for heat transfer.

hyperemia Presence of an increased amount of blood in part of the body.

hyperplasia An increase in the size of a tissue; in the skin, an increased thickness of the epidermis.

hyperstimulation analgesia See stimulus-produced analgesia.

hypertonicity Exhibiting excessive tone or tension.

hypothalamus An area of the brain that provides regulating autonomic control of vital body functions.

Ia afferents Nerve fibers carrying impulses from the muscle spindle to the spinal cord.

impedance Resistance of the tissue to the passage of electrical current.

indication The reason to prescribe a remedy or procedure.

indifferent or dispersive electrode Large electrode used to spread out electrical charge.

induction electrodes Electrical current is passed through a coil that in turn gives off eddy currents of electromagnetic energy. This energy is absorbed by the tissues and heating occurs as a result of the resistance of the tissues.

infrared A portion of the electromagnetic spectrum between the visible and microwave regions. Infrared wavelengths range from 780 to 100,000 nm.

innervate To supply a body part (e.g., muscle or skin) with nerves.

innocuous stimuli Painless stimuli.

interface Where two tissues meet.

intermolecular vibration Movement between molecules that produces friction and thus heating.

interneurons Neurons contained entirely in the central nervous system. They have no projections outside the spinal cord. Their function is to serve as relay stations within the central nervous system.

inverse square law The intensity of radiation striking a particular surface varies inversely with the square of the distance from the radiating source.

ion A positively or negatively charged particle.

iontophoresis The use of constant direct current to drive heavy metal ions into and through the skin.

joint capsule Ligamentous structure that surrounds and encapsulates a joint.

joint swelling The accumulation of fluid within the joint capsule.

keratin The fibrous protein that forms the chemical basis of the epidermis.

keratinocytes Cells that produce keratin.

laser A device that concentrates high energies into a narrow beam of coherent, monochromatic light.

ligament deformation Lengthening distortion of ligament caused by traction loading.

low-voltage current Current in which the waveform has an amplitude of less than 150 volts.

lymph A transparent, slightly yellow liquid found in the lymphatic vessels.

lymphedema Swelling of subcutaneous tissues as a result of accumulation of excessive lymph fluid.

macroshock An electrical shock that can be felt and has a leakage of electrical current of greater than 1 mamp.

magnetic field A technique of heating the tissues in shortwave diathermy in which the patient is not part of the electrical circuit.

massage The act of rubbing, kneading, or stroking the superficial parts of the body with the hand or with an instrument for the purpose of modifying nutrition, restoring power of movement, or breaking up adhesions.

mechanical effects Ultrasonic effects that involve movement as a result of vibratory motion.

melanin A group of dark brown or black pigments that occur naturally in the eye, skin, hair, and other animal tissues.

meniscoid structures A cartilage tip found on the synovial fringes of some facet joints.

metabolites Waste products of metabolism or catabolism.

metal implants Any metal device placed within tissue.

microshock An electrical shock that is imperceptible because of a leakage of current of less than 1 mamp.

minimal erythemal dose The amount of time of exposure to UVR necessary to cause a faint erythema 24 hours after exposure.

modulation Refers to any alteration in the magnitude or any variation in the duration of an electrical current.

monochromaticity When a light source produces a single color or wavelength.

muscle spindle A sensory organ in a muscle that is sensitive to changes in length of a muscle.

myositis ossificans Inflammation of muscle tissue with bony formation of the muscle.

naloxone Drug known to antagonize the action of opiates. It is used in studies of endogenous opiates to determine effectiveness of various stimuli to cause the release of endogenous opiates.

nerve conduction velocity Speed in which an impulse travels the length of a nerve.

nerve root impingement Abnormal encroachment of some body tissue into the space occupied by the nerve root.

neurotransmitter Substance that passes information between neurons. It is released from one neuron terminal (presynaptic membrane), enters the synaptic cleft, and attaches (binds) to a receptor on the next neuron (postsynaptic membrane). Substance P, enkephalins, serotonin, methionine, and leucine enkephalin are neurotransmitters.

nociceptive Pain information or signals or pain stimuli.

nociceptive neuron Afferent neuron that transmits pain signals.

nociceptive pain fibers Neurons that have their cell bodies in the dorsal root ganglion and conduct noxious stimuli. Unmyelinated C and myelinated A delta fibers are such neurons.

nonnoxious Painless.

norepinephrine A neurotransmitter that may enhance pain. When it is inhibited, analgesia is increased. Increased levels in the central nervous system decrease analgesia.

noxious Painful.

nutrients Essential or nonessential food substance.

Ohm's law The current in an electrical circuit is directly proportional to the voltage and inversely proportional to the resistance.

opiate receptors Neurons that have receptors that bind to opiate substances.

osmotic pressure The pressure for movement of a solvent across a membrane that is permeable to that solvent.

osteophytes A bony outgrowth.

overuse syndromes Injury to a tissue by working it harder than it is prepared to work over a period of time.

pad electrodes Capacitor type electrode used with shortwave diathermy.

paraffin bath A combined paraffin and mineral oil immersion technique in which the paraffin substance is heated to 126° F for conductive heat gains; commonly used on the hands and feet for distal temperature gains in blood flow and temperature.

pathology Abnormal anatomic or physiologic deviations resulting from injury or disease.

percutaneous injection Fibrous covering of bone.

periosteum A highly vascularized and innervated membrane lining the surface of bone.

petrissage Massage technique that is a kneading manipulation. Consists of repeatedly grasping and releasing the tissue with one or both hands or parts thereof, in a lifting, rolling, or pressing movement. The outstanding characteristic of this movement as contrasted to stroking movements is that the pressure is applied intermittently.

phagocyte A cell that consumes foreign material and debris.

phonophoresis Driving of medication into tissue by ultrasound.

photokeratitis An inflammation of the eyes caused by exposure to UVR.

photon The basic unit of light; a packet or quantum of light energy.

piezoelectric effect Vibration of a crystal as a result of receiving electrical current.

pitting edema A type of swelling that leaves a pitlike depression when it is compressed.

plica Thickened synovial fold.

polymodal nociceptors Small unmyelinated afferent fibers that have high threshold axons and respond only to cutaneous stimulation (i.e., pain, deep pressure, and temperature). C fibers are examples of these.

population inversion A condition in which more atoms exist in a high-energy, excited state than in a normal ground state. This is required for lasing to occur.

proprioception The reception of stimulus produced within an organism, in this case relating to positional changes or sense.

proprioceptive nervous system System of nerves that provide information on joint movement, pressure, and muscle tension.

prostaglandins Irritants that are synthesized locally during injury in tissues from a fatty acid precursor (arachidonic acid). They act with bradykinin to amplify pain by sensitizing afferent neurons to chemical and mechanical stimulation. Aspirin is thought to be capable of interrupting the process. Prostaglandins are powerful vasodilators. They induce erythema, increase leakage of plasma from vessels, and attract leukocytes to an injured area.

psoralens Methoxypsoralen, trimethylpsoralen, and other chemicals of similar make-up. These are used as dermal pigmenting agents.

pulsed ultrasound Method of administering ultrasound in which the conduction of sound waves is intermittent.

radiation The process of emitting energy from some source in the form of waves. A method of heat transfer through which heat can either be gained or lost.

radiograph Record produced on a photographic plate, film, or paper by the action of roentgen rays or radium; specifically x-rays.

raphe nucleus Part of the brain that is known to inhibit pain impulses being transmitted through the ascending system.

referred pain (referred myofascial pain) When nociceptive impulses reach the dorsal gray matter they converge and their summation can depolarize internuncial neurons over several spinal segments, causing the individual to feel pain in distal areas innervated by these segments.

reflection The bending back of light or sound waves from a surface that they strike.

refraction The change in direction of a sound wave or radiation wave when it passes from one medium or type of tissue to another.

repolarize To return to a polarized state after a depolarizing event.

resting capillaries Small patent blood vessels.

rheobase The intensity of current necessary to cause observable tissue excitation, given a long current duration.

RNA Ribonucleic acid; an acid found in the cell cytoplasm and nucleolus. It is intimately involved in protein synthesis.

sclerotomic A segment of bone innervated by a spinal segment.

secondary vasodilation Dilation following exposure to cold to sustain viable tissues.

sensitization Prolonged depolarization of nociceptive neurons that results in continuous stimulation. Most sensory receptors are rendered less sensitive after prolonged stimulation. This is not the case with nociceptive neurons.

sepsis A pathologic state that involves toxic substance in the bloodstream.

serotonin A neurotransmitter that may block noxious stimuli through descending neurons that block ascending neurons. It is found in the vesicles in nerve endings that bind when released to postsynaptic membranes. Its action is terminated by reuptake into presynaptic membranes. It is probably involved in both endogenous pain control and opiate analgesia. Increased levels of serotonin in the central nervous system are generally associated with increased analgesia.

spasmotic Marked by spasm (involuntary muscle contraction).

spondylolisthesis Forward displacement of one vertebra over another.

spontaneous emission When an atom in a high-energy state emits a photon and drops to a more stable ground state.

stellate ganglion Ganglion (group of nerve cell bodies) formed by the first thoracic ganglion and the inferior cervical ganglion.

sterile technique Maintenance of a sterile environment; aseptic; free from all living microorganisms; preventing contamination.

stimulated emission When a photon interacts with an atom already in a high-energy state and decay of the atomic system occurs, releasing two photons.

stimulus-produced analgesia (SPA) Pain relief created by stimulation of portions of the central nervous system, either directly or indirectly. Common methods are electrical stimulation, needle, pressure, or extreme cold applied to acupuncture points, trigger points, or motor points.

strength-duration curve A graphic illustration of the relationship between current intensity and current duration in causing depolarization of a nerve or muscle membrane.

subepithelial tissue Lying beneath or making up the innermost part of the epithelium.

substance P A peptide believed to be the neurotransmitter of small-diameter primary afferents. It is released from both ends of the neuron.

substantia gelatinosa Located in the dorsal horn of the gray matter; thought to be responsible for closing the gate to painful stimuli.

summation of contractions Shortening of muscle myofilaments caused by increasing the frequency of muscle membrane depolarization.

suprahumeral impingement Shoulder lesion in the space between the superior aspect of the head of the humerus and the coracoacromial ligament.

synchrony All muscle fibers contracting at the same time and rate.

synovial fringes Folds of synovial tissue that move in and out of the joint space.

T-cell Transmission cell or neuron in the dorsal horn of the cord that is an interneuron or internuncial neuron. Principal location may be lamina V.

tapotement A percussion massage technique; any series of brisk blows following each other in a rapid alternating fashion: hacking, cupping, slapping, beating, tapping, and pinching. It is used when stimulation is the objective.

tetanization A muscle contraction in which the muscle fibers are in a continuous state of contraction.

tetany Muscle condition that is caused by hyperexcitation and results in cramps and spasms.

thermal Pertaining to heat.

thermopane An insulating layer of water next to the skin.

thermotherapy The use of heat in the treatment of pathology or disease.

thrombophlebitis Inflammation of a vein with a blood clot formed within a blood vessel.

traction Drawing tension applied to a body segment.

transducer A device that changes energy from one type to another.

transmission To pass through some medium.

trigger point Localized deep tenderness in a palpable firm band of muscle. If the muscle is stretched, a palpating finger can snap the band like a taut string, which produces local pain, a local twitch of that portion of the muscle, and a jump by the patient. Sustained pressure on a trigger point reproduces the pattern of referred pain for that site.

tumor Spontaneous growth of tissue that is not inflammatory resulting in an abnormal mass.

twitch muscle contraction A single muscle contraction caused by one depolarization phenomenon.

ultrasound A portion of the acoustic spectrum located above audible sound. Sound waves higher than the 16,000 to 20,000 Hz detectable by the human ear.

ultraviolet The portion of the electromagnetic spectrum associated with chemical changes, located adjacent to the violet portion of the visible light spectrum.

unibase r Neutral cream to which medication can be added.

unilateral foramen opening Enlargement of the foramen on one side of a vertebral segment.

vagus nerve Tenth cranial nerve; this nerve innervates cardiac muscle and some smooth and striated muscle.

vascular anastomoses A union or junction of blood vessels.

vasoconstrictions Narrowing of the blood vessels.

vasodilation Dilation of the blood vessels.

venous plexus A network of interlacing veins.

vibration A shaking massage technique; a fine tremulous movement made by the hand or fingers placed firmly against a body part and causing that part to vibrate. Often used for a soothing effect; may be stimulating when more energy is applied.

viscoelastic properties The property of a material to show sensitivity to rate of loading.

volt The electromotive force that must be applied to produce a movement of electrons.

voltage sensitive permeability The quality of some cell membranes that makes them permeable to different ions based on the electric charge of the ions. Nerve and muscle cell membranes allow negatively charged ions into the cell while actively transporting some positively charged ions outside the cell membrane.

watt A measure of electrical power. Mathematically: watts = volts × amperes.

waveform The shape of an electrical current as displayed on an oscilloscope.

wavelength The distance from a peak to the same point on the next peak of an electromagnetic or acoustic wave.

Wolff's law Bone remodels itself and provides increased strength along the lines of the mechanical forces placed on it.

Appendix A

The illustrations in this appendix show the locations of the motor points located on the extremities and the torso. (Courtesy Mettler Electronics Corporation, 1333 S. Claudina Street, Anaheim, CA 92805.)

LOCATIONS OF THE MOTOR POINTS

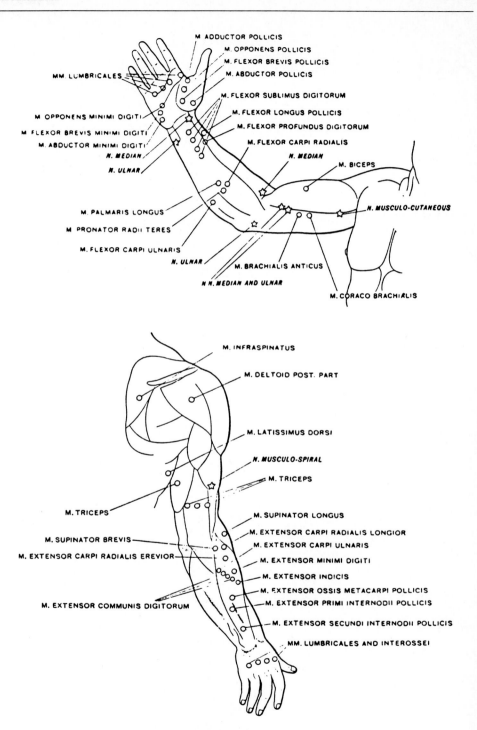

Figure A-1.

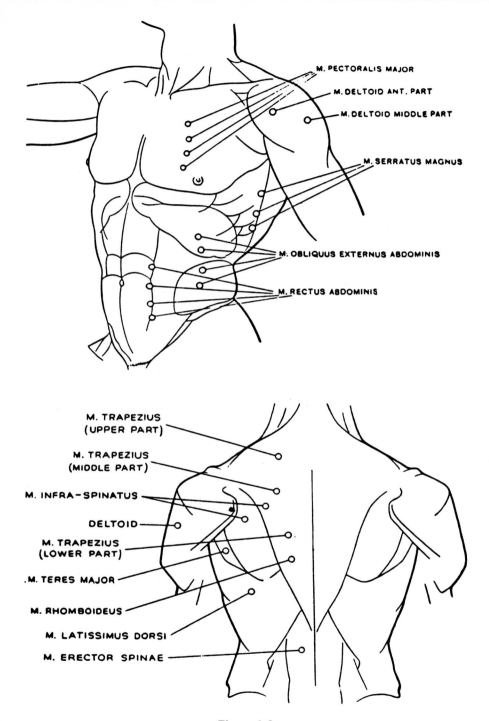

Figure A-2.

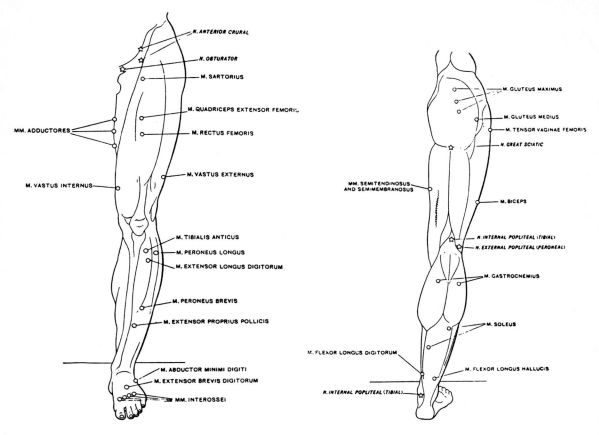

M = Muscle
N = Nerves

Printed in U.S.A.
10M/6/83

Figure A-3.

Appendix B

Clinical Decision Making on the Use of Various Therapeutic Modalities in Treatment of Acute Injury

Stage	Time Frame	Clinical Picture	Possible Modalities Used	Rationale for Use
Acute	Injury–Day 3	Swelling Pain to touch Pain on motion	CRYO ESC IC LPL Rest	↓ Swelling, ↓ pain ↓ Pain ↓ Swelling ↓ Pain
Postacute	Day 2–Day 6	Swelling subsides Warm to touch Discoloration Pain to touch Pain to motion	CRYO ESC IC LPL Range of motion	↓ Swelling, ↓ pain ↓ Pain ↓ Swelling ↓ Pain
Regeneration	Day 4–Day 10	Pain to touch Pain to motion Swollen	THERMO ESC LPL IC Range of motion Strengthening	Mildly ↑ circulation ↓ Pain—muscle pumping ↓ Pain Facilitate lymphatic flow
Repair	Day 7–Recovery	Swollen No more pain to touch Decreasing pain or motion	ULTRA ESC LPL SWD MWD Range of motion Strengthening Functional activities	Deep heating to ↑ circulation Increase ROM, ↑ strength, ↓ Pain ↓ Pain Deep heating to ↑ circulation Deep heating to ↑ circulation

CRYO = cryotherapy; ESC = electrical stimulating currents; IC = intermittent compression; LPL = low-power laser; MWD = microwave diathermy; SWD = shortwave diathermy; THERMO = thermotherapy; ULTRA = ultrasound.

Appendix C

Clinical Decision Making on the Use of Various Therapeutic Modalities in Treatment of Chronic Injury

Clinical Picture	Possible Modalities Used	Rationale for Use		
Pain on motion	Ultrasound	Deep healing to ↑ circulation		
Pain to touch	Shortwave and microwave diathermy	Deep healing to ↑ circulation		
Swelling	Cryotherapy	↓ Pain		
Warm to touch	Electrical stimulating currents	↓ Pain		
Possible crepitus	Low-power laser	↓ Pain	Strength	Range of motion
	Anti-inflammatory medication	↓ Pain		
	Range of motion			
	Strengthening			

Appendix D

Indications and Contraindications for Therapeutic Modalities

Electrical Stimulating Currents	Indications for Use		Contraindications and Precautions
High voltage	Pain modulation Muscle reeducation Muscle pumping contractions Retard atrophy	Muscle strengthening Increase ROM Fracture healing Acute injury	Pacemakers Thrombophlebitis Superficial skin lesions
Low voltage	Wound healing Fracture healing Iontophoresis		Malignancy Skin hypersensitivities Allergies to certain drugs

Shortwave diathermy and microwave diathermy	Increase deep circulation
	Increase metabolic activity
	Reduce muscle guarding/spasm
	Reduce inflammation
	Facilitate wound healing
		Analgesia	Metal implants
			Pacemakers
			Malignancy
			Wet dressings
			Anesthetized areas
			Pregnancy
			Acute injury and
			  inflammation
			Eyes
			Areas of reduced
			  blood flow

Cryotherapy Cold packs Ice massage	Acute injury Vasoconstriction—decreased blood flow Analgesia Reduce inflammation Reduce muscle guarding/spasm		Allergy to cold Circulatory impairments Wound healing Hypertension
Thermotherapy Hot whirlpool Paraffin Hydrocollator Infrared lamps	Vasodilatation—increased blood flow Analgesia Reduce muscle guarding/spasm Reduce inflammation Increase metabolic activity Facilitate tissue healing		Acute and postacute trauma Poor circulation Circulatory impairments Malignancy
Low-power laser	Pain modulation (trigger points) Facilitate wound healing	Pregnancy Eyes	

(Continued.)

Indications and Contraindications for Therapeutic Modalities—cont'd

Electrical Stimulating Currents	Indications for Use		Contraindications and Precautions

Ultraviolet	Acne
	Aseptic wounds
	Folliculitis
	Pityriasis rosea
		Tinea
		Septic wounds
		Sinusitis
		Increase calcium
		   metabolism
			Psoriasis
			Eczema
			Herpes
			Diabetes
			Pellagra
			Lupus erythematosus
			Hyperthyroidism
			Renal and hepatic
			   insufficiency
			Generalized
			   dermatitis
			Advanced
			   atherosclerosis

Ultrasound	Increase connective tissue extensibility
	Deep heat
	Increased circulation
	Treatment of most soft tissue injuries
	Reduce inflammation
	Reduce muscle spasm
			Infection
			Acute and postacute
			   injury
			Epiphyseal areas
			Pregnancy
			Thrombophlebitis
			Impaired
			   sensation
			Eyes

Intermittent compression	Decrease acute bleeding Decrease edema		Circulatory impairment

Appendix E

LIST OF THERAPEUTIC MODALITY EQUIPMENT MANUFACTURERS AND DISTRIBUTORS

Acuscope Co.
4340 Redwood Hwy., Suite 400
San Rafael, CA 94903

Amrex-Zetron, Inc.
12583 Crenshaw Blvd.
Hawthorne, CA 90250

Arjo Hospital Equipment, Inc.
6380 Oakton Street
Morton Grove, IL 60053

Bernlit Enterprises, Inc.
5800 Ellwood Ave.
Bristol, PA 19007-3498

Biomark, Inc.
6925 216th S.W.
Lynnwood, WA 98036

Biostim, Inc.
PO Box 3138
Princeton, NJ 08540

Birtcher Corporation
4501 N. Arden Dr.
El Monte, CA 91734

Robert Bosch Corporation
Flower Field Bldg #17
Mills Pond Rd.
St James, NY 11780

Brandt Industries, Inc.
4461 Bronx Blvd.
Bronx, NY 10470

Chattanooga Corporation
PO Box 4287
Chattanooga, TN 37405

Codman & Shurtleff, Inc.
Randolph Industrial Park
Randolph, MA 02368

Conrad Precision Industries, Inc.
100 Chestnut St.
Newark, NJ 07105

Dynatronics
450 West 1700 South
Salt Lake City, UT 84115

Dynawave Corporation
2520 Kaneville Rd.
Geneva, IL 60134

Electro Acuscope/Myopulse—Electro
    Medical, Inc.
18433 Amistad
Fountain Valley, CA 92708

Electro-Med Health Industries, Inc.
6240 N.E. 4th Ct.
Miami, FL 33138

Elmed Inc.
60 W. Fay Ave.
Addison, IL 60101

Empi, Inc.
261 S. Commerce Circle
Minneapolis, MN 55432

Ferno Ille
P.O. Box 3007
Williamsport, PA 17701-0007

Fluidotherapy Corporation
Henley International, Inc.
6113 Althea Lane
Houston, TX 77081

Gebauer Chemical Co.
9410 St. Catherine Ave.
Cleveland, OH 44104

General Physiotherapy, Inc.
1520 Washington Ave.
St. Louis, MO 63103

Graham-Field Surgical Company
415 Second Avenue
New Hyde Park, NY 11040

Hausmann Industries, Inc.
130 Union St.
Northvale, NJ 07647

Henley International Incorporated
6113 Aletha Lane
Houston, TX 77081

Hill Laboratories Co.
445 Lincoln Hwy.
Philadelphia, PA 19344

Huntleigh Technology, Inc.
103 Church St. #1A
Aberdeen, NJ 07747

International Medical Electronics,
    Ltd.
2805 Main
Kansas City, MO 64108

I-Rep, Inc.
504 N. Spring St., #C
Elsinore, CA 92330

Jacuzzi
298 N. Wiget Lane
P.O. Drawer J
Walnut Creek, CA 94596

J.A. Preston Corporation
60 Page Road
Clifton, NJ 07012

Joanco USA
RD 2, Box 503
Hanover, PA 17331

Jobst Institute, Inc.
653 Miami St.
Toledo, OH 43605

Logan, Inc.
3041 S. Shannon St.
Santa Ana, CA 92704

Lossing Orthopedic
2217 Nicollet Ave S.
Minneapolis, MN 55404

LTI-Dynex
11558 Sorrento Valley Rd.
San Diego, CA 92121

Medco Products, Inc.
P.O. Box E
31 Park Road
Tinton Falls, NJ 07724

Medical Devices, Inc.
833 Third St., S.W.
St. Paul, MN 55112

Medtronic, Inc.
6951 Central Ave., N.E.
Minneapolis, MN 55432

Medtronic, Inc.
PO Box 1250
Minneapolis, MN 55440

Mentor Corporation
1499 W. River Rd. N.
Minneapolis, MN 55440

Mettler Electronics Corporation
1333 S. Claudina St.
Anaheim, CA 92805

G.E. Miller, Inc.
484 S. Broadway
Yonkers, NY 10705

Nemectron Medical, Inc.
28069 Diaz Rd., Unit A
Temecula, CA 92390

Neuromedics, Inc.
c/o Intermedics, Inc.
PO Box 617
Freeport, TX 77541

Ntron
PO Box 7000
San Rafael, CA 94912

Nu-Med, Inc.
333 N. Hammes Ave.
Joliet, IL 60435

Parker Laboratories, Inc.
307 Washington St.
Orange, NJ 07050

Pharmaceutical Innovations, Inc.
897 Frelinghuysen Ave.
Newark, NJ 07114

Physio Technology, Inc.
1925 W. 6th St.
Topeka, KS 66606

R.A. Fisher Co.
517 Commercial St.
Glendale, CA 91209

Rehab Medical Specialties, Inc./
   Soken
1910 Silver St.
Garland, TX 75042

Rich-Mar Corporation
Box 879
Inola, OK 74036

School Health Supply Co.
300 Lombard Rd., PO Box 409
Addison, IL 60101-0409

SFC-Orthopod
10870 Talbert Ave.
Fountain Valley, CA 92708

Staodynamics, Inc.
1255 Florida Ave.
Longmont, CO 80501

Sutter Biomedical, Inc.
3940 Ruffin Rd.
San Diego, CA 92123

Tag-Med
6595 Odell Place
Suite B
Boulder, CO 80201

Talcott Laboratories, Inc.
301 E. Barr St.
McDonald, PA 15057

Theradyne Corporation
21730 Hanover Lane
Lakeville, MN 55044

Thermo-Electric Co.
1948 Columbus Rd.
Cleveland, OH 44101

Tri W-G, Inc.
PO Box 905
Valley City, ND 58072

Tru-Trac Manufacturing Co., Inc.
27635 Diaz Rd., PO Box 880
Temecula, CA 92390

Ultraviolet Products, Inc.
5100 Walnut Grove Ave.
San Gabriel, CA 91778

Verimed Marketing Group
3560 S.W. Third St.
Fort Lauderdale, FL 33312

Whitehall Electro Medical Co., Inc.
100 Temple Ave., PO Box 701
Hackensack, NJ 07602-0701

WR Medical Electronics Company
1995 West County Road B2
St. Paul, MN 55113

Appendix F

<table>
<tr><td>**UNITS OF MEASURE**</td><td>Milliseconds (msec)</td><td>$= \frac{1}{1000}$ of a second</td></tr>
<tr><td></td><td>Microseconds (μsec)</td><td>$= \frac{1}{1,000,000}$ of a second</td></tr>
<tr><td></td><td>Nanosecond (nsec)</td><td>$= \frac{1}{1,000,000,000}$ of a second</td></tr>
<tr><td></td><td>Milliamp (mamp)</td><td>$= \frac{1}{1000}$ of an amp</td></tr>
<tr><td></td><td>Microamp (μamp)</td><td>$= \frac{1}{1,000,000}$ of an amp</td></tr>
<tr><td></td><td>Angstrom (A)</td><td>$= \frac{1}{10,000,000,000}$ of a meter</td></tr>
<tr><td></td><td>Nanometer (nm)</td><td>$= \frac{1}{1,000,000,000}$ of a meter</td></tr>
<tr><td></td><td>Hertz (Hz)</td><td>$= 1$ cycle per second</td></tr>
<tr><td></td><td>Kilohertz (KHz)</td><td>$= 1,000$ cycles per second</td></tr>
<tr><td></td><td>Megahertz (MHz)</td><td>$= 1,000,000$ cycles per second</td></tr>
</table>

Index